Acknowledgements

The Course Team and the authors wish to thank the following who, as contributors to previous editions of this book, made a lasting impact on the present volume.

Dr A. Batty Shaw, Nick Black, David Boswell, Robert Dingwall, Gerald Elliot, Alastair Gray, David Hunter, Deborah McGovern, Kevin McConway, Perry Morley, Jennie Popay, Steven Rose, Emilie Savage-Smith, Clive Seale, Phil Strong.

Cover images

Background: Nebulae in the Rho Ophiuchi region (Source: Anglo-Australian Observatory/Royal Observatory Edinburgh). *Middleground*: Globe (Source: Mountain High Map™, Digital Wisdom, Inc). *Foreground*: Section of the fresco 'The History of Medicine in Mexico: The People's Demand for Better Health' painted in 1953 by Diego Rivera in the Hospital de la Raza, Mexico City. Reproduced by permission of Biblioteca de las Artes (Archivo CENIDIAP/INBA), Centro Nacional de las Artes, Mexico. Copyright 2001 Banco de Mexico, Diego Rivero & Frida Kahlo Museums Trust, Av. Cinco de Mayo No. 2., Col. Centro, Del. Cuauhtemoc, 06059, Mexico, D.F.

Open University Press, Celtic Court, 22 Ballmoor,
Buckingham, MK18 1XW.

e-mail: enquiries@openup.co.uk

website: www.openup.co.uk

and

325 Chestnut Street, Philadelphia, PA 19106, USA.

First published 1985. Completely revised second edition
published 1993.

This revised full-colour third edition published 2001.

A catalogue record of the book is available from the
British Library.

Library of Congress Cataloging-in-Publication Data is
available.

Edited, designed and typeset by the Open University.

Printed and bound in the United Kingdom by the
Alden Group, Oxford.

ISBN 0335 208401

This publication forms part of an Open University level 2
course, U205 Health and Disease. The complete list of
texts which make up this course can be found on the
back cover. Details of this and other Open University
courses can be obtained from the Call Centre,
PO Box 724, The Open University, Milton Keynes
MK7 6ZS, United Kingdom: tel. +44 (0)1908 653231,
e-mail ces-gen@open.ac.uk

Alternatively, you may visit the Open University website
at http://www.open.ac.uk where you can learn more
about the wide range of courses and packs offered at all
levels by the Open University.

3.2

Caring for Health:
History and Diversity

Edited by Charles Webster

Published by Open University Press

Produced by The Open University

Health and Disease Series, Book 6

OPEN UNIVERSITY PRESS

Philadelphia

The U205 *Health and Disease* Course Team

The following member of the Open University teaching staff has collaborated with the authors in the production of this book, and accepts responsibility on behalf of the Open University for its overall academic and teaching content.

Basiro Davey (Course Team Chair, Senior Lecturer in Health Studies, Department of Biological Sciences)

The following people have contributed to the development of particular parts or aspects of this book.

Sheila Dunleavy (editor)

Phil Gauron (BBC producer)

Rebecca Graham (editor)

Celia Hart (picture researcher)

Pam Higgins (designer)

Carol Komaromy (critical reader, Lecturer in Health Studies, School of Health and Social Welfare)

Jean Macqueen (indexer)

Jennifer Nockles (designer)

Harriet Pacaud (BBC producer)

Denise Rowe (course secretary)

Jenny Spouse (critical reader, Lecturer in Work-based Learning, School of Health and Social Welfare)

John Taylor (graphic artist)

Joy Wilson (course manager)

Authors

The following external academics have acted as principal authors for the chapters listed below, or have contributed material on certain historical periods or geographical areas as indicated, and have also contributed extensively to the structure and philosophy of the book as a whole.

Chapters 1, 7 and 10, the structure of the National Health Service in Chapter 6 and Academic Editor for the book

Charles Webster, Fellow of All Souls College, University of Oxford.

16th–19th-century health care in Britain, in Chapters 2–4; editor for Chapters 2–4

Margaret Pelling, Reader in the Social History of Medicine, Modern History Faculty, University of Oxford.

16th–mid-20th-century health care in continental Europe, in Chapters 3–5

Paul Weindling, Wellcome Trust Research Professor in the History of Medicine, Oxford Brookes University, Oxford.

16th–mid-20th-century health care in the European colonies, in Chapters 2–5

Mark Harrison, Acting-Director and Senior Research Fellow, Wellcome Unit for the History of Medicine, University of Oxford.

20th-century health care in Britain, in Chapters 4–6; editor for Chapters 5–6

Virginia Berridge, Professor of History and Head of Unit, Health Promotion Research Unit, Department of Public Health and Policy, London School of Hygiene and Tropical Medicine.

Chapter 8, and 20th-century health care in developing countries, in Chapter 6

Gill Walt, Professor of International Health Policy, Department of Public Health and Policy, London School of Hygiene and Tropical Medicine.

Chapter 9

Alastair Gray, Reader in Health Economics, and Director, Health Economics Research Centre, Institute of Health Sciences, University of Oxford.

External assessors

Course assessor for third edition

Professor John Gabbay, Professor of Public Health Medicine, University of Southampton, and Director of the Wessex Institute of Health Research and Development.

Book 6 assessors for third edition

Professor Virginia Berridge, Professor of History and Head of Unit, Health Promotion Research Unit, Department of Public Health and Policy, London School of Hygiene and Tropical Medicine.

Dr Carol Barker, Nuffield Institute for Health, Leeds University, and the British Council's Technical Advisor for Health Sector Reform, Ministry of Health and Population, Malawi.

Dr Ruairi Brugha, Senior Lecturer in Public Health, London School of Hygiene and Tropical Medicine.

We gratefully acknowledge the contributions made by the external assessors for the previous edition of this book:

Professor David Arnold, Professor of the History of South Asia, School of Oriental and African Studies, University of London.

Professor Anne Crowther, Director, Centre for the History of Medicine, University of Glasgow.

Professor Jane Lewis, Barnett Professor of Social Policy, Department of Social Policy and Social Work, University of Oxford.

Professor James McEwen, Henry Mechan Chair of Public Health and Head of Department of Public Health, University of Glasgow.

Professor David Parkin, Professor of Health Economics, Department of Economics, City University, London.

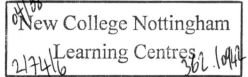

CONTENTS

A note for the general reader 6

Study guide for OU students 8

1 History and diversity 10
Charles Webster

2 Pre-industrial health care, 1500 to 1750 31
Margaret Pelling and Mark Harrison

3 The Industrial Revolution, 1750 to 1848 61
Margaret Pelling, Mark Harrison and Paul Weindling

4 The era of public health, 1848 to 1918 97
Margaret Pelling, Virginia Berridge, Mark Harrison and Paul Weindling

5 The impact of war and depression, 1918 to 1948 133
Virginia Berridge, Mark Harrison and Paul Weindling

6 Mobilisation for total welfare, 1948 to 1974 167
Virginia Berridge, Charles Webster and Gill Walt

7 Caring for health in the UK, 1974 to 2001 197
Charles Webster

8 Health care in the developing world, 1974 to 2001 253
Gill Walt

9 International patterns of health care, 1960 to 2001 295
Alastair Gray

10 Conclusions 327
Charles Webster

References and further sources 340

Answers to questions 355

Acknowledgements 368

Index 371

A note for the general reader

Caring for Health: History and Diversity takes a critical look at health care, tracing the historical development of health-care systems in Europe (with particular emphasis on Britain), and in the colonies controlled by European states, from 1500 to the start of the new millennium. The authors also examine the diversity of health-care systems and the political policies and economic circumstances that have shaped the patterns we see today. The book contains ten chapters, all of which address the following five main themes to some degree (the prominence given to each theme varies between chapters):

- Informal and formal aspects of health care, and reliance on lay carers, particularly women;
- Environmental health problems and the public-health movement;
- The professionalisation of health-care occupations;
- The welfare state and health care; the rise of acute hospitals and high-technology medicine;
- The impact of European models of health care on the rest of the world, and reciprocal influences.

After a substantial introduction to the scope of the book in Chapter 1, Chapters 2 to 6 follow an historical sequence from 1550 to 1974, arriving in modern times in Chapters 7 to 9, which deal with three different portraits of contemporary health care: British health care in Chapter 7; health care in the developing world in Chapter 8; and international health care in Chapter 9. Chapter 10 concludes the book by drawing together and reflecting on the main themes.

The book is fully indexed and referenced and contains a list of abbreviations and an annotated guide to further reading and to selected websites on the Internet. The list of further sources also includes details of how to access a regularly updated collection of Internet resources relevant to the *Health and Disease* series on a searchable database called ROUTES, which is maintained by the Open University. This resource is open to all readers of this book.

Caring for Health: History and Diversity is the sixth in a series of eight books on the subject of health and disease. The book is designed so that it can be read on its own, like any other textbook, or studied as part of U205 *Health and Disease*, a level 2 course for Open University students. General readers do not need to make use of the Study notes, learning objectives and other material inserted for OU students, although they may find these helpful. The text also contains references to a collection of previously published material and specially commissioned articles (*Health and Disease: A Reader*, Open University Press, second edition 1995; third edition 2001) prepared for the OU course: it is quite possible to follow the text without reading the articles referred to, although doing so will enhance your understanding of the contents of *Caring for Health: History and Diversity*.

Abbreviations used in this book

AIDS	acquired immune deficiency syndrome
ASH	Action on Smoking and Health
BMA	British Medical Association
BSE	bovine spongiform encephalopathy
CAM	complementary and alternative medicine
CHI	Commission for Health Improvement
CHW	community health worker
DHSS	Department of Health and Social Security
EIC	East India Company
EU	European Union
FHS	Family Health Services
FPA	Family Planning Association
FSEs	former socialist economies of Europe
GDP	Gross Domestic Product
GMC	General Medical Council
GNP	Gross National Product
GOBI	growth monitoring, oral rehydration, breast-feeding, immunisation
GP	general practitioner
HCHS	Hospital and Community Health Services
HDA	Health Development Agency
HImP	Health Improvement Programme/Plan
HIV	Human Immunodeficiency Virus
HMO	Health Maintenance Organisation
ILO	International Labor Organization
IMF	International Monetary Fund
IMR	infant mortality rate
MOH	Medical Officer of Health
NGO	non-governmental organisation
NHI	National Health Insurance
NHS	National Health Service
NICE	National Institute for Clinical Excellence
NSF	National Service Framework
OECD	Organisation for Economic Cooperation and Development
OPEC	Organisation of Petroleum Exporting Countries
ORS	oral rehydration solution
PAF	Performance Assessment Framework
PCG	Primary Care Group
PCT	Primary Care Trust
PFI	Private Finance Initiative
PHC	primary health-care approach
PPP	purchasing power parity
R&D	research and development
RCT	randomised controlled trial
TB	tuberculosis
UKCC	United Kingdom Central Council for Nursing, Midwifery and Health Visiting
UNDP	United Nations Development Programme
UNICEF	United Nations Children's Fund
VAD	Voluntary Aid Detachment
vCJD	variant Creutzfeldt–Jakob Disease
VD	venereal diseases
WHO	World Health Organisation

Study guide for OU students

(total of around 64 hours, including time for the TMA, spread over 4 weeks)

Chapter 7 is the longest in the book, but Chapter 10 is very short, so pace your study accordingly. All but four of the Reader articles associated with this book were set reading earlier in the course and are revised here, or are optional reading if you have time.

1st week

Chapter 1	**History and diversity** revise Reader article by Engels (1845); optional Reader article by Porter (1997)
Chapter 2	**Pre-industrial health care, 1500 to 1750**
Chapter 3	**The Industrial Revolution, 1750 to 1848** revise Reader articles by McKeown (1976) and Szreter (1988)

2nd week

Chapter 4	**The era of public health, 1848 to 1918** Reader article by Stevens (1976)
Chapter 5	**The impact of war and depression, 1918 to 1948**
Chapter 6	**Mobilisation for total welfare, 1948 to 1974** revise Reader article by Stevens (1976)

3rd week

Chapter 7	**Caring for health in the UK, 1974 to 2001** Reader article by Young and Cullen (1996)
Chapter 8	**Health care in the developing world, 1974 to 2001** Reader articles by Werner (1978), and Bloom and Xingyuan (1997); TV programme 'Catching the good health train'

4th week

Chapter 9	**International patterns of health care, 1960 to 2001** TV programme 'Catching the good health train'; revise Reader article by Bloom and Xingyuan (1997)
Chapter 10	**Conclusions**
TMA completion	

Caring for Health: History and Diversity introduces the subject of health care, using an historical and comparative approach to demonstrate the widest possible definition of what constitutes 'caring for health'. The structure of the book is outlined in 'A note for the general reader' (p. 6), and is developed extensively in Chapter 1.

Study notes are given at the start of every chapter. These primarily direct you to important links to other components of the course, such as the other books in the course series, the Reader, and audiovisual components. Major learning objectives are listed at the end of each chapter, along with questions that will enable you to check that you have achieved these objectives. The index includes key terms in orange type (also printed in bold in the text), which can be looked up easily as an aid to revision as the course proceeds. There is also a list of further sources for those who wish to pursue certain aspects of study beyond the scope of this book, either by consulting other books and articles or by logging on to specialist websites on the Internet.

The time allowed for studying *Caring for Health: History and Diversity* is around 64 hours spread over 4 weeks. The schedule (left) gives a more detailed breakdown to help you to pace your study. You need not follow it rigidly, but try not to let yourself fall behind. Depending on your background and experience, you may well find some parts of this book much more familiar and straightforward than others. If you find a section of the work difficult, do what you can at this stage, and then return to reconsider the material when you reach the end of the book.

There is a tutor-marked assignment (TMA) associated with this book; about 5 hours have been allowed for writing it up, *in addition to* the time spent studying the material it assesses.

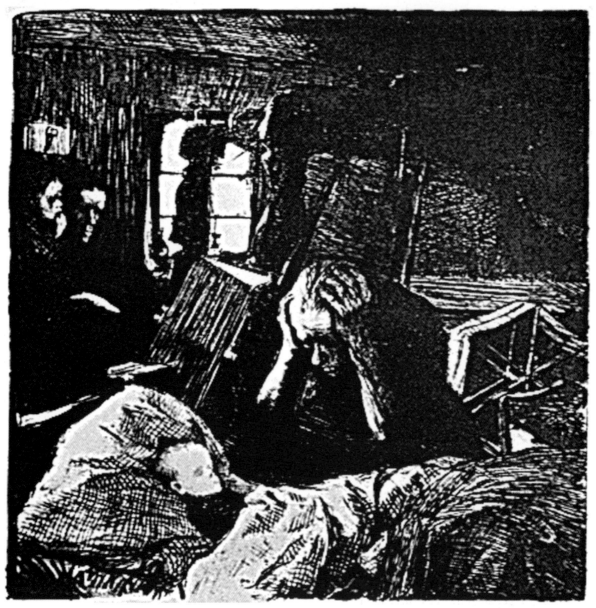

Figure 1.1 *Käthe Kollwitz, 'Destitution' from a series dealing with the weavers' sufferings produced between 1893 and 1897. (Source: Plate 1 from the lithograph cycle Ein Weberaufstand, Weavers' Revolt, Käthe Kollwitz Museum, Berlin)*

CHAPTER 1

History and diversity

1.1   Introduction   12

1.2   The scope of *Caring for Health: History and Diversity*   13

   1.2.1 Informal and formal aspects of care   14

   1.2.2 Environmental and public health   15

   1.2.3 Professionalisation of health-care occupations   15

   1.2.4 Medical advance and the health-care system   15

   1.2.5 Europe and the developing world   16

1.3   Why 'history and diversity'?   16

   1.3.1 Convergence   16

   1.3.2 Divergence   17

   1.3.3 The historical landscape of health care   18

1.4   Relentless progress?   19

   1.4.1 The triumphalist fallacy   19

   1.4.2 The problem of inequality   22

1.5   The modern world system   24

   1.5.1 Legacies from the Industrial Revolution   24

   1.5.2 Modernisation   25

   1.5.3 Hierarchies in health care   26

   1.5.4 In conclusion   27

Objectives for Chapter 1   28

Questions for Chapter 1   28

Study notes for OU students

This book builds on the discussion of the growth of medical knowledge and medical technology in an earlier book in this series, *Medical Knowledge: Doubt and Certainty* (Open University Press, second edition 1994; colour-enhanced second edition 2001), which also introduced the concepts of lay care, traditional or folk systems of health care, and complementary and alternative therapies — subjects to which we return in this book. During Section 1.5.1, we suggest that you read again the article by Friedrich Engels, entitled 'Health: 1844', which appears in *Health and Disease: A Reader* (Open University Press, second edition 1995; third edition 2001), and was set reading for *World Health and Disease* (Open University Press, third edition 2001), Chapter 5. You may also wish to read an optional article 'Hippocrates' by Roy Porter, which also appears in the Reader (but only in the third edition), and is referred to briefly in Section 1.4.1.

1.1 Introduction

This first chapter serves as an introduction to *Caring for Health: History and Diversity*. It performs a set of general but essential functions. We start by explaining the grounds for an historical approach to health care and providing some basic orientation. Then we set out general guidelines for the scope and organisation of the subsequent chapters. And finally we explain some social science concepts that will be used at various points in the book.

This book establishes a basic chronological framework for trends in **health care** over the last five hundred years.[1] For practical purposes, health care is taken as describing those interventions that most directly relate to maintaining health or curing disease. Health care therefore includes caring for the sick or disabled in the home, social support for health-disadvantaged groups within the community, as well as health promotion and curative services provided by a wide range of health professionals. Since virtually every social intervention affects health in some way, health care is not readily separated out from other social influences; for instance, health is much affected by the physical environment or living standards.

On account of the many factors that impinge on health, it is not surprising that developments in health care over the last five hundred years are tied up with the more general process of economic, social and political change. As the following chapters indicate, this period has witnessed revolutionary social changes, including major shifts in the centre of gravity of health-care interventions.

In this book, we recognise that interpretations of change based on the notion of 'inevitable progress' provide an impoverished understanding of past events. This approach overlooks the many socio-political determinants of health care, and it ignores important phenomena such as lay care, traditional or folk systems of health care, and complementary and alternative therapies. *Caring for Health: History and Diversity* therefore undertakes a more critical look at the major historical shifts that have occurred in health care, with the aim of showing that this approach to history is more intellectually satisfying. Indeed this is a constructive contribution to the understanding of dilemmas in health care in general.[2]

Figure 1.1 (the frontispiece to this book) reminds us of the immense human cost of poverty and ill-health. Although inspired by historical events of 1844, the artist Käthe Kollwitz was also drawing on her direct experience of Berlin in the 1890s, where her husband practised medicine among the poor. She was in fact reflecting on the conditions of the urban masses everywhere. This depiction of poverty illustrates that even Germany — the European power experiencing the greatest economic advance in the nineteenth century, and Berlin, the capital city of a new empire — left a substantial body of its population in abject poverty, entailing a legacy of incapacity and premature death.

● By what means has the artist in Figure 1.1 built up an impression of conditions debilitating to the health of this working class family?

[1] The usefulness of the historical approach is illustrated in *Medical Knowledge, Doubt and Certainty* (Open University Press, 2nd edn 1994; colour-enhanced 2nd edn 2001), which includes a group of chronological case studies of medical ideas, examined in the context of more general intellectual change.

[2] This book also sets the historical context for contemporary health issues explored in the next volume in the series, *Dilemmas in UK Health Care* (Open University Press, 3rd edn 2001).

■ Käthe Kollwitz has drawn attention to the lack of ventilation or sunlight and the cramped living conditions, suggesting that the family live and work in a single room, in which the weaving machinery is the dominant element. The oppressive, polluted atmosphere is conducive to lung diseases, including tuberculosis (TB) from which the child is probably dying. Kollwitz powerfully suggests that the struggle for subsistence has drained the health and energies of the family. You will notice that she places the focus on the mother as the main carer in the family and on the mother's anguish owing to the helplessness of their situation.

Even after a century of further economic and social progress, the tragic situation depicted by Kollwitz is the commonplace of the developing world; and it would not be difficult to find parallel examples in the inner cities of any Western country. Women in particular often carry the heaviest load of caring for their families in societies where inbuilt discriminations impose adversely on the health of the most disadvantaged. The historical roots of many of these forms of discrimination will be evident from the following chapters.

1.2   The scope of *Caring for Health: History and Diversity*

In this book, we aim to provide a review of health care in the United Kingdom in particular, but more generally in Western Europe and the European colonial sphere of influence, from 1500 to the present. Within the UK, in order to avoid repetition of detail, most of the specific examples will relate to England, but reference is also made to other parts of the UK where differences are significant to our themes. The overarching aim is to shed light on the system of health care evolved in modern Western industrialised society and the impact of this system in the wider world.

'Western society' is the term applied here to the general sphere of European culture, consciously embodying traditions and institutions influenced by Greek and Roman civilisation, but also incorporating much from Rabbinic and Arab culture, and from sources even further afield. The values of modern Western society extended to regions dominated by settlers from Europe, and they were imposed on indigenous inhabitants where Europeans chose to colonise. Western society provided the environment for the development of modern industrialised economies. As indicated below, advanced Western economies drew the entire world into their orbit of influence.

European colonial expansion began in the sixteenth century, as did the revolution in science, technology and medicine. Thus the foundations for European domination and the beginnings of modern knowledge and institutions can be traced back to an early date. Nevertheless, the period before 1750 was essentially a pre-industrial age. Consequently, consideration of the period between 1500 and 1750 in Chapter 2 provides an insight into health care before the great changes that took place during the Industrial Revolution.

Chapter 3 embraces the catastrophic impact on health care brought about by the first phase of industrialisation in Western Europe, from 1750 to 1848. Chapter 4 covers the long period from 1848 to 1918, during which control of the environment constituted the first priority in the field of health intervention. Chapter 5 deals with the phase of expanding competence of curative medicine; it includes the shock of two World Wars and the intervening depression. This period from 1918 to 1948 involved some consolidation of the commitment to positive welfare policies.

Chapter 6 is concerned with the vast expansion of state-sponsored forms of health care within the context of rising expectations and general support for the substantial development of social welfare services during the period from 1948 to 1974. Chapters 7, 8 and 9 consider the changed situation of health care following the oil crisis of 1973, which precipitated reversal of policies concerning state support for social welfare services. This new phase of retrenchment coincided with a radical critique of the medical establishment emanating from all political angles, and associated with the more general growth in appeal of complementary and alternative medicine.

Chapter 7 describes the impact of these changed circumstances on health services in the UK. Chapter 8 considers the troubled process of evolving appropriate forms of health care in the vulnerable context of countries of the developing world. Chapter 9 examines trends in health service provision worldwide from the quantitative and economic perspective. Chapter 10 draws together the themes of the book as a whole and reinforces the argument for the value of the historical approach.

Five themes have been selected for special attention in this book. They will occur to some extent in all the chapters, and are the subject of separate sections in Chapters 2–6. In the following introductions to each theme, we introduce some key definitions for terms and concepts that underpin the detailed discussions in later chapters.

1.2.1 Informal and formal aspects of care

Health care has always involved a multiplicity of formal and informal agencies. At the start of the twenty-first century, the most visible are the elaborate and expensive facilities, comprising hospitals, health centres, ambulances and so forth, staffed by doctors, nurses and a whole host of supporting professions and occupations — which is collectively called the **formal health-care system**. This formal provision is complemented by an **informal health-care system** drawing on family and community, and also a variety of alternative healers and complementary therapists.

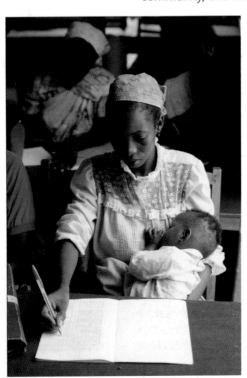

The importance of informal agencies of health care has persisted regardless of the expanding capacities of modern medicine and the extension of curative health services. If anything, the strains imposed by health services on modern economies, and the difficulties of recruiting the huge numbers of health-care personnel required for comprehensive health services has increased the incentives for reliance on informal carers. In every period of history women have played a crucial role in informal care. Opportunities for improving the status and education of women are recognised as major factors in the improvement of family health and in the reduction of infant mortality (see Figure 1.2).

Figure 1.2 *An adult literacy class in the Cameroon. Rising female literacy is closely associated with falling infant mortality and birth rates, and improved nutrition. But in some of the poorest countries of the world, female literacy rates are below 30 per cent. (Source: Giacomo Pirozzi/Panos Pictures)*

1.2.2 Environmental and public health

The term **public health** was coined in the Victorian period and became the object of the first major popular health campaigns, and the focus of state intervention for the second part of the nineteenth century. Public-health interventions are those directed at reducing the health problems of the community as a whole, in contrast to the medical treatment of individual illness. Some aspects of public health care (e.g. immunization and vaccination) are medical in character, but they are preventive rather than curative; many others (e.g. environmental health, water supply, and sewerage disposal) seem far removed from conventional notions of 'health care'. These environmental services form a blurred boundary between the formal health-care system and the many other agencies (such as education, employment or housing) which impinge on health, but are not normally included as forms of health care.

On account of its special characteristics, public health is an area of activity in which both lay and medical specialists engage according to their skills. Chapters 5–7 describe how this unusual situation contributed to a crisis of identity in the medical specialism of public health in the twentieth century.

1.2.3 Professionalisation of health-care occupations

As the formal sector of health care has expanded, the occupations involved have successively aspired to achieve professional status. A **profession** is an occupational group that is granted formal control over the education and training of its members, and over the application of a body of specialised knowledge. **Professionalisation**, the ongoing and complex process by which professional recognition is attained, is unlikely ever to be complete, owing to the urge to professionalise within each new sub-specialism or evolving occupational grouping. Every stage in professionalisation is contentious because established groupings resist the breaking away of sub-specialisms or the loss of authority over rival occupations.

The escalation of professionalisation within health-care occupations has primarily been driven by two forces: the desire of non-medical staff to gain greater parity with medical personnel, and the efforts of specialists to secure their position in competition with entrenched generalists. As noted elsewhere[3], and re-emphasised at the end of this chapter, professionalisation has entailed benefits for patients, for example in establishing standards of training and competence, but its advance has also accelerated the erosion of lay controls over medical practice. Some critics have seen this process as one aspect of **medicalisation** — the expansion of medical influence into ever widening spheres of social life — and they have accused the medical profession and the health-care system more generally as having become instruments of social control.

1.2.4 Medical advance and the health-care system

In this book, advances in medical knowledge, innovations in medical technology, and the impact of mortality, morbidity and malnutrition, take their place alongside social, economic and political forces, as determinants of the character of formal systems of health care. Translating advances in medical knowledge into health-care benefits is a high cost activity, which has inevitably drawn 'the state' into the financing and planning of health care. This has occurred especially under the modern

[3] Professionalisation is also discussed in *Medical Knowledge: Doubt and Certainty* (Open University Press, 2nd edn 1994; colour-enhanced 2nd edn 2001), Chapter 2.

welfare state — a term that was coined to denote the substantial increase in state spending and state supervision in all fields of welfare, which took place throughout the Western economic system, especially after World War II.

The complex hierarchical systems of health care we see today have developed over a very long period. In the twentieth century, by analogy with education, health-care systems came to be described in terms of three levels of organisation: *primary, secondary,* and *tertiary*. **Primary health care** is nearest to the community. In the UK, this level comprises multidisciplinary primary health-care teams led by general practitioners (GPs); the analogous teams in developing countries have less conspicuous medical-practitioner involvement. **Secondary health care** relates to the activities of district hospitals, which provide acute care services for the local population. **Tertiary health care** is centred on regional hospitals, which are concerned with more advanced specialist treatment, teaching and research, and to which patients may be referred from some distance.

1.2.5   Europe and the developing world

This theme deals with the escalation of Western dominance, beginning with minor trading relations, continuing into colonisation, and culminating with exercises in integration under imperialism. In order to give sufficient prominence to the attempt to evolve appropriate forms of health care since independence from colonial rule, the whole of Chapter 8 is an expanded treatment of health care in the developing world from the mid-1970s. It will be seen in this chapter, and in the final sections of Chapters 2–6, that the relationship of Europe with other continents has never been a one-way process. For instance, with respect to particular infectious diseases or the training of health-care personnel, the Europeans and their developing-world partners have always been bound together in a reciprocal relationship.

The remainder of Chapter 1 introduces or reminds you about some important sociological concepts and terminology that will reappear in later chapters, or that are taken as assumed knowledge. It is useful to begin by explaining briefly the reason for selecting 'history and diversity' as the organising framework for this book.

1.3   Why 'history and diversity'?

When considered in all of its dimensions, the modern health-care system is notoriously complex and difficult to understand. This difficulty is in part due to a constant process of change, as the mechanisms are adapted to meet rising expectations, the altering pattern of disease, the new capacities of medicine, or shifts in political and social policy. Of course, all of these influences have been exacting their effect over a long period. Present systems of health care are therefore the end product of a long process of accretion and modification. This book will examine the process of change in the health-care system in the light of the economic and political determinants that have fashioned the institutions of advanced capitalism as a whole. You will see that present arrangements for health care are the product and to some extent the captive of a long history.

1.3.1   Convergence

The process of historical change has brought about the dominance of the Western industrial economies and associated value systems, within which Western biomedical science is an important component. Western medicine has therefore gradually become predominant, even in regions where traditional medicine preserves some form of co-existence. Consequently, history shows the emergence of increasing uniformity. This process is termed *convergence*.

- ● Think for a moment about modern Western health-care systems. What evidence do you see that they are converging into what some have called a 'global' health-care system?

- ■ They are all primarily focused on 'disease management' rather than on 'health promotion' or 'health maintenance'. Accepted best practice among Western-trained doctors, for instance in the use of drugs employed or forms of treatment for specific diseases, also tends to be similar. This uniformity is being accelerated by the development of global networks of information made possible by computerisation and the Internet.

For example, **evidence-based medicine** collates evidence from intervention trials conducted everywhere in the world, with the aim of drawing up codes of best medical and nursing practice for universal use. In general the technology of medicine has become standardised; indeed drug companies are predominantly multinational businesses. Finally, in the dominant Western sphere of influence, the formal training of health-care personnel is everywhere largely similar and based on common scientific and technical principles.

The above factors represent powerful incentives to the breakdown of national barriers. The term **globalisation** is increasingly invoked to describe the operation of these supra-national imperatives. Gobalisation is of course a development of universal scope, which affects developing as well as developed countries. We give it further consideration in the final part of this chapter.

1.3.2 Divergence

While the existing evidence for convergence is compelling, and the hectic pace of globalisation promises further imposition of uniformity, it would be premature to conclude that localised characteristics of health care have largely disappeared or are about to be things of the past. Because history shows the progressive dominance of Western biomedical science, it is tempting to disregard complicating factors, yet it must be acknowledged that biomedical science is only one strand in a complex situation. It is evident that the application of technical expertise is affected by a wide range of political and economic factors, which collectively have produced diversity in the expression of health care through organised health-care systems. This is the reason for equal emphasis on 'history' and 'diversity' in the title of this book.

Even among the most closely-knit Western partners, health-care arrangements preserve a strong element of distinctiveness. As holidaymakers in continental Europe quickly discover, there are stark differences in arrangements for health care even between European Union (EU) neighbours. These distinctions reflect deep-rooted differences among social and political institutions.

You will find in the following chapters that one group of states in Europe imitated the model introduced in Germany in the late nineteenth century, in which health care was financed by compulsory contributory insurance. Notwithstanding this uniformity of principle, every state has evolved its own distinctive application of compulsory insurance. Under these systems, health services tend to be provided by independent practitioners and from facilities that are outside public ownership.

The UK and certain Scandinavian countries have followed an entirely different course, supporting their medical services from local and national taxes. In due course these states evolved towards a 'National Health Service' form of health care, in which the medical services were provided in state-owned facilities, and predominantly by state-employed personnel. Despite these similarities, the UK National Health Service (NHS) has no exact counterparts elsewhere.

The big changes in health care in the UK at the end of the twentieth century reinforced this process of differentiation. For instance, the health services of the four constituent parts of the UK — England, Scotland, Wales and Northern Ireland — have always retained special characteristics, and they are in process of diverging still further on account of the policy of devolution implemented since 1997.

1.3.3 The historical landscape of health care

Each vicinity harbours traces of evidence that can be used to constitute a history of health care extending way back into the past. For instance in any historic population centre in England it is possible that 'almshouses', often-called 'hospitals', are descendants of medieval charities. In town centres there are many former voluntary hospitals or dispensaries, often located in classical style buildings dating from the late eighteenth century. They were part of a comprehensive system of philanthropy, religious in origin, but in health (unlike education) inter-denominational. These institutions are dwarfed in scale by dingy workhouses or lunatic asylums bequeathed by the Victorians. These have now been absorbed into the outer suburbs, but were well outside population centres when they were built. Only recently have these hospitals been closed down and their sites sold off to the developers.

The sites of old voluntary hospitals are frequently used for modern District General Hospitals, the product of the hospital building plan, which began in the 1960s. On account of resource constraints, these hospitals were constructed in stages over a long period and many of them have never been completed. This led UK governments in the mid-1990s to turn to the controversial Private Finance Initiative (PFI) as a means to accelerate hospital modernisation (we discuss PFI in Chapter 7).

Smaller towns frequently contain structures surviving from the rash of cottage hospitals built by local subscription at the start of the twentieth century. Location and physical character tell us much about the original purposes of the miscellaneous collection of institutions absorbed by modern health authorities. Proposals for closure of hospitals and local authority residential homes, or other types of reorganisation, expose the deep-rooted feeling of local communities for their local hospitals. Any such change is likely to be resented and resisted not only on account of immediate practical inconvenience, but also because it erodes local autonomy in the provision of services that had been build up over a long period, and which had represented hard won gains for the local community.

- ● Look at Figure 1.3 (on pp. 20–21). Can you suggest why the workhouse and especially the two lunatic asylums were situated at a distance from the town?

- ■ You may have guessed correctly that the inmates were perceived as a danger to themselves or a bad example to their community, thereby a source of 'moral contamination' of those around them. Therefore they were subject to strict regimes of discipline in large prison-like institutions, which were necessarily located outside the town. These forbidding institutions served as a deterrent, and they suitably eliminated stigmatised groups of perceived deviants from the town. Also these institutions were designed to be almost entirely self-supporting, therefore requiring immense sites containing farms and market gardens.

The example of Norwich is a reminder of the great antiquity of some of our medical institutions, a conclusion that will be further reinforced by Chapter 2.

1.4 Relentless progress?

1.4.1 The triumphalist fallacy

The greater realism of recent decades has caused us to revise the once dominant idea of the seemingly relentless advance of health care. In the past, the history of medicine was particularly prone to the 'triumphalist' approach because medicine was one of the most obvious beneficiaries of the forward march of science. It was also believed that progress in health care was guaranteed by the priorities of the existing social and political order.

Under this construction, a special place of honour was granted to the medical profession, based on its scientific competence and dedication to higher purposes. This claim to 'Christian humanism' invited the public to regard the medical profession as heir to venerable standards of propriety, descending ultimately from Hippocrates[4] and the humanist founders of their first Royal Colleges during the Renaissance. According to this august tradition, the public was expected to suspend faculties of criticism that were applied in other spheres of experience. Also, because of the medical profession's claims to superior trust, it was subject to lax regulation and accountability.

● From the perspective of users of health services, can you think of any undesirable consequences of the **triumphalist fallacy**?

■ We are invited to believe that at any time the medical services are as adequate as could be expected and that there could be no reasonable grounds for complaint or criticism.

Although medical science has consistently gained credit for medical advances, the implicit trust and confidence inspired by the triumphalist hypothesis has proved difficult to sustain. Even recent history has been punctuated by serious hospital scandals, which have given rise to public disquiet about competence and ethical propriety within the medical profession. In response, the UK government at the turn of the millenium took urgent action to prevent the further collapse of public confidence by imposing more stringent audit and regulation on the medical profession in all of its spheres of activity.

Contrary to the impression given by the triumphalist approach, the historical record shows that governments habitually failed to respond appropriately to protect the health of their populations, while medical officialdom could not necessarily be relied upon to identify the root causes of ill-health.

---

[4] An article 'Hippocrates' by Roy Porter, appears in *Health and Disease: A Reader* (Open University Press, 3rd edn 2001), and includes a translation of part of the Hippocratic Oath; Open University students could usefully read this optional article.

Figure 1.3   *Map showing the locations of the main hospitals of Norwich to the end of the twentieth century, with the city wall (dashed line) marking the boundary of the medieval town. Photos (a) to (g) illustrate the range of hospital buildings, often converted from former uses. The **Norfolk County Lunatic Asylum** is marked on the map. Two other hospitals fall outside the area shown: the new **Norfolk and Norwich Hospital** (3 miles to the West of the city, completed 2001), intended to supplant (d) the existing Norfolk and Norwich Hospital and (g) the West Norwich Hospital; and the **Hellesdon Mental Hospital** (3 miles to the North West), built in 1880 as an asylum by the Norwich County Borough and expanded under the NHS to provide acute mental-health services for the area; this too will be supplanted by the new Norfolk and Norwich Hospital.*

(a) The **Lazar House**, founded in 1119 by Herbert de Losinga, Bishop of Norwich. Lazar houses were hostels for lepers and others with diseases perceived as infectious. These houses were generally located safely outside city perimeters. The surviving portion on Sprowston Road is the chapel (shown here), which was built on a substantial scale. (Photo: Dr A. Batty Shaw)

(b) The **Great Hospital**, founded in 1249 by Walter de Suffield, Bishop of Norwich, was originally part of a monastic institution providing hostels for pilgrims, care for the poor and treatment for the sick. The original buildings were remarkably large, the infirmary hall being 200 feet long. The hospital was divided into men's and women's wards. By 1500 it had ceased to function as a hospital for the sick. (Photo: Dr A. Batty Shaw)

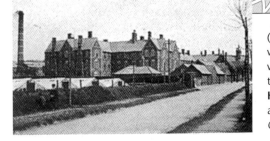

(g) The **Workhouse Infirmary** was developed for sick patients from the original workhouse established by the Poor Law authorities in 1859; (it replaced the old workhouse in the converted Blackfriars monastic buildings in the centre of town). The Infirmary was redeveloped under the NHS into the **West Norwich Hospital**, the functions of which became closely integrated with the old Norfolk and Norwich Hospital. (Photo: Standley, P. J. (1989) *Norwich: A Second Portrait in Old Picture Postcards*, S. B. Publications, Market Drayton, Shropshire)

(c) The original **Norfolk and Norwich Hospital**, completed in 1775, was representative of the hospitals established in most county towns in the mid-eighteenth century, funded by voluntary subscriptions from prosperous members of the community, and supported by various religious denominations. This voluntary hospital catered for the sick poor, largely reviving the functions of the Great Hospital. (Photo: Norfolk Museums Service, Norwich Castle Museum)

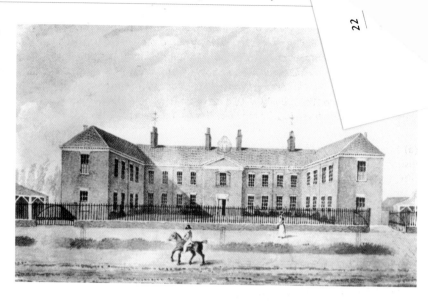

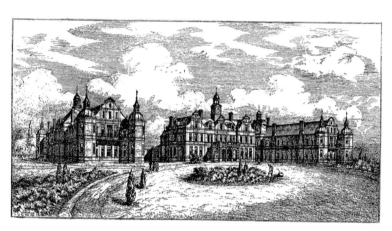

(d) The completely rebuilt Victorian **Norfolk and Norwich Hospital** was opened in 1879 on the spacious site of the original voluntary hospital. The grandiose 'Tudor' style of the Victorian voluntary hospital contrasted strangely with the bleak tower-block extensions added since 1948 under the NHS. This now congested 18-acre site has accommodated the acute hospital services for Norwich and a large surrounding area for more than two centuries. (Photo: Dr A. Batty Shaw)

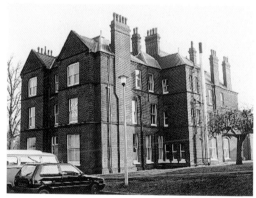

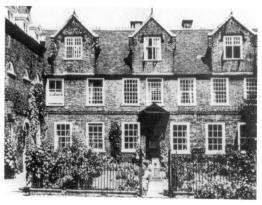

(f) The **Norwich Isolation Hospital** was built by the Norwich County Borough in 1893 opposite the Workhouse Infirmary. Under the NHS it housed various medical specialisms, until incorporated into the Norfolk Mental Health Care NHS Trust in the 1990s. In 1998 it was redeveloped as the **Julian Hospital**, a 100-bed centre for psychogeriatric services; the new name reaches back to a medieval celebrity, Juliana of Norwich, the woman mystic and hermit, who died in 1416. (Photo: Mike Levers)

(e) The **Bethel Hospital**, founded in 1724 with a bequest from Mary Chapman, was the first hospital for patients with mental disorders established outside London. It was superseded by the **Norfolk County Lunatic Asylum** 3 miles East of the town centre, one of the first county asylums built under the Lunacy Act of 1808, and by the **Hellesdon Mental Hospital** 3 miles to the North West. Under the NHS, the county asylum was renamed **St Andrew's Mental Hospital** and housed about 1 200 patients, until it closed in 1998 and was sold off for development. (Photo: Dr A. Batty Shaw)

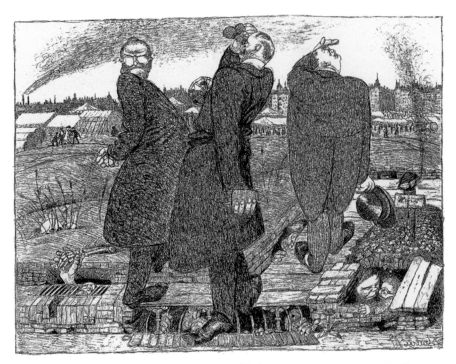

Figure 1.4 *'Aus dem Kommissionsbericht der Übersichtigen.' Draft cartoon by Ernst Barlach for the issue of the satirical magazine* Simplizissimus, *dated 25 November 1907. The caption that appeared with it was a quotation from an official report, which pronounced: 'as far as the eye can see, one is met by scenes of cheerfulness and contentment'. (Source: Courtesy of Ernst und Hans Barlach GbR, Lizenzverwaltung, Ratzeburg)*

As shown in Figure 1.4, official complacency was subjected to bitter irony by Ernst Barlach, who was responding to exactly the same social circumstances that offended Käthe Kollwitz in Figure 1.1.

● What dangers to health were the officials guilty of ignoring in Figure 1.4?

■ Barlach particularly emphases smoke pollution and homelessness, which forced the poor to live in cellars, or even improvised underground shelters constructed in cemeteries. To the left of centre, Barlach draws attention to the dangers of violent crime. In general the city is presented as a grim environment for health.

The historical record therefore warns against complacency in assessing the adequacy of the health-care system. In fact, it will be evident from the final chapters of this book that recent decades have been characterised by increasing realism about the shortcomings of modern health-care systems, and indeed a certain amount of despondency. Applause for medical advances or expectations of progress are by no means things of the past, but misguided triumphalism has slipped away into history.

1.4.2 The problem of inequality

A further potent reminder of the failure to maximise the potential benefits of medical progress and health care is provided by the continuing gap between the health of the rich and the poor. It is obvious that the problems of ill-health afflicting the poor are rooted in economic inequalities (Figure 1.5). The correction of these inequalities is clearly beyond the competence of the health services alone. Accordingly, no realistic programme for correcting *health* inequalities can be evolved without attention to

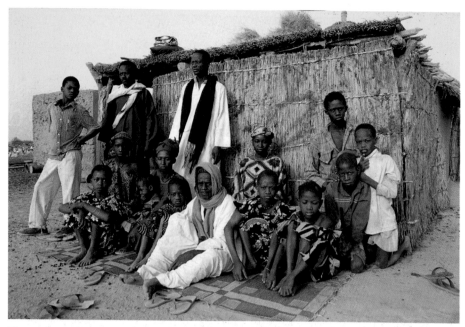

Figure 1.5 *As the counterpart of the Western urban poor (whose plight is illustrated in Figure 1.4), the poor of the developing world experience insuperable difficulties in securing the basic necessities of life and health. Three generations of the Fulani family in their compound, Senegal. (Source: Jeremy Hartley/Panos Pictures)*

reducing *social* inequalities. Therefore any meaningful conception of health care must allow for the application of correctives from any other relevant social service.

Formal **equality** — an equal share to each individual — may be a utopian goal, but this does not preclude steps being made to reduce inequalities. The effort to achieve more equal *access* to resources, employment, social security, education, housing and health care has been the major priority of the modern welfare state. Health services in the UK have therefore been provided on a more *universal* basis (that is available to everyone); they are more *comprehensive* (covering all eventualities), and they are *free at the point of delivery*.

Health services are sometimes financed through direct taxation, which maximises the redistributive effect, i.e. the poor benefit most because the rich pay the highest tax. However, events have shown that such measures have not brought proportionate benefits to the most needy. In practice, the more prosperous classes have displayed superior capacity to gain access to the resources of welfare, thereby merely exacerbating the problem of inequality.

Efforts to shift resources to give more meaningful access to services for the most disadvantaged groups began in the 1970s, when it was recognised that positive inducements were needed to provide **equity** — a share of resources according to *need*. Identified among the vulnerable groups requiring positive discrimination were working-class women, minority ethnic groups, and people who are frail and elderly, mentally handicapped, mentally sick, and physically or learning disabled. These, of course, represent a substantial segment of the population of every country, but one that possesses little purchasing power, poor command of the media, and has traditionally exercised little political influence. The final chapters of this book will consider the degree of success of efforts to achieve greater equity in health-care distribution in different parts of the world.

1.5   The modern world system

From the above remarks it is apparent that the poor in both the developed and the developing world experience analogous problems of inequality, stemming from similar economic causes. Consequently, this book strives to avoid giving any impression that societies and their health-care arrangements in the developing world have existed, like some exotic species, in a state of primitive isolation. Through international trade, colonisation and exploitation, Western capitalism rapidly extended its influence to all parts of the world. Thus, the entire world system is caught up in a process of reciprocal interaction and interdependence — in fact the forerunner of the phenomenon of globalisation that has already been mentioned as a leading theme in contemporary analysis.

1.5.1   Legacies from the Industrial Revolution

A reminder of the long-standing character of this interdependence is provided by the mills, which are such a ubiquitous feature of cotton towns in Lancashire, and which provided the basis for their prosperity. The wealth of estate owners in the West Indies and mill owners in Lancashire was gained at the cost of untold misery and disease among native populations in West Africa, imported labourers in the West Indian plantations, and workers in mills and related industries in Britain. The factory system resulting from this international transaction created a multiplicity of threats to health, stemming from conditions within the factories, the dangers associated with various occupations, or by generating adverse living conditions and poverty on a mass scale. Thus the engine of the Industrial Revolution was responsible for a health crisis in different societies separated by vast distances.

Figure 1.6 gives an impression of the wretched industrial landscape of Stockport, near Manchester, the area that inspired Friedrich Engels in 1844 to write his book *The Condition of the Working Class in England* (published in 1845).[5]

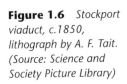

Figure 1.6 *Stockport viaduct, c.1850, lithograph by A. F. Tait. (Source: Science and Society Picture Library)*

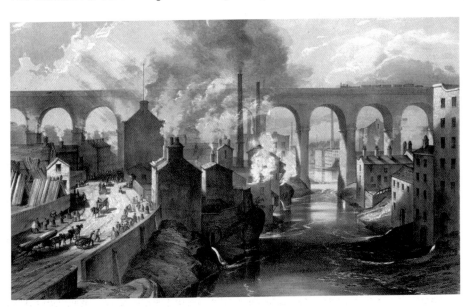

[5] An extract from Engels' book, entitled 'Health:1844' appears in *Health and Disease: A Reader* (Open University Press, 2nd edn 1995; 3rd edn 2001). It is set reading for Open University students during an earlier book in this series, *World Health & Disease* (Open University Press, 3rd edn 2001). It would be beneficial for students to read this extract again now.

- Itemise some likely threats to health illustrated in Figure 1.6.

■ Smoke; pollutants pouring into the river; obviously unhealthy working and living conditions.

Industrialisation[6], as one of the major components in the developing world economy, has added enormously to the scale of health problems. The capacity of uncontrolled industrialisation to damage health on a vast scale became apparent in Eastern Europe with the collapse of the Soviet bloc. Even the remotest regions have not been immune from the depredations of industrialisation. For instance, Donald Denoon, an Australian expert on health care in Papua New Guinea, pointed out that the supposedly enlightened colonial administration had failed to arrest the deterioration in health consequent upon industrialisation and other forms of labour exploitation:

> The mechanism for the introduction, dissemination, and redistribution of infection was the mobilisation of labour for mining, for plantation work, and for general employment by the colonists and their government. And that mechanism was much more effective than the frantic attempts of the health authorities to stamp out epidemics once they occurred … Colonialism itself was a health hazard, which colonial medical services were ill-equipped to suppress. (Denoon, 1989, pp. 31–2)

It is evident that less developed states such as Papua New Guinea are in process of importing a collection of diseases that have taken full hold in middle-income economies such as South Africa. Before the epidemic of Acquired Immune Deficiency Syndrome (AIDS) changed the health profile in Sub-Saharan Africa and Asia in the early 1990s, the common diseases in developing countries mirrored the pattern that was formally prevalent in the industrial conurbations of the West. The examples cited above demonstrate that **occupational diseases** associated with various forms of work have, since the Industrial Revolution, steadily increased their prevalence until they have become global phenomena.

1.5.2 Modernisation

The changes taking place in the Western economy and in its political and social structure in the period discussed in this book are often called **modernisation**. The Dutch social scientist Abram de Swaan identifies three important dimensions of modernisation: urbanisation, secularisation and bureaucracy (de Swaan, 1988, pp. 2–3).

Urbanisation is the drift of population from village to town communities, and from a rural to an urban way of life. Urbanisation introduces a multiplicity of threats to health, but it also provides an economical and convenient basis for organisation of such institutions as hospitals.

Secularisation involves the shift away from a social system in which religious values and institutions associated with religion perform a dominant role in all aspects of the life of the community. Secularisation also involves a move away from a charismatic and non-rational ethos, to a society where rational and routinised functions are allegedly dominant. Because religious bodies were traditionally closely bound up with the care of the poor and the sick, the escalation of these problems beyond the scope of bodies with religious affiliations created a major vacuum in welfare provision.

[6] Discussed in *World Health and Disease* (Open University Press, 3rd edn 2001), particularly Chapters 5–8.

Bureaucracy is a necessary consequence of secularisation. Bureaucrats are the lay officials and professional personnel who take on the tasks of an advanced society requiring the employment of expertise. Recruitment of bureaucrats requires a higher degree of literacy within society, adoption of universal education, training, examinations, certification, etc. The more advanced the economy, the greater the development of hierarchies of bureaucrats. The proliferation of occupations and professions associated with health care is an ideal example of the growth of a bureaucracy.

One of the striking features of modernisation has been the enormous expansion of organised provision for welfare. This process is termed **collectivisation**. The state has become increasingly involved in supervising and even directly organising the collective agencies of welfare.

It can be appreciated that acting in combination, urbanisation, secularisation and bureaucratisation, exercised a big impact in the fields of health and welfare. As de Swaan explains, these forms of rationalisation were the basis for moves towards 'a vast conglomerate of nationwide, compulsory, and collective arrangements to remedy and control the external effects of adversity' in the fields of poor relief, education and health care (de Swaan, 1988, p. 218). Chapters 3 to 7 describe the gradual, but inexorable, working out of these trends in the field of health care.

Modernisation as described by de Swaan is a complex process of rationalisation taking place over a long period. The term has long been current in the social sciences. In the UK in the 1990s, 'modernisation' came into vogue to encapsulate the drive of successive governments to reform the public sector, including the health and social services. This version of modernisation is further discussed in Chapter 7.

1.5.3   Hierarchies in health care

In this book you will find the term **elite** frequently introduced to describe the group that dominates any particular hierarchy. For instance, doctors have constituted an elite with respect to other health workers. However, within the medical profession, hospital consultants have traditionally formed an elite over general practitioners; while, among consultants, specialisms connected with general medicine or surgery have constituted an elite compared with those of gerontology, psychiatry, or public health. Structures of elitism are constantly changing, as is for instance evident in the UK in the 1990s, when the status of GPs improved at the expense of hospital doctors, owing to changes in the NHS.

Medical bureaucracies have come to dominate what is known as the **hierarchy of resort**. Most illness and infirmity is contained within the informal circle of family and friends, and it involves no steps beyond self-medication. In this sphere, women have traditionally played a dominant role. An intermediate level of care involves resort to folk medicine or complementary healers, individuals who specialise in healing, but who lie outside the officially sanctioned medical system. These healers play a leading role in developing countries, and in Western society they are more significant than is customarily assumed.

The professional or formal level of health care represents the summit of the hierarchy of resort. At this level, responsibility for care is taken over by an elaborate structure of professions, which itself has assumed an hierarchical character. This hierarchy within medicine has resulted in great coherence within the professions and occupations involved in health care, with the result that the medical bureaucracy has come to exercise enormous influence and authority.

However, as will be noted especially in Chapter 7, the hierarchy of resort is highly fluid, and relations between the various practitioners are constantly changing. For instance, it is now the case that GPs and certain classes of complementary therapists work together as equals. Certain groups of nurses are attaining specialist status that enables them to take over functions formerly performed by GPs and hospital doctors. Hospital doctors complain that their traditional autonomy has been infringed to the extent that their status is undermined and even that their profession has become 'proletarianised'.

1.5.4 In conclusion

You should already be familiar with the idea that professionalisation has entailed the emergence of *social control, medicalisation, surveillance* and *incarceration.*[7] This book will outline in more detail the historical pathways by which these developments have come about. You will see that over the last two hundred years doctors and other health professions have built up bureaucratic structures of a kind that scarcely existed before 1800. The nineteenth century witnessed the enormous growth of hospitals and asylums of many types, and the twentieth century saw both the dramatic transformation of the hospital system and the intrusion of medical values into numerous spheres of social existence.

The modern state has seen small-scale, local agencies, often with religious affiliations, dependent on the vagaries of charitable subscription, being gradually replaced by nation-wide, compulsory structures, involving a high degree of state intervention. Haphazard services, available to narrowly-entitled groups, usually conditional on means-testing or subscription, have been replaced by comprehensive services, available universally, together with less discriminatory criteria of eligibility.

The latter changes describe the features customarily associated with the welfare state, where the recognition of unrestricted *entitlement* to benefits, as a basic right of citizenship, has conferred on the community a degree of protection from the hazards of the working of the economic system and the chance effects of certain diseases. Assessment of the degree to which collectivisation and medical intervention have, in reality, fulfilled their intended purpose will be addressed in the following chapters. You will notice however that, even if trends in health care have become deeply entrenched, a changed social and economic environment is quite capable of reversing the tide. History therefore embodies no iron laws of change, even if social scientists incline to think in these terms.

---

[7] These terms and concepts are extensively discussed in *Medical Knowledge: Doubt and Certainty* (Open University Press, 2nd edn 1994; colour-enhanced 2nd edn 2001).

OBJECTIVES FOR CHAPTER 1

When you have studied this chapter, you should be able to:

1.1 Define and use, or recognise definitions and applications of, each of the terms printed in **bold** in the text.

1.2 Demonstrate the value of the historical approach towards present-day dilemmas concerning health care.

1.3 Discuss the idea that both patterns of disease and health-care systems are products of the underlying economic and political system.

1.4 Discuss the limitations of medical intervention in attempting to correct the major problems of ill-health stemming from such factors as economic inequality, urbanisation and industrialisation.

1.5 Discuss the relevance to developments in health care of the major social trends that have been introduced in this chapter: professionalisation, medicalisation, globalisation and modernisation.

QUESTIONS FOR CHAPTER 1

1   (*Objective 1.2*)

Examine Figure 1.3 again to familiarise yourself with the key hospital developments in Norwich. In particular, study the captions relating to each of the institutions pictured. What can you learn about the social, political and religious factors that influenced the foundation and subsequent relocation of these institutions, on the basis of their pattern of distribution, their size and their physical appearance?

2   (*Objective 1.3*)

Examine the following extract, in which de Swaan describes the impact of some important aspects of modernisation:

> Industrialisation and urbanization brought masses of people closely together in a new state of aggregation: the nineteenth-century industrial city. Under these conditions of physical proximity, the concomitants of poverty — squalor, malnutrition and ill health — produced novel adversities: the epidemics, which hit the poor hardest, but also threatened the established citizens, while paralyzing the city's social and economic life ... [The] response was found in the concept of urban sanitation through a 'venous-arterial system' of fresh-water supply and sewerage which would shield city-dwellers from one another by encapsulating domestic life in private homes, while connecting everyone to the grand urban service networks. (de Swaan, 1988, p. 221)

On the basis of this extract, the text and the illustrations in Chapter 1, and the Reader article by Engels, list the ways in which industrialisation and urbanisation both generated ill-health and facilitated public-health reforms.

3   (*Objective 1.4*)

The following extract comes from the 1980 report *Inequalities in Health* (widely known as the 'Black Report' after the chairman of the working group, Sir Douglas Black), which attached great importance to a 'wider strategy' for combating inequalities in health in the UK.

> While the health care service can play a significant part in reducing inequalities in health, measures to reduce differences in material standards of living at work, in the home and in everyday social and community life are of even greater importance. We have in mind not simply a general reduction of inequalities in living standards, but a marked relative improvement in the living standards of the poorest people, together with measures to prevent new technologies, new working procedures, changes in styles of urban and rural living and the emergence of new social and political associations from undermining the existing living standards of some groups. Like the strategy we propose for the health care system, the strategy to be adopted outside that system needs to be comprehensive and interlinked. (Department of Health and Social Security, 1980, p. 165)

On the basis of the above extract, your reading of Chapter 1 (and, for Open University students, your understanding of *World Health and Disease*, Open University Press, 3rd edn 2001, particularly Chapters 9 and 10), explain how some specific interventions outside the field of formal health care could be expected to reduce inequalities in health. Consider this issue with respect to both industrialised and developing world contexts.

4   (*Objectives 1.1 and 1.5*)

You are now familiar with many social science terms and concepts relevant to the interpretation of developments in health care. Summing up some of these trends, the medical sociologist Bryan Turner suggests that:

> … the emergence of the medical classification of deviance, the growing importance of the doctor as a professional man, the development of medical institutions around the hospital, the clinic and the examination, and the organization of medical surveillance of society represent components of a secularization of western cultures. Put simply, the doctor has replaced the priest as the custodian of social values; the panoply of ecclesiastical institutions of regulation … have been transferred through the evolution of scientific medicine to a panoptic[8] collection of localized agencies of surveillance and control. Furthermore, the rise of preventive medicine, social medicine and community medicine has extended these agencies of regulation deeper and deeper into social life. (Turner, 1987, pp. 37–8)

To what extent do the terms and concepts used by Turner suggest that the advance of medicine entailed negative as well as positive consequences for society as a whole?

[8] The term 'panoptic' is taken from Jeremy Bentham's idea of a panopticon, an ideal institution in which complete surveillance was possible, and which was most realised in prison building. Bentham was a nineteenth-century social reformer whose contribution to British health care is discussed in Chapter 3 of this book. A plan he produced for a panopticon appears in *Medical Knowledge: Doubt and Certainty* (Open University Press, 2nd edn 1994; colour-enhanced 2nd edn 2001), Chapter 8.

CHAPTER 2

Pre-industrial health care, 1500 to 1750

2.1 **Pre-industrial society: chances and changes 32**

    2.1.1 Population and family structure 33

    2.1.2 Death and disease 34

    2.1.3 Poverty and poor law 35

2.2 **Lay care: anxiety and expertise 37**

    2.2.1 Family and community 38

    2.2.2 Lay and formal care: blurred boundaries 38

2.3 **The cleanliness of our ancestors 39**

    2.3.1 Threats to health: public and private 40

    2.3.2 A rural society and its environment 41

    2.3.3 The responsibilities of towns 42

    2.3.4 Utopia: a healthy city 43

2.4 **Medical practitioners: many and varied 43**

    2.4.1 The tripartite division: physicians, surgeons, and apothecaries 44

    2.4.2 Specialists and itinerants 48

    2.4.3 Numbers and distribution of practitioners 49

    2.4.4 Occupational diversity: a means of living, not a way of life 49

2.5 **A health-care system outside institutions 50**

    2.5.1 The costs of medical care: community provision 50

    2.5.2 Medical poor relief 51

    2.5.3 Hospitals and other institutions 51

    2.5.4 Medicine and the 'common weal' 53

2.6 **Empires and exchanges: the first phase of expansion 54**

    2.6.1 The slave trade 55

    2.6.2 'The white man's grave' 56

    2.6.3 Indigenous medical systems 57

Objectives for Chapter 2 59

Questions for Chapter 2 59

Study notes for OU students

This and the following chapter deal with the period from 1500 to 1848. They make reference to periodisations of history according to criteria which can be mainly cultural (e.g. Renaissance, Enlightenment), religious (e.g. Reformation), or economic (e.g. Industrial Revolution). We refer to the term most relevant to our context. These terms must be used flexibly because they relate to complex developments, which vary in their character and chronology according to their location. The changing patterns of health and disease in England from 1500 to 1750 were described and discussed in *World Health and Disease* (Open University Press, 3rd edn 2001), Chapter 6, and form a useful background to the material presented here.

2.1 Pre-industrial society: chances and changes

Has contemporary society altered more rapidly than any in the past? Many of those living in the sixteenth and seventeenth centuries shared with modern populations the sense that their world was changing with terrifying speed. Europe experienced a major shift in the balance between East and West, persistent religious conflicts, emergent nationalisms, and the founding of new colonial empires.

The establishment of a Turkish European empire, by blocking the land route to India, prompted the 'discovery' of the New World of the Americas, and led to fateful biological and cultural exchanges between peoples hitherto kept apart. The fall of Constantinople to the Turks in 1453 drove the last custodians of the classical learning of the Byzantine empire to Italy and the West; these refugees, and the manuscripts they brought with them to Western Europe, encouraged new ideals of human potential based on the rediscovery of the world of ancient Greece and Rome. The new ideals, which stressed the role of the intellectual in organised society, became known as *humanism*. Though very different, all these changes proved relevant for health and disease.

Many saw this period of change optimistically, as one of 'rebirth' of the individual human spirit and rediscovery of the physical world — hence *Renaissance* — a term first applied to a broad shift in cultural outlook at its peak between about 1450 and 1550. A central aim of the Renaissance was to study and then surpass the achievements of ancient Greece and Rome. There was however a dark side of the Renaissance, of which disease represents only one aspect. This sense of a new (and perhaps final) age of corruption was balanced by fresh religious impulses and the search for greater powers over nature. Traditional beliefs in magic and astrology were reinforced at the level of *elite culture* by the rediscovery of ancient learning and 'secrets'. The period saw repeated (and conflicting) attempts to reinterpret human destiny in terms of a reconciliation of Christian and pagan philosophies.

Periods of change often lead to periods of reaction. For instance in England, following the turmoils of the Civil War period, and particularly after the restoration of Charles II in 1660, there was reduced toleration for religious differences. Society in the later seventeenth century sought to damp down 'enthusiasms' and to accentuate social and gender distinctions. At the same time religious and political divisions became institutionalised as different parties and churches. Given this kind of separate development, no single institution was likely to be able to exert an overall control. Each group in society was concerned to defend its own religious and social status, and to implement its social outlook.

The renewed growth of towns as service and leisure centres, and what has been described as a *commercialisation* of society — an accelerated shift to a cash economy, and greater consumption of material goods — reflected the increased need to express fine gradations in social differences. In the earlier half of the period, medicine can be seen as a source of consolation for all classes, like alcohol; in the latter, medicine is more obviously being bought in quantity by those who could afford a higher standard of living.

2.1.1 Population and family structure

People's chances in life can often be related to overall population distribution and demographic structure. Compared with the city-states of continental Europe, England presented the paradox of a *one-city nation*: its numerous centres of population were long-established, but small, with the sole exception of London, which by 1750 had grown to be the largest city in Europe, and the fourth largest in the world. London's population increased by immigration, particularly of young people of both sexes, many of whom travelled from remote counties and fell victim to the city's diseases.

Although English society remained predominantly rural over the period, there was a gradual shift towards *urbanisation*: the percentage living in towns rose from around 6 per cent in 1500 to around 18 per cent in 1700. The old *corporate* towns — those which had gained some control over their own affairs — were concentrated in East Anglia, the South-East, the North-East, and the West Country. The focus of economic development did not shift to the Midlands and the North until the end of the period covered by this chapter.

Population change can take many forms: for example, the age-structure of populations can vary considerably.[1] The Elizabethan period was dominated by young people; over half the population was under 25. Average life expectancy was affected by the great loss of *infant* lives: a person surviving to the age of thirty could expect to live another 30 years.

Changes in age-structure notwithstanding, the English family in the pre-industrial period followed the pattern for Northern Europe generally. Although households could be *extended* by the presence of servants, apprentices, journeymen, children being wet-nursed, and relatives temporarily accommodated, it was unusual for a family unit to contain more than two generations. Except among the elite, households were small and *nuclear*.

They could, however, be complicated by the effects of mortality — remarriage was common, especially among men — and by the driving force of poverty. The elderly poor for example often had to live alone, but also followed 'survival strategies' involving living with others who were not their own children. The population as a whole was relatively mobile, travelling to enter service or apprenticeship or to marry, for betterment, or simply in desperation. In Northern Europe generally, the supposed 'golden age' of families rooted to the soil with all duties of care carried out by extended kinship networks, turns out to be a myth.

On the other hand, though highly stratified into a hierarchical social order, this was still recognisably a 'face-to-face' society, that is, one based on communication and transactions taking place primarily person-to-person — except perhaps in London. Although it may still have had its 'neighbourhoods', London was perceived as a place of bewildering complexity in which appearances were deceiving and it was hard to know people for what they were.

---

[1] Changes in population structure are discussed in *World Health and Disease* (Open University Press, 3rd edn 2001), particularly in Chapter 2.

2.1.2 Death and disease

What diseases affected people most in the pre-industrial period? [2] If every age has its disease — as ours may be AIDS, or cancer — then this period is best represented by *syphilis*. Possibly introduced by contact with the New World and trading in slaves, syphilis was given various nicknames like 'the French pox', and 'mal de Naples', because of its association with the movement of armies in Europe. The more learned name of syphilis comes from a character in a Latin narrative poem about the disease, composed by a humanist physician in 1521. Syphilis was treated (drastically but successfully) with mercury (see Figure 2.1).

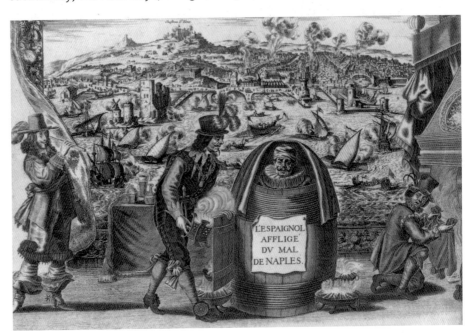

Figure 2.1 *A syphilitic suffering the dangerous treatment of fumigation with mercury. This well-known but deplorable fate is here used as a vehicle for political satire, following the revolt of Naples against Spanish domination in 1647. (Source: Bibliothèque Nationale, Paris)*

The search for alternative cures led to the trial of many novel imports from the New World, including tobacco, sarsaparilla, and the wood guaiacum (a monopoly of which by the Fugger banking family helped finance European wars). During this first outburst in Europe, syphilis prevailed in a more infectious form and caused hideous effects on the surface of the body. As a 'new disease' connected with sexual behaviour, it became a major element in satire, slander, social criticism, and fear of marginal groups in society.

Sexually transmitted disease was a major — though unquantifiable — factor affecting society from around 1500. In the early sixteenth century this sense of a crisis in public health was sharpened by the outbreak of another new disease, the 'English sweat', which alarmed because it seemed particularly to affect the elite. Victims often died within hours of onset of influenza-like illness, but by 1551 the disease seems to have died out. Dearths, or 'crises of subsistence', were probably one cause of high mortality, and were feared not least for their effects on political stability. *Plague* broke out repeatedly (Figure 2.2) until the 'Great Plague of London' of 1665–6, and travelled through rural as well as urban areas. The early-seventeenth-century epidemics, like those of the 1590s, coincided with economic decline. Although plague retreated from Europe, smallpox and then typhus seemed to increase in importance, contributing to the major peaks in English mortality in the 1680s and 1720s.

[2] The epidemiology of this period is discussed in *World Health and Disease* (Open University Press, 3rd edn 2001), Chapter 6.

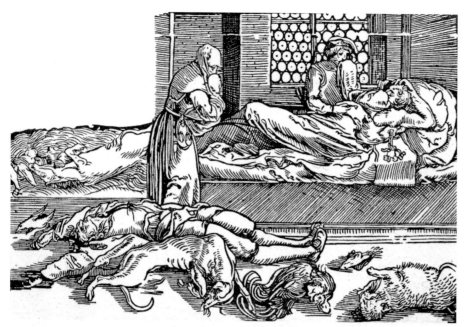

Figure 2.2 *Plague broke out repeatedly in the sixteenth and early seventeenth centuries. The first outbreaks killed rich and poor alike. In this engraving by Hans Burgkmair the elder (1473–1531), the master of a wealthy household is shown dying, the characteristic bubo in his armpit prominently displayed. His dead animals underline the point that animals were thought to carry plague (in fur and feathers) as well as suffering from it. His attendants may be grieving but they are also trying to avoid the disease by not breathing in bad odours. (Source: Mary Evans Picture Library)*

Less obvious to us, but of great concern at the time, were: scurvy; rickets (newly identified in the seventeenth century); rheumatism; eye diseases; skin diseases; parasitic infections; occupational diseases, especially rupture and infection following injury; fractures; unhealed wounds and ulcers, especially of the legs; 'the stone' (kidney and bladder stones); complications of pregnancy and childbearing; 'melancholy' (called 'the English disease'); tuberculosis; and conditions that killed infants, like diarrhoea.

2.1.3 Poverty and poor law

In the early sixteenth century, England followed other European countries in introducing ecclesiastical registration of births, marriages and deaths, primarily to detect excess mortality caused by plague. Summary **Bills of Mortality**, sometimes collating causes of death other than plague, were later instituted in London and other major centres. Surviving an epidemic also involved measuring (and increasing) available resources, so that 'numbering the people' for tax purposes intensified. Moreover, humanist ideals suggested that in a city — or 'common-wealth' — leaders should be responsible and all citizens should contribute according to their degree.

The problem of *poverty* became a major aspect of social policy, with suspicion first concentrated on the vagrant, 'sturdy' poor. Parish and town authorities subjected the vagrant poor to deterrent punishments like badge-wearing, whipping, forced labour and compulsory medical treatment, mitigated on occasion by local discretion, inefficiency, or lack of resources. 'Censuses of the poor' revealed to municipal authorities the extent of poverty and disease among 'respectable', as opposed to vagrant poor.

The quotation in Box 2.1 shows census-takers' descriptions of a few households out of 2 359 poor people identified in Norwich in 1570 — around a quarter of the English-born population of the city. The Norwich Census is the best surviving example of a 'census of the poor', but other English towns carried out similar censuses, probably after precedents set by towns in continental Europe. The references to alms (No allms.) indicate the extent of support from the *poor rate* (described below) then being levied, which the census revealed to be quite inadequate (Norwich, the second city after London, was unusually early in making the poor rate compulsory). Note especially the different compositions of the households, and the recording of sickness and disability, even among children.

Box 2.1   Entries from the Norwich Census of the Poor, 1570

Thomas Ellmere of 36 yere, laborer & in no worke, & Alyce, his wyfe, of 30 yer, that spyn & washe etc., & 4 chyldren, theldest 7 yers & is sykly, & have dwelt her 9 yer & cam from Cambrydge. *Mrs. Felixe house. No allms. Veri pore.*

John Drane of 64 yere, gardener in work, and Thannzen, his wyfe, of 40 yeris, that spyn white warpe, & a systers daughter of 15 yere that spyn also, & hath dwelt here 40 yer. (hable) [i.e. able] *The Church house. No alms. Pore.*

Thomas Barthlett of 50 yeris, with one hande, that worke nott, & Jane, his wyfe, of that age, that use to go abrode & peddle; & 3 children of 8, 6, 3 yer, and a deaf wenche that begge, and have dwelt here 7 yer, & cam from the northe. *John Goses house. No allms. Veri pore.*

Gilion Tivet of 60 yeris, wedowe, that knytt, & have dwelt here ever. (hable) *No allms. Veri pore.*

Robert Trace of 80 yere, past work & a deafe man, & Margaret, his wyfe, of 60 yere, that spyn white warpe; & a sons child of 10 yer that spyn, & hav dwelt here 6 yer, & cam from Walsham. (hable). *Ther house for lyfe. No allms. Pore.* (Pound, 1971, pp. 51, 54, 55, 61, 88)

In the context of economic difficulties, population growth, and crises of mortality it became clear not only that sickness led to poverty but that many of the poor simply lacked employment. Prompted by a range of crises including epidemic disease, dearth, and economic decline, English towns in the sixteenth and seventeenth centuries could identify as poor over 20 per cent of their populations.

Local experience of the problem of the poor accumulated during the sixteenth century and was ultimately codified in the national legislation of 1598 and 1601. This Elizabethan framework endured — eventually becoming known as the **Old Poor Law** — until the New Poor Law of 1834 (described in Chapter 3). The fundamental principle laid down by the Elizabethan law was that a parish should support its own poor on the proceeds of a compulsory **poor rate**, set by, levied upon, and administered by the parish's more prosperous householders. Elizabethan parish officials recognised both demographic and economic realities in instituting a system dependent on *community* rather than family support. In practice, even the closest relatives could be assisted by the parish to care for an infirm family member. As you will see in more detail later in this chapter, the Old Poor Law included medical care, but as one aspect of social welfare.

2.2 Lay care: anxiety and expertise

You have seen that this period was marked by the irruption of new and frightening epidemic diseases, which coincided with religious, economic and demographic changes, suggesting to contemporaries the destruction of the existing order. Some historians — Lawrence Stone and Philippe Ariès being among the most eminent — have suggested that people's response to such insecurity was fatalism, reflected in a lack of affection even within the family circle. The barrage of evidence used to counter these views, drawn from such sources as diaries, includes attitudes to health and illness. It can be shown that people worried constantly not only about major, but about minor threats to health. One reflection of this was the widespread resort to health care to monitor and maintain health, even in the absence of illness.

You will already be aware that many modern health surveys depend for their data on how much people use health services, rather than on whether people see themselves, or are seen, as ill.[3] This is a limited way of measuring health, but the information is at least accessible. For similar reasons, more historical attention has been given to *doctors* than to the sick, and the extent of *lay care* in the past has been greatly underestimated. Where historians have recognised the role of women, for example, it has been mainly in terms of the charitable role of gentlewomen among their dependants. This is seen as a redeeming feature of a situation in which skilled professional services were unavailable to most of the population. Lay care thus appears in a negative light, as a function of the *absence* of doctors.

This has particular relevance with respect to *children*: few doctors seem to have treated children in this period, and it has been inferred that parents were resigned or even indifferent to their loss. (It is worth remembering that even today up to 90 per cent of children's illnesses are dealt with by *lay* carers.) In fact, parents seem to have assumed that professional care was inappropriate and even dangerous for the majority of children's complaints. The care of children was, then as now, primarily the responsibility of women (Figure 2.3). Lay nursing care naturally played an even greater role in a medical system in which *symptoms* were treated rather than the underlying disease.

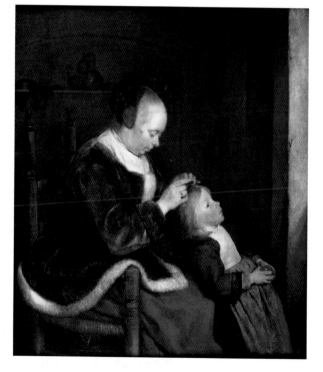

Figure 2.3 *A woman fine-combing a child's hair to remove lice, in a seventeenth-century painting by Gerard ter Borch (1617–1681). Then, as now, the care of children's health was primarily in the hands of women. The artist is showing, not the problems of poverty, but the virtues of the well-run bourgeois household and of female domesticity. (Source: Royal Cabinet of Paintings, Mauritshuis, The Hague, Netherlands)*

[3] The importance of health-service use as an indirect measure of morbidity is discussed in *Studying Health and Disease* (Open University Press, 2nd edn 1994; colour-enhanced 2nd edn, 2001), Chapter 7, and in *World Health and Disease* (Open University Press, 3rd edn 2001), Chapter 9.

2.2.1 Family and community

Until recently, it had been assumed that formal welfare systems became necessary as a result of the breakdown of the 'extended family'.

● What demographic realities (mentioned earlier) undermine the basis of this assumption for much of Northern Europe in the pre-industrial period?

■ For most of the population, extended families of the kind assumed did not exist. Families were small, especially among the poor; widows and old people often had to live alone; the population was mobile rather than settled.

Thus, although care within the family was important, we need to stress the extent of informal consultation and assistance provided *within communities* — examples being the persistence of folkloric and magical beliefs; the resort to 'cunning' (i.e. knowing) men and women; the role of clergy and parochial assistance; the passing-on of remedies by letter, word of mouth, and recipe book; the survival of local traditions such as holy wells; the origin in popular knowledge of practices as important as inoculation and vaccination (discussed later in this chapter); and the respect given in agricultural communities to those skilled in treating animals. The self-sufficient household was less and less a reality, but most forms of production were still organised on the domestic level. Thus, when historians note the importance of 'kitchen-physic', you should remember not only that the workplace was more like a kitchen, but also that the kitchen was more like a workplace, with implications for people's knowledge of processes and materials. We should, however, avoid idealising lay care, just as we should acknowledge the extent to which health care provided (and provides) a form of psychological support.

2.2.2 Lay and formal care: blurred boundaries

A more revealing historical picture of health care in the pre-industrial period has been achieved in recent years by abandoning definitions of the medical practitioner which derive from the modern idea of *professionalisation*. Modern definitions lay stress upon extensive training, academic qualifications, autonomy, vocational commitment, recognition by the state, and the restraint of groups of inferior status.[4] Even today, some of these criteria are professional *ideals*, rather than realities.

In the pre-industrial period, such levels of regulation and institutionalisation did not exist; nor was full-time salaried employment the way in which people gained their livings. As you will see later in this chapter, many practitioners of all kinds, for a variety of reasons, practised medicine on a *part-time* basis, and learned by experience. Community approval could play a decisive role in legitimating a practitioner's activities. Consequently, lay and formal care are often very difficult to distinguish.

It is also right to emphasise how difficult it was for any kind of practitioner to claim a *monopoly* of relevant knowledge. Ill people were, in general, both sceptical and discriminating in their choice of practitioner, and the relationship between practitioner and patient was more evenly balanced than it is now. One reason for this is that practitioners did not then occupy a fixed and relatively advantageous position in the social hierarchy, as they do today, but occurred in all walks of life.

---

[4] The professional status of modern medical practitioners is discussed in Chapter 7 of this book, and in *Medical Knowledge: Doubt and Certainty* (Open University Press, 2nd edn 1994; colour-enhanced 2nd edn 2001), Chapter 2.

The conventional account of the growth of medical knowledge might suggest another reason: you might expect that traditional practitioners were not cut off from their patients by a massive body of scientific information accessible only to themselves, as is the case today. There is some truth in this, but it is an over-simplification. Three objections to this interpretation can be raised. First, 'special knowledge' is, in all health-care systems, claimed by the practitioner and/or attributed to the practitioner by the patient. Second, we should avoid the idea that there 'wasn't much to know'. There were major bodies of knowledge then seen as relevant to medicine, and at the elite as well as the popular level, relevant knowledge was not confined to practitioners. Third, a plurality of medical philosophies was available: this increased the grounds of choice between practitioners, but also threw patients back on their own judgement. All of these factors enlarged the potential for lay care, and blurred the boundaries between lay and formal care.

A good example illustrating these points is provided by **midwives** (Figure 2.4). It is rare in most formal records of the period to find women designated by the occupation of midwife, yet women prepared to *act* as midwives were possibly better distributed in both rural and urban parishes than any other class of practitioner. Women's skills in midwifery were gained on the basis of occasion, example and experience. Community — that is, lay — sanction played the major role in their definition as practitioners. Attempts at ecclesiastical regulation of midwives were uneven and inconsistent.

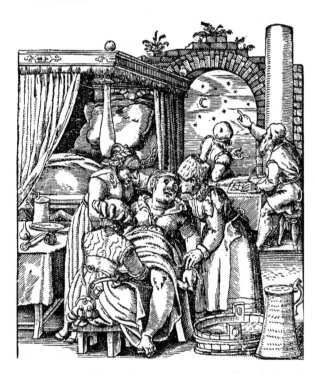

Figure 2.4 *Childbirth scene by Joost Amman, from Jakob Rueff (1500–1558),* De conceptu et generatione hominis, *1580, a well-known handbook for midwives (and for those who, in northern European towns, were officially responsible for supervising midwives), first published in German in 1554. (Reproduced from* Medicine and the Artist (Ars Medica) *by permission of the Philadelphia Museum of Art)*

2.3   The cleanliness of our ancestors

Until recently, little interest has been taken in the environment of pre-industrial societies in relation to public and personal health. It has simply been assumed that our ancestors were dirty. Increasing awareness of the environmental problems caused by post-industrial society, as well as better research, may well remove some of our easy sense of superiority about earlier standards of sanitation and personal cleanliness.

People of this period very frequently expressed disgust, either about their neighbours' habits as compared with their own, or about the habits of other nations. However, living and organic matter of all kinds — urine, for example — was, because it had practical uses, also more intrusive than now. The relationship with the natural world may have been closer and more casual, but this did not preclude cruelty, fear, or distaste (Box 2.2).

> **Box 2.2 A 'judgement of God' (recorded by the Puritan artisan, Nehemiah Wallington, in the early seventeenth century)**
>
> The Templers found tow [two] Sargents at a tavarne neare the Temple. And they toke them out. And set them in a kinde of a valt [vault] (where their felth [filth] runeth) up unto the anckels, then they drew their Swords. And said they would rune them through if they did not Shave off halfe one anothers head and halfe the other side of their beard then they did so: then they caused them to take some of the felth and rube one a others face with it then they cut a peace of their eares off and hurled them into the Theams [Thames] and dowssed them...But marke the hande of God upon on [one] of the cheefe actors of this Cruel mischife...Hee boosting of this his cruelty...at the Tavarne hee being drunke went to the house of office [latrine] and fell in to the valte and was there halfe an houre before he was mist, and when they had found him they tooke him out, and laid him upon the grasse, and there he died presently [immediately]. (Quoted in Jenner, 1991, p. 227)

In the medical theory and natural philosophies of the time, *odour* was an active substance and was consequently taken seriously both as a cause of disease, and a means of its prevention or cure. Similarly, bathing the body had high status, not as an everyday procedure, but as one with important consequences for health. Different waters had different (and potent) properties, a belief which is perhaps best known as leading to the development of spa towns — named after Spa, in Belgium, one of the most successful examples.

2.3.1 Threats to health: public and private

The German sociologist Norbert Elias, in his account of the 'civilising process' in Western Europe (1939, translated 1978), formulated a major shift in attitude from the communal habits of the Middle Ages — for example in eating and bathing — to the emergence in the eighteenth century of sharply defined distinctions between the public and private domains. Obviously such a shift can be detected only among those classes of society with the economic resources to express it, and it could be seen as an inevitable adjunct of periods of increased material consumption. One such period was the 'great rebuilding' which began to change the man-made environment of Tudor England in the later sixteenth century. Permanent materials such as brick were more widely used, and the space within dwellings gradually became more subdivided and less communal. There was also an increased acquisition of linen and textiles, furniture (including chamber pots and close stools) and items relating to personal appearance such as looking glasses.

At the same time, while their comforts and possessions increased, the Elizabethan elite saw around them a 'crowded society', threatened in an unprecedented way by population increase, social mobility, poverty, and disease. Although the 'sweating sickness', bubonic plague, and syphilis are not 'filth diseases' in the nineteenth-century sense, sixteenth-century authorities did develop a fear of situations in which disease might be engendered by putrefaction. Both people and places could be seen as dangerous — as, for example, when beggars congregated together, strangers used the same utensils in alehouses, or butchers threw offal into a town ditch. Although plague had a more obvious effect in redefining social administration — as, for example, in quarantines or the collection of mortality statistics — the contagion of syphilis was also a factor in Tudor and Stuart social policy, and may have been even more important than plague in prompting the sense of estrangement from 'other people' suggested by Elias.

After the 1660s, plague became an exotic disease in Britain, and hence an aspect of relations with other countries. Domestic policy was influenced more by endemic diseases such as typhus, smallpox and syphilis. These diseases affected relations within households and between social groups. Smallpox, for example, which particularly affected young migrants to towns, became a factor in the agreements between masters and apprentices. One of the most successful measures introduced was **inoculation** against smallpox.[5] Inoculation was practised in India, North Africa, and the Middle East, from where it was introduced into Britain in 1717 by the wife of the ambassador to Turkey, Lady Mary Wortley Montagu. The elite first took up the practice to protect their children, and soon extended it to servants and to the poor. Inoculation at this period involved the deliberate introduction of smallpox matter through the skin or mucous membrane. A variety of methods were used. This would frequently, but not invariably, result in a milder case of the disease which conferred immunity from subsequent infection.

2.3.2 A rural society and its environment

When considering environmental effects on health we tend to think of towns rather than the countryside. However, local conditions are first determined by local geography. In the pre-industrial period, classical tradition and folk experience affirmed the influence of 'airs', waters and places on health. A disease which very much underlined these traditional beliefs was *malaria* (then called ague or marsh fever), which was endemic in the fen country and low-lying parts of South-East England, as well as in similar regions throughout continental Europe. The countryside was, of course, increasingly shaped by human activity, such as deforestation. Major projects in fen drainage and water supply were begun for economic reasons in the sixteenth and seventeenth centuries.

It is important to note not only the influence of agricultural labour on health in this period, but also the effect of agricultural practices on the environment. In arable areas, according to the nature of local industries, animal hair, bone, dung, decaying fish, offal, blood, sawdust, malt dust, soot, soap ashes, leather scraps, and rags were used to condition the soil. Agriculture thus provided some incentive for the removal of wastes from towns and villages. Research is beginning to reveal the extent of 'recycling' in the economies of this period. Sometimes (as in the trade in second-hand clothes and left-over food), this would have had adverse consequences for health.

---

[5] See also the discussion of the slave trade later in this chapter. As indicated in Chapter 3, inoculation was superseded by vaccination. The terms 'vaccination' and 'immunisation' are explained there.

2.3.3   The responsibilities of towns

It would be incorrect to assume that the development of relevant services such as street cleaning and paving had to await the emergence of strong centralised government, although the piecemeal nature of improvements — like paving in main streets — carried out in the interests of 'polite' society has to be acknowledged. The changing prosperity of a town could produce considerable variation in its physical condition, and a town's representatives would complain of defects in drainage, paving and cleaning as proof of decline.

In older towns, the detailed regulation of markets included constant attention to the quality, honesty and price of provisions exposed for sale — especially staple commodities such as meat, grain, bread, and ale or beer. Fairly consistent concern was felt by parishes, trade and craft **companies**,[6] and town corporations for the effects on the public health of the activities of butchers, fishmongers, curriers, dyers, tanners, and other trades producing 'annoying' wastes, or contaminating large volumes of water. Such tradesmen were normally restricted in certain ways, for instance in being allowed to burn or transport their waste only at night, or to operate only outside city walls.

During this period, hitherto small-scale or domestic industries, such as brewing, soap boiling, distilling, and even baking, were moving on to an industrial scale of operation, and beginning to use coal or charcoal rather than wood as a fuel, thus changing the character of urban pollution. The medieval legal concept of 'nuisance', which was still a major feature of public-health legislation in the nineteenth century, enshrined the conviction that offences against the environment were injurious to neighbours or to the community at large.

Two examples follow (Box 2.3), from different levels of the legal system, of action taken to control noxious trades in seventeenth-century London. Note that James Farr provides an instance of a barber diversifying into a new branch of the food and drink trades.

> **Box 2.3   A justice giving his view in the case of Jones vs. Powell** (heard in the court of King's Bench in 1629, and concerning complaints over pollution from a brewhouse)
>
> I have known someone indicted for making candles, namely for using the trade of tallow-chandler, whereby he annoyed his neighbours; and yet that is a trade necessary for the common wealth, but because it was so obnoxious to men and so noisome, being in an inapt place for such a trade, he was indicted…one may use a trade that is lawful in itself in such a way that it shall be noxious and unlawful. Thus if a butcher (which is a trade lawful and necessary for the public good) uses his trade in Cheapside, certainly an action lies against him by those that live there. There is a lawful place for such noisome trades, as the Shambles at Newgate, and therefore no action lies against a butcher who occupies his trade there, since it is a proper place for it. The makers of hats and beavers have a lawful trade; yet one was indicted for setting up and using such a trade at Ludgate Hill. But we all know that on the back side of Bridewell there is a great number of this trade; and surely they may lawfully use it there. (Quoted in Jenner, 1991, p. 34)

[6] The companies, post-Reformation descendants of the guilds, were associations of merchants or artisans formed in self-governing or corporate towns for the maintenance of trade and manufacture, good order and fellowship, and other mutual purposes, including the control of access to a given craft or trade, supervision of standards, and the training and regulation of apprentices.

A prosecution for nuisance (by the wardmote inquest of the parish of St Dunstan's in the West, London, in 1657)

[James Farr, barber, is presented] for makeing & selling of a Drinke called Coffee whereby in making the same he annoyeth his neighbors by evill smells & for keeping of ffier for the most part night & day whereby his Chimney & Chamber hath ben set on fier to the great danger & affrightment of his Neighbours. (Quoted in Jenner, 1991, p. 37, note)

2.3.4 Utopia: a healthy city

Some of those facing the realities of human society also tried to imagine ideal states, or to find good models elsewhere. A number of writers in this period produced **utopias**, beginning with Utopia, the ideal Christian city imagined by Sir Thomas More in 1516. A noticeable characteristic of utopias is that they addressed themselves to the problems of urbanisation, postulating planned environments which ensured a high standard of hygiene and fostered the prolongation of life. More was influenced by humanist ideals of civic responsibility but also by the model architectural designs of the Italian Renaissance. There was consequently little resemblance between More's highly planned Utopia and the organic growth of the countrified towns of provincial England. More's authoritarian prescriptions for the public health are likely to have been based on the quarantine regulations and public-health boards of the cities of Northern Italy, which developed from temporary measures prompted by the Black Death in the fourteenth century.

One such board (Venice) wrote to another (Bologna) in 1630:

> With letter from Your Lordships, we received the box containing the drugs against the current disease. We shall dispatch them to the pesthouse in order to have them tested. We shall keep you informed of the results… (Quoted in Cipolla, 1976, pp. 51–2, note)

The quotation shows these boards taking an active role in medical care and investigation, yet they were an arm of civic rather than medical administration, and in time of plague had very major powers over medical personnel. Compared with this level of development, in terms of institutions, personnel, and the built environment, English public health remained in a state of nature.

2.4 Medical practitioners: many and varied

People of this period suffered a high level of anxiety about health and disease. This in turn created demand for health care, which was met, once the decision was made to look outside the resources of the family and the community, by an extremely wide range of healers. Medical practitioners existed in large numbers as well as great variety, and there is ample evidence of their activities in a broad range of sources. As you have seen earlier in this chapter, modern criteria of professionalisation are inappropriate for analysing medical practice in the pre-industrial period. To do justice to the historical picture, we adopt here the term **medical practitioner**, to cover all forms of practice, by women as well as men, and we define a *practitioner* as one whose contemporaries saw him or her as pursuing the occupation of caring for health and of healing the sick.

● Can you think of any objections that could be made to this definition?

■   You may feel that, since we are referring to an early period, the definition is too inclusive — that we should include only those practitioners who were effective, and should also exclude those who were dishonest.

These are, of course, essential issues in relation to any service provider. However, both criteria are very difficult to apply historically, and the first is not applied directly even to modern health-care workers. It is best to adopt a critical approach to the claims made in *any* historical context, and to assume also that 'gullibility' is a danger at all periods, because of patients' need to believe in their practitioners. Similarly, 'effectiveness' must be judged relative to the standards of the time.

2.4.1 The tripartite division: physicians, surgeons, and apothecaries

Medical polemics can be highly misleading. For example, in different historical contexts critics and apologists alike tended to claim the existence of a rigid (and male-dominated) **tripartite division of medicine** into *physicians*, *surgeons*, and *apothecaries* (Figure 2.5), in descending order of status (each occupation is described below). For England, however, the occupational structure of medicine, looser and more competitive than in continental Europe, meant that the divisions between types of practitioner were by no means clear cut. In the pre-industrial period, the tripartite division was an *ideal* transferred from the highly organised city-states of continental Europe. Not surprisingly, this was an ideal which appealed particularly to the physicians, who claimed pre-eminence on the ground of their lengthy formal education in humanistic learning as well as medicine. We will return to this ideal in the next section, but here we need to ask what relation it bore to the reality of the occupational structure of medicine in this period. A rough version of the tripartite structure did exist in pre-industrial towns, but had far less meaning for patients in rural areas.

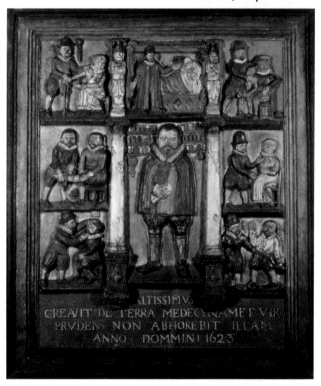

Figure 2.5 *This carved and painted signboard, dated 1623, shows the various services available from the Dorset (surgeon-) apothecary who displayed it. (Source: Wellcome Library, London)*

Many high-status university-trained **physicians** (Figure 2.6) based themselves in towns, and patients often travelled long distances to consult them. But in other ways physicians did *not* dominate urban medical practice. Their numbers were small; only two English towns possessed universities, and only London, which had no university, developed an organisation for physicians. The English elite lived as much in the country as in the town, and physicians usually had to do the same. These factors help to explain the frequent presence of academically qualified physicians in the countryside, although it is harder to determine whether such men practised extensively.

Probably more numerous, and certainly more accessible, were the *practitioners of physic*, who were rarely university-trained but saw themselves as qualified by reading or experience in this 'internal' part of medicine.

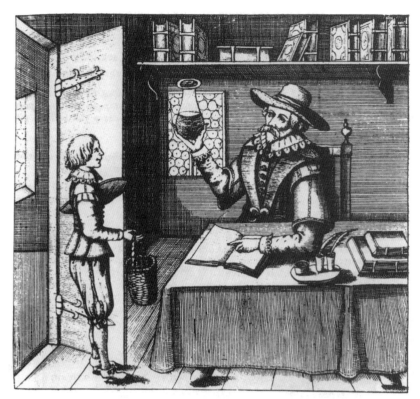

Figure 2.6 *An engraving from a work by the English physician Robert Fludd (1574–1637) shows a physician studying a specimen of urine brought by the patient's servant, who is holding a wicker case for the urine flask. (Source: from Fludd's* Medicina Catholica, *Frankfurt, 1631)*

Paradoxically, the anxiety of English physicians to maintain their status could make their practice more rigid than in countries where medicine was actually better regulated, as the report of one late-sixteenth-century traveller, Fynes Moryson, indicates:

> The Universities … espetially of Padoa … have yielded famous phisitians who in Italy are also shirgians [surgeons] and many of them growe rich for all that have any small meanes will in sicknes have their helpe, because they are not prowde but will looke upon any ordure and handle any sore, but espetially because they are carefull for their patients, visite them diligently and take little fees which make heavy purses. (Quoted in Cipolla, 1976, p. 107)

● What does the quotation suggest were the virtues of the surgeon–physicians of Italy — and, by implication, of **surgeons** in general as compared with physicians?

■ The Italian practitioners were well-trained, with a wide range of skills — but just as important, from the patient's point of view, they did not charge prohibitive fees, they provided careful attention for all but the poorest, and, rather than diagnosing or prescribing from a distance (as in Figure 2.6), they were prepared to come to the patient and with their own hands treat even the more revolting conditions. Moreover, Moryson suggests that the Italian practitioners also reaped material rewards by their absence of pride — they became rich, even though they often charged small fees.

Medical organisation in Scotland more closely resembled that in continental Europe, especially France, and surgery was consequently of higher status than in England.

The **barbers** and **barber-surgeons**, who offered the greatest range of personal services, from beard-dyeing and toothscraping to blood-letting (Figure 2.7), surgery, and the treatment of sores, were more popular than the physicians, as well as better integrated into urban life. Although of only middling status, they were among the most numerous of urban trades, and could be found even in villages (Figure 2.8). The barber-surgeon is the nearest equivalent in this period to the modern general medical practitioner (GP), and can be seen as providing the bulk of formal health care in towns. Living over (or in) 'the shop' was then the norm in medicine as in most other trades, and some barber-surgeons (as did other kinds of practitioner) took in patients as lodgers. Different notions of privacy meant that the barber-shop could offer treatment and yet be a place of semi-public resort, involving attractions such as drink, musical instruments and the exchange of news.

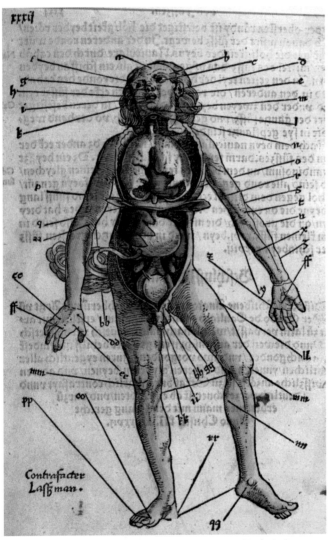

Figure 2.7   *Blood-letting man, by the German artist Hans Wechtlin (1480–1526), in a sixteenth-century manuscript, showing the points at which to let blood from veins. The body and the extremities are fairly naturalistic; the internal anatomy is somewhat behind the knowledge of the time. (Source: Art Archive/Jean-Loup Charmet Medical)*

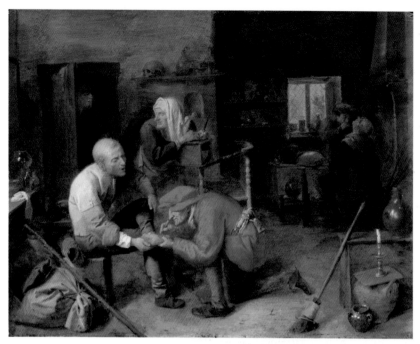

Figure 2.8(a) *Village barber-surgeon, by Adriaen Brouwer (1606–1638). Brouwer's art stressed the black comedy of the human condition. His 'low-life' version of the barber's shop shows a public setting, with a stress on pain and vulnerability — the wayfarer's feet, and, in the background, the head, teeth, or mouth. (Source: Alte Pinakothek, Munich; Photo: Artothek)*

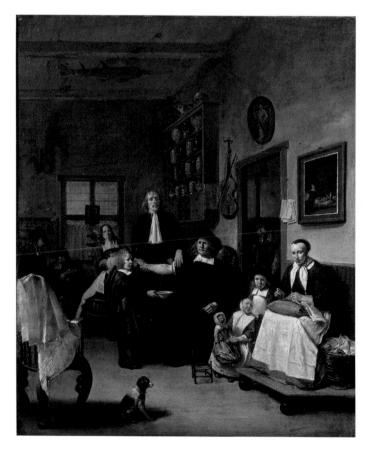

Figure 2.8(b) *The surgeon Jacob Fransz Hercules, with his family, painted in 1669 by Egbert van Heemskerck (1634/5–1704). The surgeon is letting blood, but 'barbering' is also going on in his shop. The artist has included objects characteristic of barber-surgeons' shops, such as the basin, stuffed animals, and a musical instrument, as part of the interior of a relatively prosperous household. (Source: Amsterdams Historisch Museum)*

Under such influences as the campaign for the 'reformation of manners' from the later seventeenth century — an aspect of the changing attitudes identified by Elias — and the association of barber-surgeons with the treatment of sexually transmitted disease, the barber-shop connection became, by the early eighteenth century, one which higher-status surgeons wished to shed as thoroughly as possible. At the same time, surgeons wished to retain the advantage of being seen by patients as both useful and effective.

By the early seventeenth century, some **apothecaries** as well as some barber-surgeons in towns were beginning to call themselves 'doctor', and we also see the emergence of the **surgeon-apothecary** who is usually regarded as the true ancestor of the modern GP. It is, however, mistaken to see apothecaries as humble tradesmen who climbed in status as a result of intruding into medicine. From the medieval period, apothecaries were more often traders in expensive commodities (drugs and spices), who ranked in the higher-status retail sector of urban occupations with other merchants and holders of capital, such as goldsmiths. It is at least arguable that apothecaries *lost* status as their numbers expanded and they increasingly adopted roles within medicine. As London grew as a centre of distribution, apothecaries were able to set up shops in smaller towns (look back at Figure 2.5).

2.4.2 Specialists and itinerants

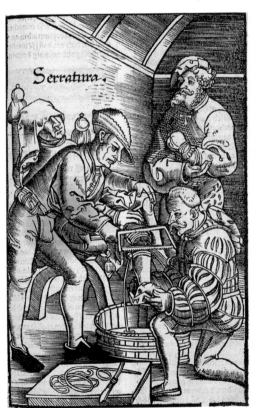

Because pre-industrial populations were comparatively mobile, and tireless in their pursuit of health care, the services of physicians, surgeons and apothecaries were not limited to those living in towns. People also travelled to resort to such specialists as bonesetters, cutters for cataract, lithotomists and specialists in such deformities as fistula and harelip. Before anaesthesia, lithotomy or 'cutting for the stone' was, after amputation, the most frequently performed major operation and a traditional specialty. It usually involved the removal of calculi or stones from the bladder via a cut in the perineum (the area between the genitals and the anus). Fistulae could occur anywhere in the body and were in effect drainage holes caused when wounds and ulcers would not heal. Before antibiotics they could be extremely difficult to treat and were a major cause of long-term distress. These specialties involved high risk and expense for the patient, but existed because the need was correspondingly great (Figure 2.9). The useful bonesetter existed in both rural and urban versions. Not surprisingly, some specialists travelled from centre to centre, but acquired as much accreditation as possible from patients to distinguish themselves from unscrupulous itinerants.

The spread of remedies associated with a particular healer began early in this period and these, whether *specifics* ('sovereign remedies' for particular diseases) or *panaceas* (cure-alls), had all the ambiguous attractions of metropolitan or continental sophistication.

Figure 2.9 *An illustration of amputation by Hans Wechtlin in the textbook by Hans von Gersdorff (c. 1455–1529), Feldtbuch der Wundartzney, 1540, first published in 1517. Note that the patient undergoing surgery appears to be unconscious. (Reproduced from* Medicine and the Artist (Ars Medica) *by permission of the Philadelphia Museum of Art)*

2.4.3 Numbers and distribution of practitioners

It does not follow, of course, that all classes of practitioner are equally visible in the historical record — or that those for whom we have the most evidence were necessarily the most numerous or even the most important in terms of contemporary health care.

● What kinds of practitioner would you expect to be least visible, and which most visible?

■ Women practitioners (including midwives), and practitioners serving small rural communities are less likely to be visible. Most visible are elite university graduates, such as royal physicians.

Intensive local surveys aimed at including all kinds of practitioner except midwives have suggested that the ratio of practitioners to population in England around 1600 may have been as high as 1:200 in major towns, and 1:400 in well-populated rural areas. By contrast, an average GP's 'list' in England and Wales in 1951 was 2 600, and in 1997, 1 800. This striking comparison might suggest that modern populations are *less* well provided for than those of the past.

● Why might such a direct comparison be misleading?

■ There are several reasons:
1 The ratio for the pre-industrial period was probably much lower for sparsely populated rural areas.
2 The ratio for the pre-industrial period refers to all kinds of practitioners: the modern GP is expected to provide *comprehensive* primary care, but with the help of the primary care team, which includes several kinds of health-care worker.
3 The modern model of effectiveness in treatment requires less time to be spent by the GP with each patient.
4 A modern GP works full-time in medicine, whereas the majority of practitioners around 1600 (and probably much later) almost certainly did not.

2.4.4 Occupational diversity: a means of living, not a way of life

Today we stress the vocational aspect of medicine, even though it is frequently chosen as a dependably lucrative career. It is important to realise that in the pre-industrial period, even for the educated elite, medicine was a useful means of subsistence and people drifted in and out of it as their needs required. For example, religious upheavals meant that many of the educated elite could find themselves unable to hold an ecclesiastical benefice and had to earn a living by other means. Medicine could also be a useful resort for those wanting to do something else that society would not pay well for, such as satirists and writers. Among the less literate, medicine could combine well with a range of other trades, especially those connected with food and drink, and the production of such substances as dyes and cosmetics.

This tendency was denounced (and exaggerated) by propagandists like the London surgeon William Clowes who, in 1585, deplored the intrusion into medicine of good trades and bad, such as painters, glaziers, tailors, weavers, cooks, bakers, tinkers, toothdrawers, pedlars, sow-gelders, horse-leeches, witches, rat-catchers, and 'such other like rotten and stinking weeds' (quoted in Webster, 1979, p. 186). Medicine, as a portable skill much in demand, was also a useful occupation for those wishing or needing to travel. These social and economic factors increased the difficulties of regulating the practice of medicine, and were one reason for the persistence of 'quacks' peddling patent medicines and magical cures (Figure 2.10).

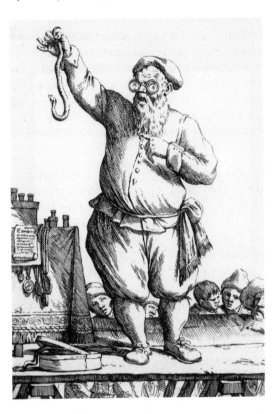

Figure 2.10   'The Quack', after Annibale Carracci (1560–1609), in a set of street characters of Bologna, published in 1660. Italy, which provided models of medical organisation, also supplied striking images of quackery — including the terms 'mountebank' and 'charlatan'. Some 'quacks' became highly successful by advertising their services in urban centres. (Source: Wellcome Library, London)

2.5   A health-care system outside institutions

In previous sections, we have outlined a health-care system that included a high consumption of medical care and a high per-capita incidence of medical practitioners of various kinds.

● From what has been said, can you suggest how pre-industrial society was able to sustain such a system?

■ Much medical care was provided by family or community members on an exchange basis; most medical practitioners did not practise full-time but followed other occupations as well.

2.5.1   The costs of medical care: community provision

Practitioners in pre-industrial England offered a scale of treatments, and a scale of charges, according to what the patient was likely to be able to pay. With respect to adolescents and young adults, the potential burden was spread in that masters were expected to take responsibility for servants or apprentices if they fell ill.

Nonetheless, families could be rendered destitute by the high cost and protracted nature of medical care, and this was also a factor in the gradual breakdown of apprenticeship. Recognition of the catastrophic effects of ill-health or disability, together with the community's fear of disease, produced a range of systems in which the community contributed to the costs of medical care.

2.5.2 Medical poor relief

In England the basis of most of these systems was the *parish*, although major towns evolved a more elaborate and centralised system of **medical poor relief** involving payments (sometimes on a 'retainer' or contract basis) to a wide range of both male and female practitioners. By the eighteenth century, parishes were also employing practitioners on a contract basis. This was in addition to occasional payments by towns or parishes for individual parishioners to seek expensive cures, 'go to the Bath' (i.e. Bath Spa), or be sent to 'Bedlam' (Bethlehem), London's hospital for the insane.

As we noted earlier, the financial basis for poor-law provision (also known as *poor relief*) was the *poor rate*, although charitable doles and endowments made an important contribution in many parishes. Parish officials decided on pensions to single-parent families, the infirm elderly, and those too disabled to work, and made temporary grants in time of sickness and to large families. These officials also provided for improved levels of clothing, heating, and nutrition, paid the expenses of childbirth or burial, and supported children into service or apprenticeship. Single payments for medical treatment could be extremely high, and officials certainly saw medicine as a worthwhile investment, transforming the impotent into the able-bodied, that is, able to work. Overall, however, the bulk of parish expenditure on poor relief was in the form of *income support*.

Most forms of support for the sick poor involved an expedient which was to prove very enduring: the able poor were employed to look after, nurse, or even treat the sick poor. Typically, a woman needing support herself would be paid as a nurse, 'watcher' (i.e. night-nurse or sick-minder), or child-minder. Although sometimes coercive, this practice can be seen, in this period at least, as increasing the resources of informal care within the community.

The importance of lay care notwithstanding, it may seem from this account that the poor were offered only a very 'second-class' service. The evidence suggests the contrary: town and parish authorities did, according to need, select medical practitioners from among the whole range of those available, including high-status physicians. Notable aspects are first, the lack of reference by such authorities to any system of licensing or regulation of practitioners, and second — since parish officials were laymen — the primacy of lay control.

2.5.3 Hospitals and other institutions

It may have surprised you that we have made little mention so far of hospitals, almshouses, or other institutions. Except for London, the hospitals familiar today date only from the 1730s, and will be dealt with in the next chapter; but, in general terms, hospitals were not central to health care in Britain until the twentieth century (unlike the rest of Europe; Figure 2.11, overleaf).

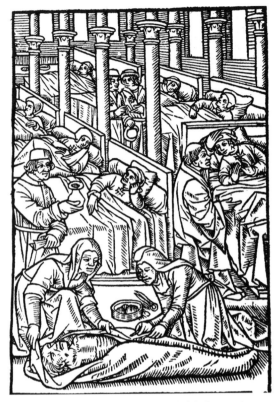

Figure 2.11 *Woodcut from Saint-Gelais,* Le vergier d'honneur, *c. 1500. This rare depiction is not so much a literal representation of a hospital interior, as an image of the cycle of life and death which took place there. (Reproduced from* Medicine and the Artist (Ars Medica) *by permission of the Philadelphia Museum of Art)*

The poor-relief system just described was gradually built up following the Reformation,[7] although its roots go back much earlier. As a one-city nation, England was unusual even before the dissolution of the monasteries in its lack of major institutions for the sick poor, just as it was unusual in the elaboration of its system of parish administration. Even in major centres, like London and Norwich, this was primarily a system of *out-door* relief, so-called because it involved forms of community care that did not entail entering an institution.

In the mid-sixteenth century, the City of London refounded five monastic hospitals for the custody and regulation of the poor (all were originally established in the twelfth or thirteenth centuries), but only three of them (St Thomas's, St Bartholomew's, and Bethlehem) had any major responsibility for the *sick* poor. Christ's Hospital was refounded for orphans; Bridewell for the summary punishment and work-training of rogues, prostitutes, and vagabonds. London also used, in a more *ad hoc* way, an outlying circle of smaller institutions, once leperhouses, to treat or segregate chronic or threatening cases (in this respect it mirrored the pattern of provision already established for Norwich; look back at Figure 1.3).

Other towns seem at times to have made equivalent use of the same range of institutions but, as in London, the numbers institutionalised were very small compared with the scale of need, and the initiatives involved were often short-lived. Sick people (including lunatics) crop up in almshouses, prisons, 'houses of correction' or 'bridewells' (named after the London institution), and (especially from the early eighteenth century) **workhouses**, and relief could be provided for these individuals on an occasional basis. As the names suggest, the primary aim of houses of correction and workhouses was to instil work-discipline or, more positively, to provide work and train the poor to be self-supporting (Figure 2.12).

● Overall, what would you see as the disadvantages and advantages of these provisions for the sick poor?

■ Relief was not systematic or comprehensive; it could be punitive; and it depended upon the presence and goodwill of prosperous householders. But, especially at the parish level, it could also have the flexibility to meet individual needs possible only in a 'face-to-face' society; and it did not require massive investment in institutions such as hospitals.

[7] The Reformation refers to the fragmentation of the church which occurred in Europe in the first half of the sixteenth century. The breakaway movement is known as Protestantism. Acceptance or rejection of Protestantism in any state usually involved a lengthy power struggle. Only gradually were the dominant traditions of Protestantism, linked with such figures as Calvin or Luther, consolidated into national and international church organisations.

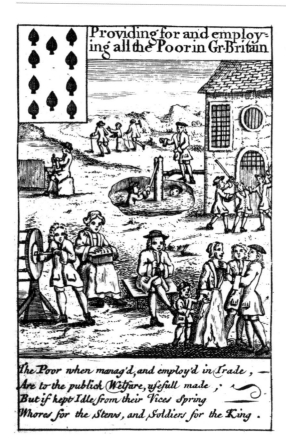

Providing for and employ=
ing all the Poor in Gr.Britain

The Poor when manag'd, and employ'd in Trade,
Are to the publick Welfare usefull made;
But if kept Idle from their Vices spring
Whores for the Stews, and Soldiers for the King.

Figure 2.12 *A workhouse depicted on a playing card of 1720. Note the emphasis on productive forms of labour. The late seventeenth century brought renewed interest in work training and workhouses for the poor. (Source: Hulton Getty Picture Collection)*

2.5.4 Medicine and the 'common weal'

What responsibility did society take for the *quality* of medical care? In this period, relations between patient and practitioner seem often to have been governed by conditional contracts, including an element of payment by results. What was bargained for was not cure, but 'a cure', a balance between what the ill person wanted and what the practitioner was prepared to predict as the outcome of his or her treatment. Pre-industrial society was highly litigious and dissatisfied patients readily took legal action. Both the highest- and the lowest-status practitioners tried to bypass this system — physicians by stressing their role in prognosis and by charging standard fees for advice, and quacks by minimising follow-up contact with their patients.

Even in a highly competitive situation, in an emergent capitalist economy, 'buyer beware' was not the only law. By around 1600, the medieval town guilds had evolved into *companies*, controlled and manipulated according to changing economic and social conditions by civic authorities — a form of devolved economic planning. Companies supervised training, inspected merchandise, and exerted a 'right of search' over premises, apprentices and journeymen. These standard functions could take different forms according to the trade in question: for example, a responsibility of the officebearers of barber-surgeons' companies was to supervise contracts for 'cures' made with dangerously-ill patients by less-experienced members. Separate barber-surgeons' companies, which could include physicians, existed in the largest towns. Apothecaries were commonly in companies that included grocers and other merchants.

The nearest approach to a *national* system regulating medicine was represented by the licences to practise issued by bishops, after 1511, to physicians, surgeons and midwives, but this system was only patchily administered. The humanist *College of Physicians of London*, founded in 1518, differed from the *London Barber-Surgeons' Company* (reorganised in 1540) and the *Worshipful Society of Apothecaries of London* (separated from the Grocers' Company in 1617) in aspiring to national control. However, although it sought to prosecute unlicensed practitioners, the College was limited in its effectiveness, even within London. Municipal authorities, and under them the companies, seem to have been the most effective regulators of crafts and trades in the pre-industrial period, including the different branches of medicine.

Later in this book, we will compare this situation with that in developed modern societies, in which the ideals of professionalisation are firmly established. Expectations at the start of the twenty-first century tend to be high, but a successful outcome of medical care is not guaranteed, and redress for the individual is often a lengthy and much-obstructed process.

2.6 Empires and exchanges: the first phase of expansion

Systems of health care in Western Europe did not develop in isolation. The beginnings of European expansionism mentioned at the outset of this chapter, and the increasing frequency of maritime trade with distant parts of the globe, resulted in a series of exchanges of pathogens and cultural practices which proved deadly to both colonisers and colonised, and which had lasting consequences for the development of both Western and indigenous medical systems. In the pre-industrial period the establishment of territorial and commercial interests overseas was central to the consolidation of European nation-states referred to earlier.

The impulse for English overseas expansion began during the reign of Henry VIII and gathered momentum under Elizabeth I, with the voyages of Drake, Frobisher, and Ralegh. By the mid-seventeenth century, England had established colonies and trading posts in Ireland, the Americas, and in India, but England was still in its infancy as a colonial power. Foremost among the expansionist powers were Spain, which held sway over much of South and Central America, and Portugal, with footholds in South America and the East Indies.

The medical and demographic impact of European expansion is one of the darkest but now, also, one of the best-known chapters in imperial history. The unparalleled savagery of the Spanish *conquistadores*, in particular, has attracted a good deal of attention from historians.[8] So too has the decimation of the native American population by epidemic diseases, like smallpox, brought from the Old World — a process which the American historian Alfred Crosby has referred to as the 'Columbian exchange' (Crosby, 1986). The horrific effects of smallpox were chronicled in accounts written by the Spanish and depicted in illustrations such as Figure 2.13. The importation of these diseases, which might more generally be referred to as an **epidemiological exchange**,[9] precipitated a demographic decline which greatly facilitated the European conquest of the Americas, although the role of technology and military force in establishing European domination should not be underestimated.

[8] The effects of European colonisation on the patterns of infectious diseases in Asia, Africa and the Americas are discussed in *Human Biology and Health: An Evolutionary Approach* (Open University Press, 3rd edn 2001), Chapter 5.

[9] The concept of an 'epidemiological exchange', which caused epidemics in 'new' host populations, is discussed in *Human Biology and Health: An Evolutionary Approach* (Open University Press, 3rd edn 2001), Chapter 5.

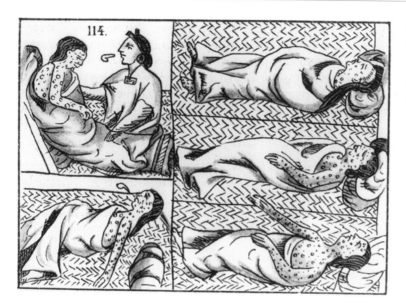

Figure 2.13 *Various stages of smallpox among Aztec victims of the disease in the sixteenth century, illustrated in a manuscript, 'Historia de las Cosas de Nueva España'. (Source: Peabody Museum, Harvard University)*

2.6.1 The slave trade

The birth of the Atlantic slave trade in the seventeenth century also had terrible medical consequences for those black Africans who were enslaved, and for those who were left behind. The slave trade, which involved the capture of indigenous peoples in West Africa for work on European plantations in the Americas, and which in turn provided the raw materials for industrial expansion in Europe, provides one of the most vivid examples of the pervasive and deadly influence of Western capitalism. By forcibly bringing together slaves from all over Western Africa, the slave trade blended the varied and hitherto distinct disease environments of different parts of Africa with 'new' European diseases. In overcrowded 'barracoons' on the African coast, and in the cramped and ill-ventilated conditions on slave ships, smallpox, dysentery, and eye diseases spread like wildfire. Just how crowded slaving vessels were can be appreciated from Figure 2.14.

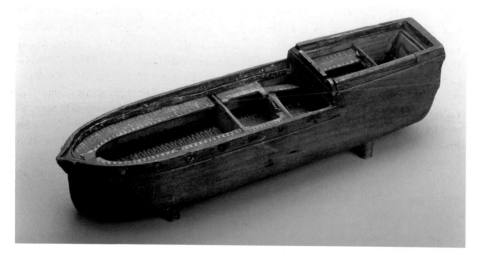

Figure 2.14(a) *Model of the slave ship* Brookes *used by William Wilberforce in the House of Commons, 1788, to demonstrate the conditions in which slaves were transported from Africa to the West Indies. (Source: The Bridgeman Art Library) (Figure 2.14b is overleaf.)*

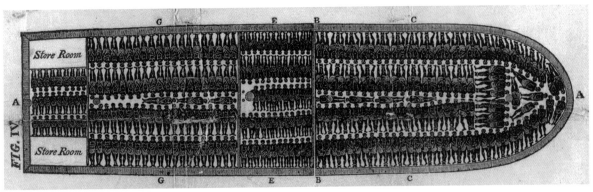

Figure 2.14(b)   *Plan of the lower deck of the slave ship* Brookes. *The space allowed is 'To the Men 6 feet by 1 foot 4 inches. Women 5 feet 10 in. by 1 foot 4 in. Boys 5 feet by 1 foot 2 in. Girls 4 feet 6 in. by 1 foot', providing room for 482 slaves. The actual numbers carried by this ship were 351 men, 127 women, 90 boys and 41 girls, a total of 609; the report to the House of Commons also notes how the men were chained together, and the 'horrible mortality. ... the slaves are from six to eight weeks on their passage from thence to the West Indies...when to a long passage are added, inhuman treatment, scanty and bad provisions, and rough weather, their condition is miserable beyond description'. (Source: The Bridgeman Art Library)*

On arrival, conditions at the plantations were little better, with people, plants and animals concentrated in lowland areas ridden with vector-borne diseases such as malaria and yellow fever, imported from Africa by the slave trade. This trade, then, not only facilitated the geographical spread of infectious disease, but greatly favoured its multiplication. Initially, little thought was given to the health of slaves, but the appallingly high mortality among them led to some attempts to contain disease — for example, inoculation against smallpox — in order to increase the profitability of the trade and the plantations.

The same desire to increase economic efficiency lay behind other medical provisions for slaves on plantations, including the establishment of 'slave hospitals' staffed mainly with black attendants, and the occasional employment of European doctors in cases of last resort. Western medical care and the slave hospitals were usually distrusted by slaves, who had good reason to be suspicious of the intentions behind such arrangements, and who generally preferred to consult practitioners of African medicine, which was closely intertwined with their religious and cultural practices. Given this cultural distance, 'the white doctor could only practise medicine as if he were a veterinarian' (Sheridan, 1985, p. 355). Limited medical provisions on plantations had little effect on the health of slaves while they continued to be subject to over-work, poor diet, and poor housing.

2.6.2 'The white man's grave'

Yet the 'epidemiological exchange' was not as one-sided as Alfred Crosby and others have suggested.

● Can you recall an example given earlier in this chapter?

■ It was widely believed that syphilis was introduced into Europe from South America or Africa.

The first English writer on so-called *tropical medicine*, Thomas Trapham, believed that syphilis was a form of divine punishment for the 'sexual transgressions' of black and native American peoples, and that its increasing incidence among the Spanish was a sign that they were becoming morally and physically unfit to rule their vast conquests. Equally, in the colonies, and especially in West Africa (the 'white man's grave'), Europeans experienced levels of mortality far higher than indigenous peoples. In the early eighteenth century, troops stationed in the colonies suffered much higher death rates than those who remained in Britain, as Table 2.1 shows.

Table 2.1 Death rate of British troops stationed in Britain in the early eighteenth century, compared with those stationed in the colonies.

Troops stationed in:	Death rate per 1000
Britain	just over 15
India	30–75
West Indies	85–138
West Africa	483–668

Data from Sheridan, R. B. (1985) *Doctors and Slaves: A Medical and Demographic History of Slavery in the British West Indies 1680–1834*, Cambridge University Press, Cambridge, p. 12

2.6.3 Indigenous medical systems

European medical practitioners, having made only limited progress in alleviating the burden of sickness in their own countries, found themselves virtually powerless in the face of 'new diseases' and more familiar afflictions which seemed to increase in virulence in the tropics. It was not long before they began to solicit information from indigenous practitioners of medicine, who had a superior knowledge of local medicinal plants. This was particularly true of Europeans in India, who were confronted by two highly-sophisticated traditional medical systems: the Hindu or *ayurvedic* system, and the Islamic *unani-i-tibb*. Surgeons of the English East India Company (the EIC) incorporated many Indian drugs into their pharmacopoeia, and practitioners of Hindu and Islamic medicine (*vaidyas* and *hakims* respectively) found employment with the Company as apothecaries and, from the 1660s, as assistants in its hospitals.

The Spanish, too, employed Aztec medical practitioners to tend their sick and wounded, while some European practitioners in the West Indies and North America were intrigued by the folk medicine of slaves and native Americans. Indeed, indigenous medical practitioners, or 'medicine men', frequently captured the imagination of Europeans, and were often depicted in illustrations accompanying travellers' accounts (see Figure 2.15 overleaf).

The use of indigenous medical knowledge by Europeans was by no means confined to the colonies. As trade with the Americas and the Indies became more frequent, indigenous remedies were transported to Europe and were employed increasingly against the maladies of the Old World. The 'voyages of discovery' were bound up with a new spirit of investigation in science and medicine, associated with the rediscovery of ancient learning and 'secrets' mentioned earlier in this chapter.

Trade with the colonies fuelled this new approach to medicine by supplying exotic new remedies attractive to innovative practitioners. The 'new disease' of syphilis, as already mentioned, was treated with the wood guaiacum from South America; while the bark of the Peruvian cinchona tree (from which quinine was later derived) was widely employed in the treatment of various fevers. Opium, together with cinnamon, ginger, cumin, nutmeg and other spices became popular remedies for a wide range

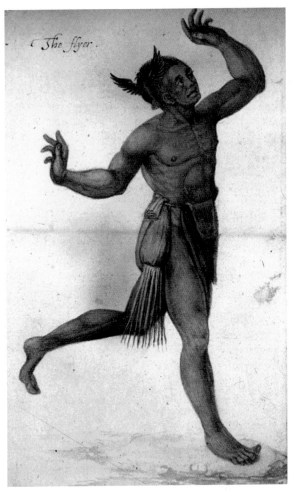

Figure 2.15   *A medicine man of Roanoke, North Carolina, 1585. Watercolour by John White. (Source: British Museum)*

of diseases — cinnamon water, for instance, in the treatment of intestinal disorders. Thus, increasing contact with America and the Orient opened up exciting new therapeutic possibilities as well as testing the resourcefulness and resilience of European practitioners.

In the long run, however, the most profound consequences for health stemmed from the importation of the potato and of tobacco. The potato (originally cultivated in South America) became one of the principal sources of nutrition for the poor of European countries such as Ireland; tobacco (originally from the West Indies and North America) — a subject of medical controversy from the start — was identified as a major cause of certain cancers and of heart disease in the later twentieth century.

By the end of the seventeenth century, European medical practitioners in India and the colonies were becoming more confident of their ability to treat and to combat diseases in the tropics. Having imbibed considerable local knowledge, their dependence on indigenous practitioners decreased, though cross-cultural consultation did not cease altogether. This tendency was perhaps most marked in Portuguese India, where the municipality of Goa attempted to ban the practice of indigenous medicine.

●   What does the decision of the Goa municipality tell us about the attitude of Europeans to indigenous medical practice?

■   European practitioners exploited indigenous medical knowledge but saw their own system as fundamentally superior to indigenous systems. They may also have been concerned about competition from indigenous practitioners.

European expansion, then, brought only a gradual extension of European systems of health care, but the medical problems and opportunities presented by the encounter with India, Africa, and the New World fuelled important developments in medical knowledge and practice. The fatal consequences of the epidemiological exchange between Europeans and indigenous peoples was matched by an exchange of medical knowledge and expertise.

However, this exchange was, in both pathogenic and cultural terms, an unequal one. The incidence of disease among European colonisers may have been as high as, if not higher than among indigenous peoples, but the devastation of the latter was far more extensive, and played a major part in the process of European domination. Equally, while European practitioners freely plundered indigenous medical knowledge, the benefits of Western health care were distributed only selectively, and with little effect, upon their colonial subjects. This state of affairs was to alter little in the next century of colonial expansion, considered in Chapter 3.

OBJECTIVES FOR CHAPTER 2

When you have studied this chapter, you should be able to:

2.1 Define and use, or recognise definitions and applications of, each of the terms in **bold** in the text.

2.2 Illustrate the difficulties of distinguishing between lay and formal care in the pre-industrial period.

2.3 Briefly describe the principal epidemic diseases and environmental threats to public health in this period and estimate the extent of concern about them.

2.4 Explain what is meant by the tripartite division of health-care occupations in this period, indicate the limits of its applicability, and give reasons for the limited role of physicians compared with practitioners of other types.

2.5 Discuss the ways in which the problem of poverty was related to the development of poor-relief systems of health care, supported by public expenditure.

2.6 Demonstrate, by use of appropriate examples, an understanding of the relevance for health of the increasing European domination of the 'New World' of the colonial empires.

QUESTIONS FOR CHAPTER 2

1 (*Objective 2.2*)

Look back at Figures 2.3 and 2.4, and consider them together with the following. In 1601, Lady Margaret Hoby of Hackness, Yorkshire, recorded in her diary:

> This day, in the afternone, I had a child brought to me that was born at Silpho, one Talliour sonne, who had no fundament [anus] and had no passage for excrementes but at the Mouth; I was ernestly intreated to Cutt the place to see if any passage could be made, but, although I Cutt deepe and searched, there was none to be found. (Quoted in Wyman, 1984, pp. 31–2)

In what ways do women occupy the roles of both formal and lay practitioners in the pre-industrial period?

2 (*Objective 2.3*)

The following is a lease of property agreed in late sixteenth-century London:

> This daie order is taken by this courte that Humfrey Morrey Inholder shall have the house in Goldinge Lane...being bound to all reparacions with condition he suffer no butchers to dwell in any parte thereof or usuallye take any sicke people into the house which shalbe diseased of the plague or pox [venereal disease]. (St Bartholomew's Hospital Journal, H/a 1/2, fd. 165 [1581])

What does this tell us about efforts at this time on behalf of the public health?

3   (*Objective 2.4*)

The different behaviour of practitioners in the plagues of the late sixteenth and early seventeenth centuries had a considerable effect on popular opinion at the time. Recalling the crises of the 1590s, the self-taught astrological practitioner of physic, Simon Forman, wrote:

> And in the time of pestilent plague When Doctors all did fly, And got them into places far From out the City, The Lord appointed me to stay To cure the sick and sore, But not the rich and mighty ones But the distressed poor. (Quoted in Rowse, 1974, pp. 56–7)

Forman's 'poem' says something about the individual sense of religious pre-ordination characteristic of the period. What does it also suggest about the activities and reputations of the different types of practitioner?

4   (*Objective 2.5*)

The historian Paul Slack has estimated for pre-industrial England that 'five per cent was the normal background level of poverty in urban societies'. This however was a minimum. Among other, higher contemporary estimates he mentions that:

> The crisis level could go higher still. A listing taken in Sheffield in 1616 counted at least 20 per cent and perhaps as many as 33 per cent of the population as 'begging poor', and there were other householders who '(though they beg not)…are not able to abide the storm of one fortnight's sickness but would be thereby driven to beggary'. When sickness in the form of plague hit Cambridge in 1630, 2,858 people — 36 per cent of the population — were thought to require relief. (Slack, 1988, p. 72)

What does this suggest to you about the connections between poverty, disease, and poor relief?

5   (*Objective 2.6*)

Writing of his experiences in the East Indies in 1658, the Dutch physician Jacobus Bontius extolled the medicinal virtues of local plants and medical practitioners; if he himself was ill, he preferred to 'trust himself to one of them' rather than to a European practitioner (quoted in Patterson, 1983, p. 460). What does this tell us about the nature of the medical exchange which took place in this period between European and indigenous practitioners?

CHAPTER 3

The Industrial Revolution, 1750 to 1848

3.1 The first industrial nation 62
3.1.1 Industrialisation and health 62
3.1.2 Class divisions 64

3.2 The New Poor Law 67

3.3 Lay care: urbanisation and self-help 68
3.3.1 Useful knowledge 68
3.3.2 Druggists: further steps in the commercialisation of self-help 69
3.3.3 Friendly Societies 70

3.4 Public health: a shared environment? 71
3.4.1 Old corruption 71
3.4.2 Fever: the diagnosis of social evils 71
3.4.3 New arms of government 72
3.4.4 Benthamism and sanitary reform 72

3.5 Partly professionalised: the general practitioner 75
3.5.1 Regular and irregular practitioners? 76
3.5.2 Medical reform: internal struggles 77

3.6 Philanthropy: the role of bricks and mortar 80
3.6.1 Voluntary hospitals 80
3.6.2 Dispensaries 84
3.6.3 Medical poor relief and the Old Poor Law 85
3.6.4 Health care and the New Poor Law 86
3.6.5 Lunacy 86

3.7 Continental Europe: medical police or social medicine? 87
3.7.1 Medical police 88
3.7.2 Medicine and revolution 88

3.8 British India: the costs of colonialism 89
3.8.1 Medicine and military considerations 90
3.8.2 Medical practice in India 91
3.8.3 The health of Indians 91
3.8.4 Public health in India 92
3.8.5 Tropical hygiene 92

Objectives for Chapter 3 94

Questions for Chapter 3 95

Study notes for OU students

This chapter builds on knowledge of the rate and underlying causes of population growth in the Industrial Revolution in Britain, and the shifts in patterns of disease associated with profound changes in the structure of an industrialising society, discussed in *World Health and Disease* (Open University Press, 3rd edn 2001), Chapters 5 and 6. The article by Friedrich Engels, which was set reading for Chapter 6 of that book (see *Health and Disease: A Reader*, Open University Press, 3rd edn 2001), is particularly relevant here.

3.1 The first industrial nation

During the Industrial Revolution, Britain seems to have escaped the Malthusian trap of the pressure of population on resources.[1] The heading of this section, 'the first industrial nation', reflects the essentially optimistic idea that Britain was the first to experience dramatic economic and demographic changes which will, sooner or later, be repeated in the 'undeveloped' world, just as they were in nineteenth-century mainland Europe. In simple terms this view assumes that progress, in the form of unrestricted economic growth, can always be expected to 'trickle down' to raise the standard of living even of the poorest.

Commentators are, however, increasingly noting that this process of *modernisation* (defined in Chapter 1) is *not* being duplicated in developing countries. This is one reason for the continued interest in the 'standard of living' debate about conditions in Britain in the period after 1750, when modernisation first occurred. Some historians (the so-called 'optimists') point to certain measurable factors such as economic growth, rising incomes, and falling mortality rates, and conclude that other historians (the so-called 'pessimists') have greatly exaggerated the ill-effects of industrialisation on the condition of the British people at this time. The pessimists, say the optimists, have paid too much attention to impressionistic evidence, such as the 'horror stories' publicised by reformers, or the claims put forward by working-class protesters.

3.1.1 Industrialisation and health

Particularly important in the context of health care is a counter-argument put by one of the pessimists, the social historian E. P. Thompson:

> The controversy as to living standards during the Industrial Revolution has perhaps been of most value when it has passed from the somewhat unreal pursuit of the wage-rates of hypothetical average workers and directed attention to articles of consumption: food, clothing, homes: and, beyond these, health and mortality. (Thompson, 1975, p. 347)

Thompson's main point is that rapid urbanisation and the uncontrolled exploitation of the labouring poor during industrialisation caused a drastic deterioration in living and working conditions. For many the most basic necessities of life — air, water, food, rest, and shelter — degenerated to an appalling degree (see Figure 3.1), and these evils could not be remedied by the poor themselves — at least not under the existing system. The effects on the health of the urban poor are graphically illustrated by the death rates in one of the most intensively industrialised areas of England — Stoke-upon-Trent (Figures 3.2a and 3.2b; now Stoke-on-Trent).

● How do the crude death rates shown in Figure 3.2a compare with that for England and Wales today?[2]

■ The crude death rate is currently about 11 per 1 000 population, compared with 20–25 per 1 000 in England and Wales in 1840–1880; in Stoke and Wolstanton it was above 25 for most of this period and reached 32 at its worst.

---

[1] The theory of Thomas Malthus (1766–1834) that population size would be limited by the shortage of resources is discussed in *World Health and Disease* (Open University Press, 3rd edn 2001), Chapter 5.

[2] Crude death rates are discussed in *Studying Health and Disease* (Open University Press, 2nd edn 1994; colour-enhanced 2nd edn 2001), Chapter 7; and also in *World Health and Disease* (Open University Press, 3rd edn 2001), Chapter 6.

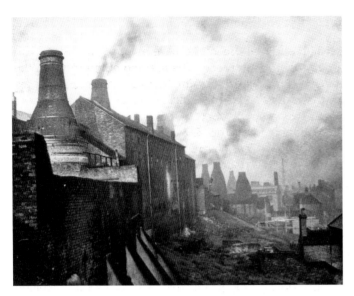

Figure 3.1 *This photographic record provides a startling reminder of the grim state of the environment in the potteries, which constituted one of the areas of greatest density of industrial activity in the UK. In any such district, kilns, mines, foundries and factories were polluting the atmosphere, land surface and water courses with their smoke, effluents and spoil heaps. You will notice that the hapless families of the workers were forced into slum housing sandwiched between industrial developments. (Source: The Potteries Museum and Art Gallery, Stoke-on-Trent)*

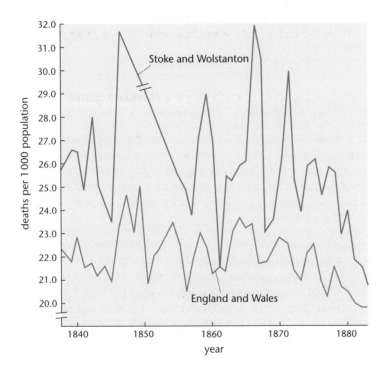

Figure 3.2(a) *Crude death rates for Stoke-upon-Trent and Wolstanton Registration Districts, and for England and Wales, 1838–1883 (data not available for 1847–54). (Sources: data on death rates for England and Wales, 1838–1883 from Mitchell, B. R. and Deane, P., 1971,* Abstract of British Historical Statistics, *Cambridge University Press, Cambridge,* **316**; *other data from the* Annual Reports of the Registrar General; *graphs redrawn from originals in Dupree, M. W., 1995,* Family Structure in the Staffordshire Potteries, 1840–1880, *Clarendon Press, Oxford, p. 83)*

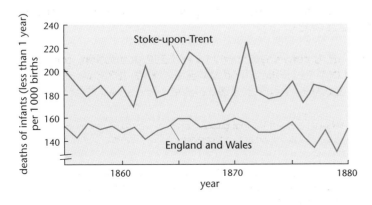

Figure 3.2(b) *Infant mortality rates for Stoke-upon-Trent and Wolstanton Registration Districts, and for England and Wales, 1855–80. (Sources: as Figure 3.2a)*

● How do the infant mortality rates (IMR) shown in Figure 3.2b compare with that for England and Wales today, and with contemporary developing countries?[3]

■ The IMR in all high-income countries, including England and Wales, is about 6 per 1 000 live births; in 1855–1880 it fluctuated between 140–160 infants dying per 1 000 births in England and Wales, and a staggering 160–220 per 1 000 births in Stoke-upon-Trent (almost a quarter of all babies died in infancy in the worst years). This compares with an average of 62 infant deaths per 1 000 live births in today's lowest-income countries.

Neither the optimists nor the pessimists would see medical advance as making much difference at this time (a point we return to in Chapter 4). The only innovation of note was the replacement of inoculation (see Chapter 2) with *vaccination*, a similar procedure using cowpox, a related but lesser disease which experience had shown to confer immunity against smallpox.[4] The comparative unimportance of medical progress gives added prominence to the role of nutrition and environmental regulation.

3.1.2 Class divisions

Some people, as you will see, gave early warning of the effects of industrialisation. However, the humanitarian principles that inspired some reformers in the later eighteenth century were severely set back by the depressed economic conditions and political repression of the period around the Napoleonic Wars. The term *working class* was first used in the revolutionary 1790s, and was applied by middle-class reformers from around the end of the wars with France in 1814. Many saw a solution in political action, as remembered by one middle-class observer, the mathematician, de Morgan: 'From 1815 to 1830 the question of revolution or no revolution lurked in all our English discussions' (de Morgan, 1915, p. 187). The fear of popular unrest was one motive behind upper-class support of social policies aimed at 'improvement' adopted in the wake of industrialisation.

What no historian involved in the 'standard of living' debate would deny is the *magnitude* of the changes over this period. The Census of 1851 showed that, for the first time, more people (in Wales as well as England) lived in towns than in the country. In Scotland, the shift of population to the major industrial centre of Glasgow was particularly rapid.

Eighteenth-century *urbanisation* produced different kinds of town, many of which would not be described as industrial. This point is made especially clearly by considering pairs of different towns — as for example, Wakefield and Huddersfield, contrasted by the historian Hilary Marland. Of these adjacent centres in the industrialising North, Wakefield was the county town, the favoured residence of gentry and the prosperous middle classes (particularly doctors and lawyers), while Huddersfield was industrial, highly productive but at the cost of poor conditions among its burgeoning working-class population. There was, however, no simple contrast between such towns in terms of economic growth or mortality: Wakefield had its poor, but they were hidden away in alleys and subdivided tenements.

[3] Infant mortality rates and comparisons between low-, middle- and high-income countries are discussed in *World Health and Disease* (Open University Press, 3rd edn 2001), Chapter 7.

[4] Edward Jenner published the account of his first experiment with vaccination in 1798. The term 'vaccination' originates from the Latin for 'cow' — hence *variolae vaccinae*, cowpox. 'Vaccination' was later applied to a similar preventive treatment for tuberculosis; for other infectious diseases the term 'immunisation' was generally applied in the twentieth century.

Much the same point can be made about the debate over the effects of *enclosure of common land* and *agricultural improvement*: these effects varied enormously according to region. Forced emigration from rural Ireland, for example, not only devastated that country but had consequential effects for major industrial ports in England such as Liverpool. It was not only regionally that experience varied. The 'cellar-dwellers' of Liverpool became a by-word for squalor and depravity — yet Liverpool was also 'the city of millionaires across the Mersey'.

In the previous chapter, we noted a trend towards *social differentiation*: this trend greatly accelerated during the Industrial Revolution, and increasingly came to be expressed in physical terms, so that the poor were even seen as racially distinct. In rural society, the breakdown of the system of 'live-in' service in husbandry increased estrangement between the classes. Even those seeking to understand rural decline could describe the rural labourer as 'a physical scandal, a moral enigma, an intellectual cataleptic' (the *Morning Chronicle*, 1850, quoted by Snell, 1987, p. 7).

Towns enlarged at first by 'in-filling', leading (as in Wakefield) to hidden pockets of poverty; and then by sprawling new terraces, where contact between the different social classes was minimised, and amenities non-existent. In both town and country, the face-to-face society gave way, in the terms of the time, to a society in which one half did not know how the other half lived. Pompous urban architecture expressed social distance as well as civic pride, although there were attempts, as with the voluntary hospitals (discussed later in this chapter), to bring the classes together in a hierarchical way within new institutions.

By the 1830s and 1840s, it could come as a profound shock to the comfortably off that they shared an environment with the 'labouring population', and that the environment in which the poor lived was so physically degraded as to pose a greater threat to society than the 'moral' (or political) condition of the poor. Different ways of seeing the poor and their conditions are represented in Figures 3.3a and 3.3b.

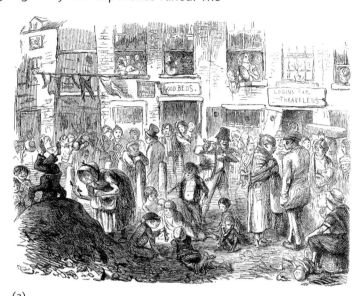

(a)

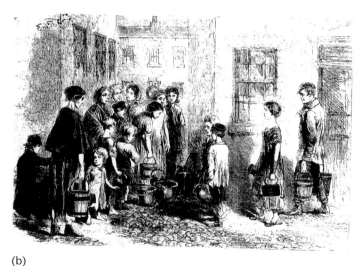

(b)

Figure 3.3 *Two ways of seeing: the 'undeserving' and the 'deserving' poor. (a) 'A Court for King Cholera', a* Punch *cartoon by John Leech. (b) Queuing for water in Bethnal Green. In (a), Leech shows the poor as almost sexless, full of low cunning, and as matched to their conditions of life. At the same time he depicts particular targets of sanitary concern: lodging houses, muck heaps, and the 'court' itself — a crowded courtyard squeezed between buildings and almost hidden from the street — a classic 'fever nest' as well as a focus for cholera. In (b), the poor are made to look pitiable rather than depraved, the women are more feminine, and the emphasis is placed on the inappropriateness of the physical burden being imposed on women and children in particular. (Sources: (a)* Punch, *25 September 1852; (b) Mary Evans Picture Library)*

In 1832, while investigating the cotton operatives, Dr Charles Turner Thackrah of Leeds, the pioneer of 'industrial hygiene' — the study of health and safety at work — glimpsed the working poor *en masse*:

> I saw, or thought I saw, a degenerate race — human beings stunted, enfeebled, and depraved — men and women that were not to be aged — children that were never to be healthy adults.
> (Quoted by Thompson, 1975, p. 364)

Thackrah was looking at factory workers, but he was well aware that the conditions for those working long hours in slum housing or in cramped workshops could be equally disabling.[5] Reformers first expressed this revelation in terms of different class-related and district-related mortalities, using local surveys and then the information provided by the *Registrar-General's Office* instituted in 1836 (for an example, see Table 3.1; Figures 3.2a and 3.2b also testify to the effect on death rates).

Table 3.1 Life expectancies for different classes in different localities, 1839–40, as set out by Edwin Chadwick.

Number of deaths		Average age of deceased/years
	Bethnal Green	
101	Gentlemen and persons engaged in professions and their families	45
273	Tradesmen and their families	26
1 258	Mechanics, servants, labourers and their families	16
	Leeds Borough	
79	Gentlemen, etc.	44
824	Tradesmen, farmers, etc.	27
3 395	Operatives, labourers, etc.	19
	Liverpool	
137	Gentlemen, etc.	35
1 738	Tradesmen, etc.	22
5 597	Labourers, mechanics, servants, etc.	15
	Unions in the County of Wilts.	
119	Gentlemen, etc.	50
218	Farmers, etc.	48
2 061	Agricultural labourers, etc.	33
	Kendal Union	
52	Gentlemen, etc.	45
138	Tradesmen, etc.	39
413	Operatives, labourers, servants, etc.	34

Data from Flinn, M. W. (ed.) (1965) *Report on the Sanitary Condition of the Labouring Population of Great Britain, by Edwin Chadwick, 1842*, Edinburgh University Press, Edinburgh, pp. 224–5, based on the earliest returns of the Registrar-General's Office. Note, however, that in all areas each class is present in very different proportions, and that the table has not been corrected for the age-structure of the population in question.

[5] Such conditions are graphically described in the article by Friedrich Engels, 'Health: 1844' in *Health and Disease: A Reader* (Open University Press, 2nd edn 1995; 3rd edn 2001), which could usefully be consulted again, even if you read it during your study of Chapter 1.

However, it is as well to stress that *mortality* is only a rough index to health experience. The argument over the effects of industrialisation can be explained not only in terms of the radically different experiences of different groups in society, but also in terms of *our* inability to measure *morbidity* as accurately as we can mortality. Extreme disadvantage, even protracted suffering — suggested by the quotation from Thackrah — may occur without being reflected in mortality statistics.

It is necessary too to take note of what people themselves regarded as making the difference between subsistence and despair. In the rural context, this could be the loss of such entitlements as bed-and-board, gleaning and the right to keep livestock. A similar point can be made about the abandonment in towns of controls on the price and quality of staple foodstuffs such as bread (which we mentioned in Chapter 2) — what has been referred to as the displacement of the *moral economy* by the rise of *economic liberalism* during the eighteenth century.

3.2   The New Poor Law

Above all, it is issues of *entitlement* that are at stake with respect to the Poor Law. The **New Poor Law** of 1834 targeted the *able-bodied*; it stressed *deterrence* rather than entitlement, *institutionalisation* rather than 'out-door' mechanisms of relief such as pensions, and sought to replace haphazard localism with the ugly principle of **'less-eligibility'**.

The main aim behind the New Poor Law was to reduce public expenditure, and in particular to reduce the supplementation of depressed wages in the agricultural South of England. In order to eliminate this form of out-door relief, the **workhouse test** was instituted: to obtain assistance, the poor person had to be desperate enough to enter the workhouse (*in-door relief*). In-door relief had to be 'less eligible' (more distasteful) than any work available *outside* the workhouse — and there were no minimum standards governing conditions of employment at this date.

The 15 000 autonomous parishes of the Old Poor Law could not be expected all to have workhouses, so economies of scale were achieved by creating fewer and larger organisational units, the *Poor Law Unions*, which were accountable to a central administration, and which were better able to provide large institutions (see Figure 3.4).

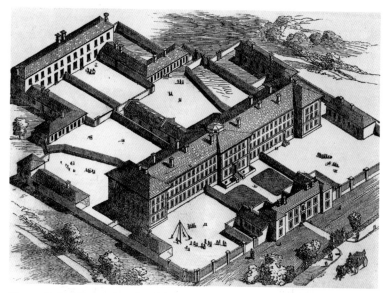

Figure 3.4   *'Economies of scale': an aim of the New Poor Law, in amalgamating 15 000 very different parish units into fewer than 600 Poor Law Unions, was to make it possible to construct large workhouses with purpose-built infirmaries. Some Unions did so (though many did not, especially in rural areas): this vast new workhouse, opened on 4 August 1849, was for the united parishes of Fulham and Hammersmith. The largest workhouses not only segregated the poor according to age, sex, and health, but provided separate accommodation for each of the sexes according to 'good' and 'bad' character. (Source: Hulton Getty Picture Collection)*

Rather than appearing to the poor as a source of assistance at times of their lives when they needed it most, the New Poor Law created a new underclass, the *paupers*, which the poor had to join before any assistance was offered. While designed to reduce the dependency of the poor by deterrence, the harshness of the New Poor Law was intended to be balanced by the preventive principles of *sanitary reform*, and by a system of *medical poor relief*. We will look at these later in this chapter.

3.3   Lay care: urbanisation and self-help

Many aspects of lay care show remarkably little change into the industrial period and beyond, in spite of major social and economic dislocations. The wealth of sources (letters, diaries, pamphlets) produced by a literate (male) population, and the flourishing of a less-restricted press, increased the 'noise level' of lay interest in health, but it should not be assumed that such interest was new. Charles Waterton, eccentric naturalist and Squire of Walton Hall, near Leeds in Yorkshire, for example, came from a long line of busy gentry, advocating long-established remedies as well as adapting to new emergencies:

> [Waterton] recommended that travellers should carry with them bark [cinchona, the source of quinine], laudanum [tincture of opium], calomel [chloride of mercury] … and, most important, a lancet…He had his own prescriptions and Mr Waterton's Pills were famous in Walton and the neighbourhood. During the 1849 cholera epidemic Waterton gratuitously distributed amongst the poor of Leeds and adjoining townships a powder which he claimed was highly beneficial in cases of cholera. (Marland, 1987, pp. 214–15)

The example of Squire Waterton suggests that it is not necessarily the case that lay knowledge was falling behind professional knowledge. This is partly because medical practice itself continued to be traditional in content. The interconnected phenomena of *population growth*, *social dislocation*, and *class differentiation* did, however, create a mass of conflicting claims affecting the possession and diffusion of knowledge. This is one aspect of what is called **the Enlightenment** — a set of ideas and political beliefs stressing the power of reason (and therefore of information) and the perfectibility of 'man'. The Enlightenment particularly expressed the interests of the middle classes, speaking on behalf of the working class.

3.3.1   Useful knowledge

Although the ideas behind it seemed mainly to have spread from other countries — especially France, America, and Scotland — the Enlightenment in England was also a revival of grievances left over from the Civil War period (approximately 1640–60). These grievances had included criticism of the monopoly of knowledge by doctors and lawyers, as well as assertions of the unity of spiritual and physical life. Thus we find that much lay interest in health and healing was allied to movements in popular religion — just as, for more established denominations, subscribing funds to a hospital had religious as well as medical justifications.

These different trends are illustrated in this period by the two most successful medical manuals written for the laity — *Primitive Physick* (1747) by John Wesley, the founder of Methodism, and William Buchan's *Domestic Medicine* (1769), which was based on a French handbook. These provided new resources for local figures traditionally inclined to take an interest in medicine, such as the clergy and schoolmasters.

Here is a nineteenth-century writer recalling a late-eighteenth-century Scottish schoolmaster:

> He was very useful in the parish, for he could let blood, and was a daily reader of 'Buchan's Domestic Medicine', all whose instructions he rigidly, and often successfully, practised. (Quoted by Lawrence, 1975, p. 32)

By the time editions of Buchan's book ceased appearing, in the early nineteenth century, the four major movements in popular medicine were well-established: *medical botany* or *herbalism, homoeopathy, hydropathy* (a system of cure based on water), and *mesmerism* (a form of hypnotism combined with magnetism). In this period these 'alternatives' are best seen as self-help systems, appealing to a wide range of classes in society (including medical men), and offering a rich mixture of traditional concepts, modern science, and spirituality. These eclectic systems were essentially urban growths, imported from mainland Europe or America. They were not simply updated versions of traditional indigenous folklore about herbs, magic, and holy waters, although there was a stress on a 'return to nature' which we also hear today. The proliferation of spas in this period further shows how readily the traditional could combine with the scientific, the fashionable and the entrepreneurial.

In addition, provincial towns experienced, on a variety of scales, the diversity — and insecurities — of urban life as it was previously known only in London and the provincial capitals. The irrepressible lay interest in health and disease had many new outlets for its expression, as well as new sources of concern. The outlets included book clubs, circulating libraries, publication by subscription, mechanics' institutes, and lectures on such subjects as chemistry and phrenology.

It is characteristic of this period's methods of communication — and of the difficulty of separating lay care from qualified practice — that both medicines, and information about practitioners, were sold and distributed by booksellers, circulating libraries, printers, and publishers (who could also be the proprietors of newspapers carrying medical advertisements). These links were *in addition to*, rather than instead of, medicine's older occupational diversifications, such as those involving traders in food and drink, or farriers, blacksmiths, and others dealing with animals.

3.3.2 Druggists: further steps in the commercialisation of self-help

Two other developments can be mentioned to illustrate the theme of self-help. The first is the rise of the **druggist**, who in this period displaced the apothecary and the grocer as the shopkeeping source of medication and advice. The apothecaries were tending to run practices rather than shops. By the 1840s, according to Census information, there were in England and Wales about two druggists to every three qualified medical practitioners. Like the barbers' shops in pre-industrial towns, the druggists were well-distributed, and could be up-market or down, able to cater for high levels of self-medication among the better-off as well as the poor. Here is a druggist targeting the middle-class market in Wakefield:

> Those Families who may honor him with their Commands, may depend upon having every Article in the Medical Department, as Genuine as at the Apothecary's Hall, London. (Quoted in Marland, 1987, p. 217)

● The druggists were very like today's pharmacists — but does the quotation suggest any differences?

■ Their main business in medicine was not filling the prescriptions of doctors, but filling the orders and making up the recipes brought to them by their (lay) customers.

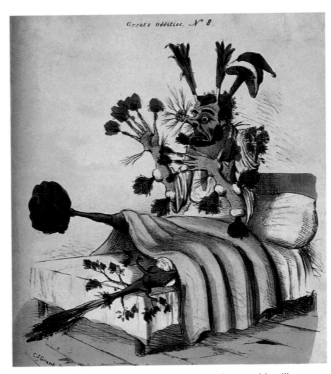

Figure 3.5 *'Singular effects of the universal vegetable pills on a green grocer!' Coloured lithograph by C. J. Grant, 1831. One of a series of skits on the philosophy of health of James Morison (1770–1840), who successfully advocated a simplified self-help approach based on purging the blood of impurities by means of large doses of vegetable pills. (Source: Wellcome Library, London)*

Druggists also sold *proprietary remedies* (Figure 3.5), which began to be patented in the seventeenth century, and had swelled to become a useful source of tax revenue by the late eighteenth. The better-known of these medicines differed little in composition from the official versions listed in pharmacopoeias. Many of them, patented and otherwise, also dated from the seventeenth century rather than the eighteenth, although they multiplied during the period of industrialisation according to increased demand, improved distribution, and the beginnings of the pharmaceutical industry — an area in which Nonconformists such as Quakers were highly successful, as they were in the food industry.

3.3.3   Friendly Societies

The second development in this period is the emergence of the **Friendly Societies** — self-help organisations which first developed in the industrial North to meet the three main threats to working people and their families: sickness, unemployment, and death. A society might maintain a subscription to an institution such as a hospital, but its main function was to pay out benefits to members according to their contributions. Unlike the guilds and their successors the companies, which had been broader organisations, taking some responsibility for sick and aged members, the Friendly Societies were organised by wage-earners for wage-earners. They were often the only safety-net for working men and women affected by long-term, seasonal, and chronic illnesses; they remained so until well into the twentieth century, and still exist in modified form today.

● Can you think of factors likely to limit the success of Friendly Societies dependent upon the contributions of wage-earners?

■ The societies could be affected by: the age-structure of their membership; prolonged slumps in employment; a decline in mortality not associated with a decline in morbidity. Dependants could benefit only indirectly.

In this section we have concentrated upon lay care as an aspect of self-help (and self-expression) in an urbanising society. We should also stress here how elites among the laity not only continued to control previously established systems of health care, such as the Poor Law, but also dominated the new urban systems, such as the hospitals, the dispensaries, and other forms of medical charity. This will be further examined later in the chapter.

3.4 Public health: a shared environment?

Most public health issues involve a practical idea of the common good. Listen to Samuel Johnson, condemning schemes to pipe water from Plymouth to the adjacent industrial sprawl of Dock (now Devonport):

> No, no! I am against the *dockers*; I am a Plymouth man. Rogues!
> let them die of thirst! (Quoted by Corfield, 1989, p. 46).

3.4.1 Old corruption

Johnson's hyperbole encapsulates the successes and failures of the impulse to environmental improvement in this period. Local initiatives and Improvement Acts — enabling legislation specially applied for by a locality — achieved benefits for certain parts of certain towns, but the public good tended to be very narrowly defined. This reflected the extremely inconsistent and undemocratic structure of eighteenth-century English local government, which was only partially rectified by Bills passed in the 1830s aimed at eliminating corruption and extending the franchise.

The idiosyncrasies of local custom were an impossible basis for managing social and economic crises of mounting scale. Population growth and industrialisation could mean gross mismatches between changing local needs and traditional political structure and representation. Local bodies such as Boards of Commissioners multiplied on an *ad hoc* basis to take separate responsibility for services like street paving, nuisance removal, lighting, highways, sewerage, and burial grounds, but only for limited areas and with minimal accountability.

All such services were dependent upon a narrow rate base, restricted borrowing powers, or on local philanthropy. Above all, they were dependent upon the honesty and goodwill of a few individuals, in a situation where conflict of interest was inevitable. Gas lighting and the extension of water supplies were left to market forces: private water companies were active in this period, but tended to compete for the same few profitable customers. Industrial change provided potential for improvement but new standards had to be enforced: for example, iron rather than wooden piping for water systems was made compulsory in 1827.

3.4.2 Fever: the diagnosis of social evils

The disease that lay at the heart of the dominant approaches to public health in this period was *fever* — in particular, *typhus* (an infection carried by the body louse), with an increasing admixture of *typhoid* (a water-borne disease), and *relapsing fever* (a disease exacerbated by famine). These diseases were only gradually distinguished from each other during the first half of the nineteenth century. They were known collectively as 'continued fever' (as distinct from ague or intermittent fever — that is, malaria).

During the eighteenth century, typhus became recognised as a disease of the poor and of crowding — notable outbreaks occurred in ships, prisons, and military camps. Hospitals and factories were also observed to become foci of infection. Hospitals generally excluded fever cases for fear of concentrating infection. Investigators, for example the prison reformer John Howard, concluded that these epidemics could be prevented by such measures as improving ventilation, reducing overcrowding, and strengthening the constitutions of those at risk.

An even broader diagnosis of the causes of continued fever was made by Thomas Percival (1740–1804), a Unitarian physician and intellectual, who was central to pioneering initiatives undertaken in England's 'first industrial city', Manchester. Percival and his associates saw children as especially sensitive to industrial conditions; they condemned child labour and advocated universal education. Percival's comprehensive reforms included local boards of health given wide regulatory powers by national legislation. The hostility of industrialists blocked most of his ideas; one of the model institutions to survive — mainly as a version of the voluntary hospital specialising in infectious cases — was the *fever hospital*. The major outbreaks of fever in Ireland in the early nineteenth century also led to some experimentation with institutions like fever hospitals.

3.4.3 New arms of government

As you have seen, health-related administration was at its most fragmented just when the environmental crises of industrialisation and population growth became most acute. Apart from quarantine and other emergency provisions, no responsibility was taken for public health at the national or even regional level. Late in the period, the Unions of the New Poor Law in England and Wales provided for the first time a national system of larger units of civil administration; Poor Law authorities, notably the *Board of Guardians* elected by each Union's ratepayers, were subsequently expected to take on other responsibilities — civil registration, sanitary improvement, and vaccination, for example.

● Can you see a disadvantage in this use of the Poor Law authorities for public health administration and health education?

■ Health-related functions became linked in people's minds with the New Poor Law — and could acquire negative associations as a result of its unpopularity.

As already suggested, the connection between sanitary reform and the New Poor Law goes even deeper than this.

3.4.4 Benthamism and sanitary reform

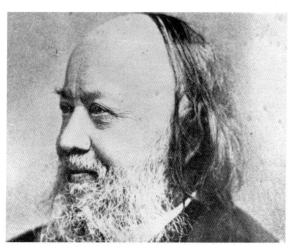

Figure 3.6(a) *Edwin Chadwick, the lawyer and lifelong campaigner for sanitary reform, died in 1890 at the age of 90 years. (Source:* The Londoners, *The Pilot Press)*

The **sanitary movement**, launched in the 1820s, became a broadly-based campaign aimed at cleansing, watering, sewering, and rehousing — and thus preventing disease among — neglected human populations, especially in large towns. Britain was the first country in Western Europe to approach the urban environment in this way, because it was the first to impose unrestricted industrial development on an entirely inadequate system of local administration.

The immediate inspiration of the sanitary movement was provided by the **Benthamites** — followers (notably Edwin Chadwick, see Figure 3.6a) of the lawyer and philosopher Jeremy Bentham (1748–1832) (see Figure 3.6b). Bentham's ideas became the main means by which the Enlightenment belief in reason and the perfectibility of man was preserved for nineteenth-century reformers. Bentham's

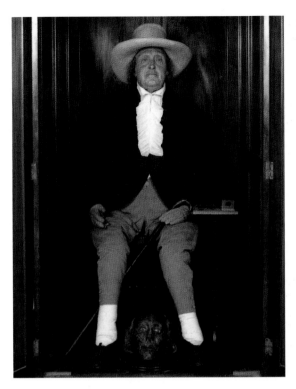

Figure 3.6(b) *Jeremy Bentham died in 1832, aged 84 years. In his will he left his body for public dissection by his friend and fellow-campaigner for sanitary reform, Thomas Southwood Smith, 'with the desire that mankind may reap some small benefit in and by my decease'. Bentham's private papers included a pamphlet on 'Auto-Icons' — dehydrated human corpses, preserved for posterity and recognisable as individuals. Southwood Smith had an Auto-Icon (pictured here) made from Bentham's skeleton and stuffed to fit his clothes, but his attempt to dehydrate the head did not preserve the features and it was replaced by a wax model. (Source: University College London)*

'constitutional code' placed considerable stress on health and *disease prevention* as responsibilities of the state, along with complementary functions such as education and the gathering of statistics.

The Benthamites emphasised the need for the role of the qualified expert in the service of government — for example, in factory inspection. In economic matters, they saw the function of government as one of regulation, rather than direction. In practice, Bentham's view of the collective functioning of individual self-interest tended to be taken out of context and combined with the prevailing climate of liberalism or *laissez-faire*, which minimised the role of government with respect to the economy. In 1842 Chadwick wrote with typical trenchancy:

> The expenses of local public works are in general unequally and unfairly assessed, oppressively and uneconomically collected, by separate collections, wastefully expended in separate and inefficient operations by unskilled and practically irresponsible officers. (Quoted by Simon, 1897, p. 193)

●   What features of the Benthamite approach does this suggest to you?

■   Particularly characteristic are the stresses on: efficiency; equity of taxation and representation; co-ordination of administrative functions; accountability; and professional qualifications.

Both the New Poor Law and sanitary reform were designed to reduce wasteful expenditure, to induce labour to move to where there was employment, and to prevent the diseases which so reduced the earning capacity of the labouring classes. A major point of the Benthamite inquiries was to establish that epidemic disease struck *unnecessarily* at the *able-bodied breadwinner*, rather than 'conveniently' removing the weak and unproductive (see Table 3.2 overleaf).

Table 3.2 'Pecuniary burdens created by neglect': the top and the bottom of a table of Poor Law returns for a lead-mining area in Cumberland as presented by Chadwick in the 1842 Report, highlighting the deaths of breadwinners.

Alston with Garrigill Parish Number of widows, and children dependent upon them, in receipt of relief in the above parish; age of husband at death; and the alleged cause of death					
Initials of widows	No. of children dependent at husband's death	Occupation of deceased husband	Age at death	Years' loss by premature death	Alleged cause of death
R.W.	–	miner	83	–	decay of nature
M.B.	–	miner	73	–	not stated
M.L.	–	miner	64	–	influenza
J.P.	–	labourer	62	–	consumption
H.T.	2	mason	62	–	asthma
S.H.	2	miner	60	–	rupture of blood-vessel
M.P.	1	turner	57	3	consumption
H.S.	3	miner	57	3	influenza, terminating in dropsy
M.J.	3	blacksmith	55	5	asthma
S.M.	–	miner	55	5	inflammation of lungs from cold
J.W.	2	mner	54	6	pleurisy
H.P.	5	miner	48	12	typhus fever
E.H.	6	miner	48	12	killed in lead mines
M.A.	7	miner	48	12	consumption by bad air in the pit
H.P.	3	miner	45	15	scarlet fever
M.S.	2	miner	45	15	inflammation of bowels
H.M.	7	miner	43	17	asthma, which terminated in consumption
A.J.	2	miller	42	18	found drowned
M.R.	–	shoemaker	40	20	injury from fall of a cart
E.R.	7	joiner	38	22	affection of the liver
J.B.	5	miner	38	22	consumption
A.P.	7	miner	37	21	asthma
E.H.	3	miner	35	25	killed in coal-pit
M.L.	2	miner	35	25	water of the head
S.H.	7	miner	34	26	accident in coal-mine
E.A.	2	miner	30	30	consumption
A.W.	2	miner	28	32	cholera
J.M.	2	miner	21	39	small-pox
89	**242**	–	**4418**	–	**totals listed in unedited table**
	average age at death of each below 60 years of age: } 45			total no. of orphans by deaths caused below 60 years of age: } 236	

Chadwick added: 'This premature widowhood and orphanage is the source of the most painful descriptions of pauperism … it is the source of a constant influx of the independent into the pauperised and permanently dependent classes'. (Data from Flinn, M. W. (ed.) 1965, *Report on the Sanitary Condition of the Labouring Population of Great Britain, by Edwin Chadwick, 1842*, Edinburgh University Press, Edinburgh, pp. 258–60, 255)

The *preventable* diseases were traced to the influence of local causes of pollution — impure or inadequate water supply, accumulated sewage, contaminated air, overcrowded housing, overcrowded graveyards, industrial waste and decaying organic matter generally. Other commentators pointed to the broad range of factors behind poverty; still others blamed the conditions in which the poor lived on their own habits or lack of moral education.

For the Benthamite sanitarians, moral effects were defined as having physical causes. Intervention in 'social wrongs' was seen as imperative; the most efficient way of intervening in this case was to remove the physical causes of preventable disease, and the most efficient means of intervention was by government action. In this, as in other areas of social policy, the Benthamites formed a model pressure group committed to national legislation.

As you might be thinking, not even the Benthamites could move the mountains of filth by themselves. **Sanitarianism** became a broadly-based creed, having as its unifying principle the reduction of environmental pollution in the interests of human health. The 'health of towns' was a major political and social issue in the 1830s and 1840s, leading to local initiatives such as the appointment of the first *Medical Officer of Health* or MOH in Liverpool, 1847 (Chapter 4 discusses how the role of the MOH developed), national pressure groups such as the Health of Towns Association, and national legislation, culminating in the Public Health Act of 1848. This Act set up England's first central health department — the shortlived *General Board of Health*, of which Chadwick was the dominant member.

In continental Europe as well as in Britain, public health reformers increasingly saw *infectiousness* — and therefore 'excess' or preventable disease — as dependent upon environmental factors, rather than being a fixed property of a given disease. The 'sanitary idea' pushed by the Benthamites from the late 1820s onwards was based on experience of *fever nests* — pockets of urban degradation, inhabited by the poorest, from which disease could spread, not by the movement of infected individuals, but through the widespread prevalence of insanitary conditions. (Look again at Figure 3.3.)

These ideas were adapted to include *cholera*, which first extended to Europe in the 1820s, reaching Britain in 1831. Cholera gave impetus to sanitary reform, but being an occasional invader it was not the most important cause of death. One effect of cholera was to limit initiatives to temporary or emergency provisions.[6]

Sanitarians continued to stress the cost to society of endemic, indigenous disease, with continued fever as the best example, and called for a central, permanent Board of Health. But Chadwick's General Board foundered in 1854, owing to pressure from vested interests and political opposition to centralised health administration.

3.5 Partly professionalised: the general practitioner

Medicine lagged well behind the Church and the law in its achievement of middle-class respectability. Whether this status was gained during the process of 'gentrification' in towns in the eighteenth century, or as a result of the 'multiplication of intellectual callings' in the nineteenth, has been a matter of debate. Historians

---

[6] The work of John Snow (1813–1858) in mapping the spread of cholera in Soho, London, in the 1848 epidemic is discussed in *Studying Health and Disease* (Open University Press, 2nd edn 1994; colour-enhanced 2nd edn 2001), Chapter 7.

have also suggested that medical practitioners in this period were 'marginal men' who took on a range of high-profile social roles in provincial institutions and societies in order to establish their professional position.

3.5.1 Regular and irregular practitioners?

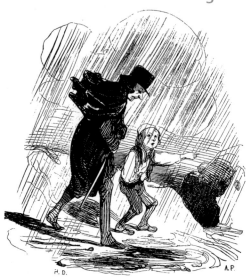

Figure 3.7   *The country doctor: copper engraving after Honoré Daumier. (Source: A. F. H. Fabre,* Némésis médicale illustrée, *revised edition, Paris, 1840)*

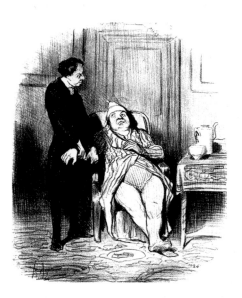

Figure 3.8   *'Oh, doctor, I'm sure I'm consumptive': lithograph by Honoré Daumier. (Reproduced from a series by Daumier,* Tout ce qu'on voudra *('everything one would want'), Paris, 1847)*

What does seem clear is, *first*, that the rank-and-file 'regular' practitioners managed to redefine themselves somewhat — a change signified by the deployment of the term **general practitioner** around 1820. *Second*, the new ideals of respectability increased the pressures of competition for 'respectable' patients among regular practitioners, even though middle-class demand for medical services also increased (Figure 3.7 suggests the working conditions that many were trying to get away from, and Figure 3.8 that even middle-class practice could be less than rewarding, at least intellectually).

Third, medical practitioners remained extremely various, and critical of each other. *Finally*, it is unhistorical to regard medical practitioners even of this period as behaving first and foremost as medical personnel, defined in their outlook only by purely professional considerations — as if, for example, they were not also motivated, like their contemporaries, by different religious or political beliefs, which determined their alliances and position in society.

Doctors, in effect, did not 'hang together' just because they were doctors. It might be more important to an individual practitioner that (for instance) he was Unitarian in his religious beliefs, or that he had read an influential philosophical work at an impressionable age. Religion was important for a variety of reasons — for example, many able Nonconformists went into medicine, because their religion debarred them from other means of advancement.

The sporadic attempt at national regulation of physicians, surgeons and midwives, made through the ecclesiastical licensing system of the sixteenth century, faded out during the eighteenth century, as did the provincial barber-surgeons' companies, except where they became small, privileged enclaves dominated by certain families. Apprenticeship for barber-surgeons and apothecaries continued, but on an individual basis, as the system of apprenticeship in general was broken down. Personal knowledge was more than ever the patient's best security in choosing a practitioner. In an urbanising society such knowledge was harder to come by, and so was valued accordingly; this helped to shape, for the middle classes at least, new ideals of the private relationship between practitioner and patient.

At the same time, in the urban setting, if a practitioner did not have good connections he might gain acceptance by other means (for example, a striking physical presence, or public appearances, such as lectures), which could equally well be exploited by his rivals. As you will recall from earlier discussion, the necessary techniques of self-assertion, such as advertisement in newspapers, were also increasing.

Consequently it is difficult to define a 'regular' practitioner in this period, although this adjective (and its opposite, 'irregular') were beginning to be used (perhaps derived from military service). It should not surprise you that itinerant practitioners were probably more numerous (in proportion) before 1800 than at any other time; and that the laity were still ready to assume the medical role — even though, for example, the aspiring middle-class family might decide to patronise a *man-midwife*, rather than a more traditional female attendant (compare Figure 2.4 in Chapter 2 with Figure 3.9).

The first of the nineteenth-century national Censuses to include detailed occupational information (1841) showed that, even when only main occupations were asked for, the *regular* practitioners — defined by then in terms of formal qualifications — were still considerably out-numbered by the *irregulars*, by a ratio of 1 : 3. The irregulars included particularly the druggists, whom we discussed earlier.

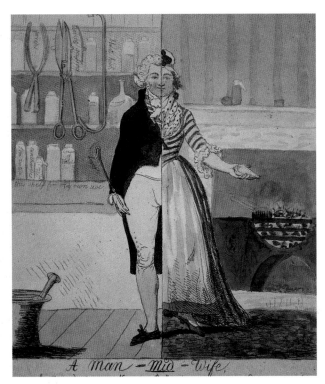

Figure 3.9 *Cartoon from S. W. Fores,* Man-Midwifery Dissected, *1793. The term 'man-midwife' was in use in England by 1625, and such work seemed for a time likely to become a largely male preserve (as it did in the USA). Behind the male half-figure are bottles of 'love water' and other potions allegedly used as sexual stimulants. (Source: Wellcome Library, London)*

As in the pre-industrial period, the numbers of regular practitioners actually practising only physic, or only surgery, were extremely small, even in the London hospitals, where you might expect demarcation lines to be most precise. The hospitals offered an opportunity for professional self-definition, but were also an arena for religious, political and professional conflicts. A hospital connection, for reasons we shall look at later, was honorary or unpaid, but it offered rewards to be competed for in the form of social contacts, which increased private practice, and large fees or premiums from pupils.

3.5.2 Medical reform: internal struggles

Regular medicine at this time was hierarchical but far from orderly. Entry to the pinnacles of practice was guarded in London by the *Royal College of Physicians* and the *Royal College of Surgeons* (which had abandoned the Barbers in 1745, and obtained new charters in 1800 and 1843). These two London medical colleges, by withholding recognition of the courses offered by private or provincial medical schools — while recognising pupilage in the London hospitals, or degrees from Oxford or Cambridge — also restricted access to the higher levels of qualification (the medical colleges' licentiateships, memberships, or fellowships).

● What general strategy for maintaining professional dominance is exemplified by this action of the medical colleges?

■ They were using 'exclusion' tactics to ensure that entry to the highest status positions in medicine was limited to practitioners with specified qualifications.[7]

Pressure on the London medical colleges, especially the Surgeons, came from the increasing minority of regular practitioners who were university-trained — not by Oxford and Cambridge, which produced only tiny numbers of medical graduates throughout the period and imposed religious tests — but in the Netherlands (especially Leiden), in Scotland (especially Edinburgh and Glasgow), in Dublin, and, from 1828, by the non-denominational University College London (which became the nucleus of the University of London). A minimum qualification by examination was first introduced with the LSA — *Licence of the (London) Society of Apothecaries* — in 1815.

The favoured credentials for the ambitious new 'general practitioner' (GP) were *'College and Hall'*, meaning respectively the MRCS (Membership — not Fellowship — of the Royal College of Surgeons), and the LSA ('Hall' because the Apothecaries' Society, being one of the old London companies, still had its 'guild hall'). Box 3.1 shows how, by 1847, the emergent GP could make his credentials contrast with those of some of his competitors in the medical directories of the period.

Box 3.1   Selected entries from the *Provincial Medical Directory*, 1847, London, John Churchill (pp. 20, 23, 98, 200)

BARRETT, John, Orange-grove, Bath — Surg.; F.R.C.S. (by exam.) 1846; Surg. to Western Dispensary; to St Michael's Lying-in Charity; to Great Western Railway (Bath District); Vaccinator, and Registrar of Births and Deaths for Abbey District.

BATTEN, Thos., Coleford, Monmouthsh. — General Pract.; M.R.C.S. 1827; L.S.A. 1826; Surgeon to eight collieries in the district.

BEASLEY, John, Oadby Blaby, Leicester — Gen. Pract.; In practice prior to the Act of 1815.

BEDINGFIELD, James, Stowmarket, Suffolk — Gen. Pract.; M.D.; In practice prior to the Act of 1815; formerly Apoth. to the Bristol Infirmary; Surg. to the Hundred of Stow, and the Dorcas Society; Mem. of the Council of the Prov. Med. and Surg. Association, and of the Nat. Instit.; Author of "The Enemy of Empiricism", and of a "Compendium of Medical Practice"; Contributor of numerous Papers to the *Lancet, Provin. Med. and Surg. Journal*, and *Dublin Med. Press*, on Medicine, Surgery, and Midwifery, on Medical Reform, and on the New Poor Law.

FERNELEY, Charles, Denton, near Grantham, Lincolnshire — Gen. Pract.; M.R.C.S. 1833; Med. Officer to Grantham Union. Author of "Lectures on Nutrition of Plants". Contributed to *Med. Gaz.* a paper "On certain Medical Laws which obtain in the Animal Economy", Jan. 1840.

MOTT, William Hadley, Kemp Town, Brighton — Surgeon; in practice prior to the Act of 1815; formerly Surgeon in the Army.

---

[7] The medical profession's strategies for maintaining professional dominance over other health care practitioners (e.g. nurses, osteopaths, radiographers), are discussed in *Medical Knowledge: Doubt and Certainty* (Open University Press, 2nd edn 1994; colour-enhanced 2nd edn 2001), Chapter 2.

Although inspired by the *Medical Reform* movement, the 1840s medical directories were essentially commercial enterprises which preceded the Medical Register resulting from the Act of 1858. The publisher put together the *Directory* of 1847 from Census-related information collected by the District Registrars, supplemented with other sources. Note that not all those who might have done so, wished to call themselves 'General Practitioner'; and that those giving themselves this description were still very diverse. Note also that publications on almost any scientific subject could be regarded as improving a practitioner's status, and that practitioners already lived on connections with a wide range of institutions (the army, mines, the Poor Law, etc.).

However, because educational options had multiplied, and there was no effective overall regulation, even formal credentials remained very confusing. 'The legal titles of medical practitioners', as one experienced critic put it, 'were as various as the names of snuffs or sauces' (Simon, 1897, p. 269). In the period from around 1800 to the Medical Act of 1858, between 15 and 20 bodies could offer different qualifications to someone wishing to practise in England.

This, the period of the Medical Reform movement, was one of campaigning and conflict. The main ingredients were attacks by rank-and-file practitioners on the London royal colleges and the London medical elites (Figure 3.10), and the founding in 1832 of a rival pressure group representing general practitioners — the Provincial Medical and Surgical Association (PMSA, re-established in 1855 as the *British Medical Association* or BMA).

Crucial to the success of the medical profession in gaining status and influence was its effective use of medical journalism. The two most famous examples were *The Lancet*, founded by the twenty-eight-year-old Thomas Wakley in 1823, which was the first medical weekly ever published, and the *British Medical Journal* (the *BMJ*), another weekly which dates from 1857, but began life under a different name in 1840. Whereas Wakley's journal was established as, and has remained, a vehicle of independent opinion, the *BMJ* was instigated by the PMSA and since 1857 has been tied up with the British Medical Association.

Wakley's journal waged a fearless and uninhibited war against incompetence and nepotism among the London medical elites, and against adulteration of foods, drinks and drugs. Wakley himself championed a range of radical causes (including the Tolpuddle martyrs, transported for the equivalent of trades unionism), but his view of the profession was meritocratic, rather than democratic. He pushed the claims of the increasing numbers of well-educated medical men, particularly in the provinces, who

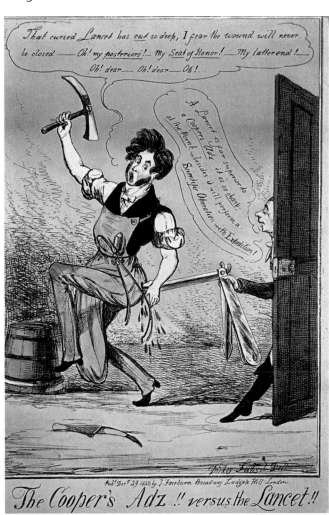

Figure 3.10 *Cartoon satirising a celebrated controversy in 1827–8, over the effects of patronage in London hospitals, involving a campaign in* The Lancet *against a 'Hospital surgeon', Bransby Cooper (nephew of Sir Astley Cooper of Guy's Hospital, London) whom* The Lancet *accused of 'bungling' operations and causing the death of his patients. (Source: Wellcome Library, London)*

reflected most credit upon the new category of general practitioner. The *BMJ*, especially during its early years, broadly echoed Wakley's campaigning approach to such issues as medical and public health reform.

3.6 Philanthropy: the role of bricks and mortar

Major changes in 'bricks and mortar' provision took place in the period covered by this chapter — in Britain, the spread of 'voluntary' hospitals and other medical charities, and in continental Europe, the reshaping of the large institutions dating from earlier periods. However we should stress that the bulk of medical care — even *formal* medical care — continued to be provided *outside* institutions. Only small select categories of poor people were treated in British hospitals. The intake of the new lunatic asylums seems to have been broader in social terms, as a reflection of demand for that kind of custodial institution from families of all classes.

3.6.1 Voluntary hospitals

The **voluntary hospitals** were 'voluntary' rather than 'chartered' because they were initially supported not by endowments but by annual donations from subscribers, who administered the institution and also had the right to sponsor patients for admission. This amounted to a system of lay control, although the medical and surgical staff normally had the same rights as subscribers, and — as another indication of a shared social outlook — gave their services free. As we mentioned in the previous section, these honorary posts rewarded their holders indirectly.

The voluntary hospitals probably owe their origins in the early eighteenth century to a new form of piety, which stressed philanthropy as a common ground on which Anglicans and Nonconformists could work in the interests of social harmony. Some founders had in mind other political and economic questions which amounted to a continued interest in what was known as 'political arithmetic', or the relevance to government of the structure, wealth, health, and earning capacity of the nation's population, particularly with reference to war and colonial expansion. Some hospitals, like the London Fever Hospital, became important sources of statistics on disease and mortality.

As they had been by seventeenth-century reformers, hospitals were advocated as only one element in systems of medical provision for the whole population. These model hospitals were intended to have a major role in the improvement of medical knowledge, and were inspired partly by continental European examples (especially in the Netherlands). In the event, no comprehensive formal health care systems were created in Britain in this period, and the hospitals — which began with the Westminster Infirmary in 1720 — were designed to be *charitable* institutions, rather than useful to the state as instruments to improve the nation's health.

Entry to the voluntary hospitals was restricted to 'deserving Objects' (i.e. objects of charity — the term often used for patients) who had managed to bring themselves to the favourable notice of a subscriber. The procedure for admission by subscriber's letter involved close personal contact between rich and poor, with the poor entirely dependent upon the goodwill of the rich. (You may like to reflect on how little, or how much, this resembles the modern system of referral to hospital by GP's letter.)

This procedure was more appropriate for paternalistic relationships within a traditional 'face-to-face' society, than for large urban populations where the different social classes were increasingly divided. Take the 'domestic' note sounded in the following advice, given as late as 1816:

> A lady visitor in an hospital or Asylum, should be to that institution
> what the kind judicious Mistress of a family is to her household,
> — the careful inspector of the economy, the integrity and the
> good moral conduct of the housekeeper and other inferior servants.
> (Quoted in Prochaska, 1980, p. 141)

This quotation illustrates the way in which the voluntary hospitals attempted to display, in a very different context, a set of social relations modelled on the traditional, pre-industrial extended household — that is, the kind of household likely to have included servants and apprentices. The geographical distribution of hospitals was also related to concentrations of middle-class medical practitioners and clergy.

(The maps shown in Figure 3.11 (overleaf) reveal in two stages the dates and places of voluntary hospital foundations in the eighteenth century, alongside population growth and urbanisation.)

● Look carefully at Figure 3.11 and note when and where the hospitals were founded, remembering that the effects of industrialisation belong to the second rather than the first half of the century. What strikes you about the pattern of foundation of hospitals in relation to industrialisation?

■ It is not closely related either to the pace or to the location of industrial change. The foundations began in London and the old corporate or county towns (mentioned in Chapter 2), which, apart from places such as Norwich and York, were located mainly in the South and West of England (Figure 3.11a), with fourteen new hospitals founded between 1720 and 1749. But the rate of opening slackened just when the demands of industrialisation began to increase in the later eighteenth century (Figure 3.11b). Only four new hospitals were founded in the last twenty years of the century, and many areas with rapid population growth remained without a hospital.

(The few hospitals that were founded in industrial centres, such as Manchester (1752) and Birmingham (1779), had huge catchment areas. As in the earlier period, many hospitals were small, even those in industrial towns. The Leeds Infirmary had only 27 beds in 1771; it had reached 128 beds by 1802, for an estimated population of about 200 000 in that part of West Yorkshire.)

(Admission policies varied, but most hospitals tried to *exclude* major categories of those in need, such as young children, pregnant women, *domestic* servants (as opposed to apprentices or journeymen), the incurable or terminally ill, consumptives, epileptics, the mentally ill, and those suffering from infectious diseases, especially sexually transmitted disease. These policies differed little from those of the poor-relief hospitals of the pre-industrial period (Chapter 2). Accident cases might obtain admission without a letter, the main problem for the patient very often being one of reaching the hospital in time.)

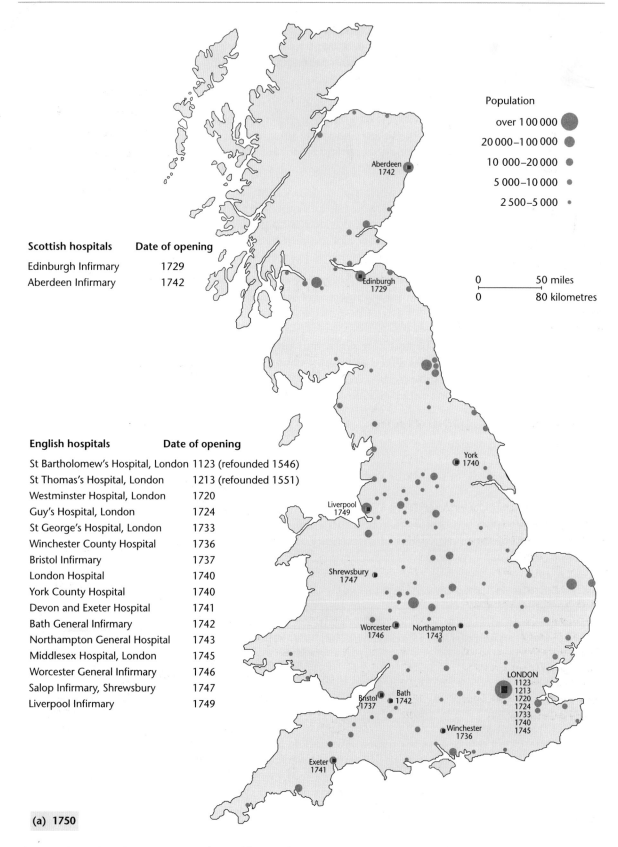

Scottish hospitals   **Date of opening**

Scottish hospitals	Date of opening
Edinburgh Infirmary	1729
Aberdeen Infirmary	1742

English hospitals	Date of opening
St Bartholomew's Hospital, London	1123 (refounded 1546)
St Thomas's Hospital, London	1213 (refounded 1551)
Westminster Hospital, London	1720
Guy's Hospital, London	1724
St George's Hospital, London	1733
Winchester County Hospital	1736
Bristol Infirmary	1737
London Hospital	1740
York County Hospital	1740
Devon and Exeter Hospital	1741
Bath General Infirmary	1742
Northampton General Hospital	1743
Middlesex Hospital, London	1745
Worcester General Infirmary	1746
Salop Infirmary, Shrewsbury	1747
Liverpool Infirmary	1749

(a) 1750

Figure 3.11   *The voluntary hospitals of the eighteenth century in England and Scotland, and towns with 2 500+ inhabitants. (a) Hospitals founded by 1750. (b) New hospitals founded between 1751 and 1801. Note that we are equating population growth with industrialisation. (Population figures from Corfield, P. J., 1982,* The Impact of English

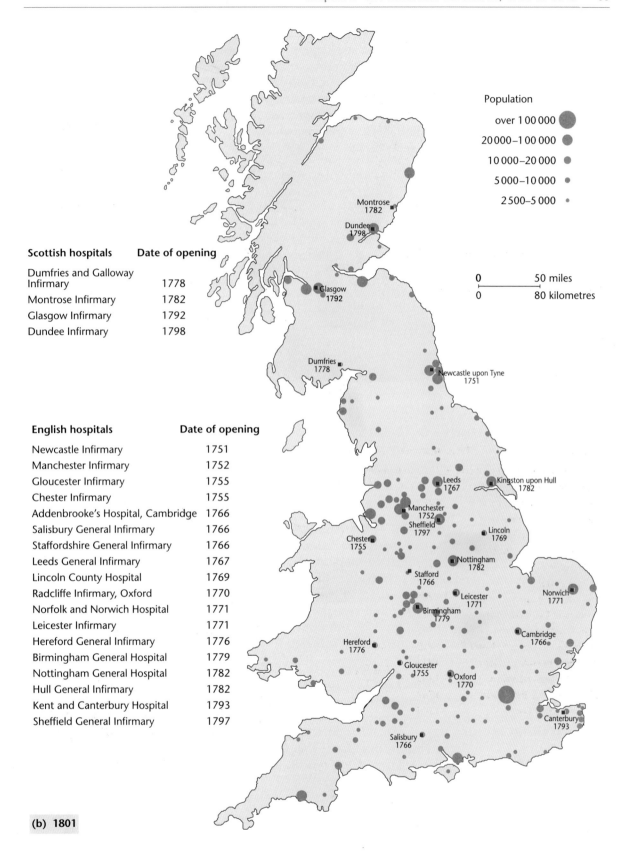

Population

- over 100 000
- 20 000–100 000
- 10 000–20 000
- 5 000–10 000
- 2 500–5 000

Scottish hospitals	Date of opening
Dumfries and Galloway Infirmary	1778
Montrose Infirmary	1782
Glasgow Infirmary	1792
Dundee Infirmary	1798

English hospitals	Date of opening
Newcastle Infirmary	1751
Manchester Infirmary	1752
Gloucester Infirmary	1755
Chester Infirmary	1755
Addenbrooke's Hospital, Cambridge	1766
Salisbury General Infirmary	1766
Staffordshire General Infirmary	1766
Leeds General Infirmary	1767
Lincoln County Hospital	1769
Radcliffe Infirmary, Oxford	1770
Norfolk and Norwich Hospital	1771
Leicester Infirmary	1771
Hereford General Infirmary	1776
Birmingham General Hospital	1779
Nottingham General Hospital	1782
Hull General Infirmary	1782
Kent and Canterbury Hospital	1793
Sheffield General Infirmary	1797

0 ⊢——— 50 miles
0 ⊢——— 80 kilometres

Montrose 1782
Dundee 1798
Glasgow 1792
Dumfries 1778
Newcastle upon Tyne 1751
Leeds 1767
Kingston upon Hull 1782
Manchester 1752
Sheffield 1797
Chester 1755
Lincoln 1769
Nottingham 1782
Stafford 1766
Leicester 1771
Norwich 1771
Birmingham 1779
Cambridge 1766
Hereford 1776
Gloucester 1755
Oxford 1770
Salisbury 1766
Canterbury 1793

(b) 1801

Towns, *Oxford University Press*, Oxford, esp. pp. 13–14; Mitchell, B. R., 1988, British Historical Statistics, *Cambridge University Press*, Cambridge, pp. 25–7; Kyd, J. G. (ed), 1952, Scottish Population Statistics, *Scottish Historical Society*, Edinburgh; data on hospitals, with amendments, from Woodward, J., 1974, To Do the Sick No Harm: A Study of the British Voluntary Hospital System to 1875, *Routledge*, London, Appendix 1)

When hospitals extended their functions, it tended to be with the aim of attracting middle-class interest and support. They therefore diversified into lunatic asylums (Figure 3.12), baths and balneotherapy (therapeutic bathing), 'medical galvanism' (a form of electrotherapy fashionable at the time), and 'pneumatic medicine' (a by-product of the growing scientific interest in gases). Some unmet need was catered for by hospitals which developed departments for large numbers of outpatients. Home visiting, however, was extremely rare, which restricted knowledge among hospital practitioners of the living conditions of poor patients.

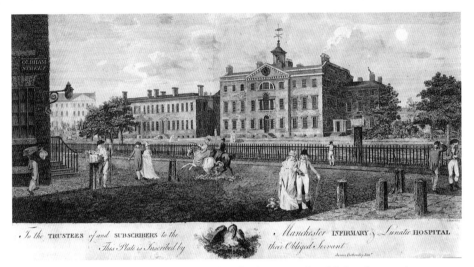

Figure 3.12 *An illustrative plate dedicated to the 'Trustees of and Subscribers to the Manchester Infirmary and Lunatic Hospital', dated 1790. (Source: Archives and Local Studies Unit, Manchester Central Library)*

3.6.2 Dispensaries

The limitations of the hospital system, as to both function and geographical distribution, led to the founding of **dispensaries**. These were more modest institutions than the hospitals, less well known, but in many ways more significant in health care terms. They gave out free medicine and advice to all comers. A few tried to provide food, by prescription. The charitable dispensary as an adjunct of a hospital or medical college had existed since the Renaissance, but the British movement, in which the dispensary was usually an independent institution, effectively began in the 1760s. The following appeal to dispensary subscribers was made in 1816:

> If it be our Duty to guard the Poor from the frequent ill Effects of defective Food and Clothing, of ill ventilated Abodes, or dangerous Callings; as well as our Interest as much as possible to arrest the spread of Infection, which commonly has its rise in the Abodes of Poverty, this Charity imperiously calls for your Support. (Quoted in Marland, 1987, p. 128)

● What does this suggest to you about the aims and concerns of the dispensaries compared to those of the voluntary hospitals?

■ The quotation concentrates on the *living conditions* of the poor, and in particular the problem of infection. The voluntary hospitals generally excluded infectious diseases.

Dispensary staff carried out home visits, and attempted to restrict the spread of infection in poor housing. Like the fever hospitals, some dispensaries tried to deal with changing epidemiological patterns. They had an important role in the measurement of disease, and in medical education. Dispensaries were diverse in character. They were often sectarian (especially Unitarian and Quaker) in inspiration, they found it hard to attract subscriptions, they could be disliked by the subscribing classes because they gave benefits to the poor with no strings attached, and they required a high degree of idealism in their medical staffs.

By the early nineteenth century, a high take-up by the lower classes of the services of the medical charities was coming to be seen, not as *success*, but as a sign of growing *dependency* or *exploitation*. In this altered political climate, 'provident' dispensaries became more popular. These required regular contributions from their beneficiaries, on the insurance principle. Some dispensaries from this period (like that of Newcastle-upon-Tyne) continued to function up to the foundation of the National Health Service, in 1948.

Besides the fever hospitals and the dispensaries, other forms of medical charity evolved to cater for some of the groups excluded by the hospitals. These included *lying-in* charities (for pregnant women), vaccination charities, children's hospitals and dispensaries, and hospitals for the control of prostitution and sexually transmitted disease. The early nineteenth century was a major growth period for small 'specialist' hospitals.

3.6.3 Medical poor relief and the Old Poor Law

The hospitals, although intended for the poor, in no way removed the need for other forms of provision. Under the Old Poor Law, many parishes paid subscriptions to hospitals, dispensaries, and Friendly Societies, as one means of providing for their sick poor. Otherwise, parish overseers continued the range of expedients adopted in the earlier period.

● Can you summarise the principal features of *medical poor relief* under the Old Poor Law (recall Section 2.5.2)?

■ You could have selected five features:
1 one-off payments to a wide range of practitioners, from lay healers, local midwives, and bonesetters, to physicians and surgeons;
2 paying the poor to care for the poor;
3 paying for the poor to be kept in private houses;
4 'buying in bulk' by contracting with practitioners;
5 paying pensions to single-parent families, the infirm elderly, and those disabled for work.

Box 3.2 (overleaf) shows payments made to one family during a particular period of need, illustrating the wide range of specific necessities which could be provided in some cases. Directly provided medical poor relief — as here, to Nathaniel Hudson and his wife Rachel — remained a *minor proportion* of total parish expenditure on the poor, but could be a *major investment* at any given time. Even before 1834, many sick, aged, or lunatic poor were accommodated in *workhouses*, which began to be purpose-built from about 1760, financed by the poor rate. By the early nineteenth century however, the Old Poor Law, 'the largest branch of public administration', had come to be seen as *creating* paupers, rather than relieving them.

Box 3.2	**Extract from an account book of poor relief payments in 1784**	
May 9	John Marshall Wife midwife for Nat. Hudson Do. [Do. = ditto, i.e. Nat. Hudson's wife]	2s 0d
May 16	Rachel Hudson Going to Church after Lying in	9d
	Rachel Hudson shoes	3s 6d
May 30	Itch Salve & Brimstone for Nat. Hudson	7d
July 25	A Godfrey Bottle for Rachel Hudson Child	6d
Aug 15	Natt Hudson to Whitworth Doctor	5s

(Quoted in Marland, 1987, p. 69)

3.6.4 Health care and the New Poor Law

The economic assumptions of the New Poor Law (1834) were deeply flawed; it assumed, for example, that there would always be enough employment to go round, and that it would be well-enough paid, since only the workless paupers 'deserved' financial support. The Law was also not as originally envisaged by the Benthamite reformers who helped to shape it. The compensating *collateral aids* envisaged by Chadwick — for example, the improvement of health by investment in housing — were dropped, and almost no attention was paid to the implications of the new Law for medical poor relief. This had to be defined in further directives in the 1840s.

True to the Benthamite belief in professionalism in the service of the state, the New Poor Law prohibited the employment of unqualified medical practitioners. Each Poor Law Union was to have a contracted, qualified surgeon, who had to supply all drugs as well as attendance, and to whom midwifery cases had also to be referred. This looks like a more powerful role for the professional practitioner – except that the Poor Law surgeon, in addition to being low-paid, was also *subordinate* to the Relieving Officer, a *lay* employee of the Guardians of the Union, who decided on all applications for relief, including medical poor relief.

In *principle*, paupers were to be admitted to a large workhouse organised on 'scientific' principles of classification: instead of the all-in-together approach of the Old Poor Law, women, children, the mentally ill, the sick, were to be catered for separately. In *practice*, many Poor Law Unions avoided building large-scale institutions and coercive segregation, because of the expense. (Look again at Figure 3.4.)

Forms of out-door relief such as pensions continued, especially in the North, where mass *seasonal* lack of employment made the New Poor Law inoperable. In sickness, the poor of the northern industrial areas continued to depend on Friendly Societies or sick clubs, and on the wide range of resources of 'irregular' medicine.

3.6.5 Lunacy

There was one major exception to the continued piecemeal approach of most Poor Law Unions. Institutional provision for the mentally ill and mentally disabled grew relatively rapidly. Under the Old Poor Law, provision for lunatics tended to be the largest single item of expenditure on medical poor relief. As you have seen, the distancing of all classes from these groups had led to the building of lunatic **asylums** in conjunction with the hospitals, as well as to the proliferation of private madhouses.

By the early nineteenth century, lunatic asylums were seen as being as much in need of reform as prisons. Counties were first permitted to build large asylums at public expense in 1808. Efforts to make such provision (and a system of inspection) compulsory finally came about as a result of legislation in 1845. As with other forms of institutional provision, the county asylums did not necessarily appear where need was greatest. Both workhouses and asylums housed an expanding population of poor people perceived as deviant. Both types of institution reflected the Victorian obsession with classification and incarceration, and as a result both became feared by the poor.

The intention of the new system was that the sick poor would benefit from organised access to qualified practitioners, and from purpose-built workhouse infirmaries. In practice, the more formalised — and more professionalised — medical services of the New Poor Law were slow to develop, even to the extent intended. The old 'out-door' practices such as payment of pensions were discouraged, but were not compensated for by enforcement of the new standards. At the same time these services fell under the shadow of the workhouse, which became a thoroughly detested institution (see Figure 3.13).

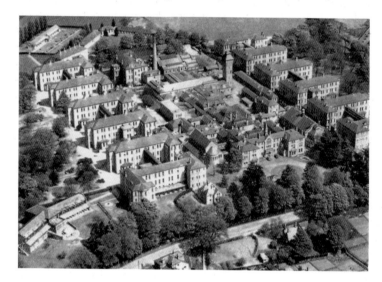

Figure 3.13 *Photograph of one of the many vast Victorian lunatic asylums, situated around the periphery of London. This one, in the North West metropolitan area, housed some three thousand patients, and these numbers persisted well into the life of the NHS. (Source:* The Report of the North West Metropolitan Hospital Board, *1968)*

3.7 Continental Europe: medical police or social medicine?

You have seen how Enlightenment ideas, current in a number of countries, combined with the social and economic factors behind Britain's status as 'first industrial nation' to produce a particular kind of health-care system. What was happening in continental Europe, which (especially in the eighteenth century) had slower rates of industrial and population growth than in Britain?

The period saw a series of confrontations (often in the same country) between two divergent models of health care. State-administered systems — in theory covering all aspects of health care — emerged under rulers who, although politically *absolutist*, harnessed the Enlightenment faith in human reason to promote educational and economic reforms. These hierarchical health-care systems conflicted with more modern notions of health care as a *democratic right*, arising from the post-1789 revolutionary movements. We will look at each system in turn.

3.7.1 Medical police

The aim of the absolutist rulers of the eighteenth century was to boost population numbers and so ensure a fit labour force and plentiful military conscripts. The notion of **medical police** was promoted from 1779 by the physician Johann Peter Frank, to assert state omnicompetence in the medical sphere. This amounted to a cohort of health inspectors with state powers to quarantine, disinfect and cleanse. That Frank was partly educated in France, but had administrative roles in various German-dominated states, is indicative of the widespread European influence of Frank's system of state-administered preventive and curative medicine. For example, a treatise on medical police was published in Edinburgh in 1808. The policing model of public health was to remain influential in Britain: for example with the factory inspectorate from the 1830s, and John Simon's vision in the 1850s of a universal system of Medical Officers of Health (MOHs) with compulsory powers under the criminal law. (We will be looking further at MOHs in Chapter 4.)

A distinctive feature of absolutist states was massive metropolitan hospitals. These were crowded institutions with vast numbers of patients (the General Hospital in Vienna, for example, had an annual turnover of 14 000) and consequent high mortality.

Enlightenment rulers like Joseph II, the Habsburg emperor, pressurised monastic religious orders to adopt a useful *secular* role, to establish hospitals and to provide nursing: indeed, the formally recognised *priest-physician* was an innovative feature of rural health care in Austria and Sweden. The elaborate state-supervised hierarchies of physicians, surgeons, and midwives were intended to eliminate unlicensed practitioners, who were branded as 'quacks'. We find here a strong contrast with Britain, where there was a greater emphasis on medicine as a free trade.

3.7.2 Medicine and revolution

Turning to the second model of health care, the French revolutionary ideals of liberty, equality, and fraternity stimulated movements for the emergence of a unified medical profession, for state control and reform of hospitals, and for the application of science to clinical medicine. An example of an innovation disseminated to the general population in the wake of the French armies was vaccination against smallpox from 1800.

The full working-out of revolutionary ideals for health care — with their inevitable clash of social interests — occurred in the period before 1850. The French Revolution of the 1780s and 1790s enhanced the prestige of the bourgeois medical profession, freed from absolutist regulation. Concepts of *social medicine*[8] were introduced in France in the 1830s and disseminated more widely in Europe, but the notion of health care as a democratic right only emerged in the German medical reform movement during the revolutions of 1848–9. Reacting against state policing systems, revolutionary doctors argued that diseases were caused by political repression, and economic and educational deprivation. In 1847, Salomon Neumann, a poor-law doctor in Berlin, defined health as 'the highest individual right of every person'.

However, the medical revolutionaries clashed over the principle of the public accountability of the medical profession. The radical German pathologist, Rudolf Virchow, resisted demands for a democratically accountable health-care system. Reflecting science's perceived role as a secular faith and source of ethical standards,

[8] The term 'social medicine' has many definitions, which have shifted over time and from place to place. Sometimes this direction in medicine was predicated on the idea that disease was caused by socio-economic factors; at other times, advocates were using various biological explanations of social class and social conditions.

he argued that the doctor's scientific credentials were a basis for professional autonomy, without need of state regulation. He was criticised by other radicals, including Neumann, who responded that doctors should be accountable to workers subscribing funds in democratically organised workers' health-care associations.

● In your view, was the doctor the 'best friend of the poor' in this period, as Virchow claimed in 1848?

■ Doctors helped the poor by showing how social and economic factors (like malnutrition and poor housing) caused the spread of disease, and by arguing the need for education. But doctors were reluctant to allow medical systems to be subjected to democratic controls.

Reviewing Virchow's influential position in the revolutionary medical reform movement, the historian Erwin H. Ackerknecht commented, 'the patient remains silent'. Ackerknecht's verdict leads us to ponder the question: did demands for professional autonomy from state regulation help legitimate a fully medicalised and coercive new form of authority over the patient? If so, what are the implications for patients' rights today?

3.8 British India: the costs of colonialism

Just as rapid and unregulated industrial development posed serious threats to health and labour efficiency in Britain, so too did British overseas expansion present a series of medical problems which threatened the profitability of colonial rule and the lives of both colonisers and colonised.

In India, which was the main focus of European expansion in this period, the London-based *East India Company* (EIC) was rapidly expanding its territorial and commercial interests in the subcontinent (Figure 3.14), bringing it into conflict with Indian princely states and its imperial rivals the French. By the end of the eighteenth century, French influence had been confined to several enclaves in the South, and

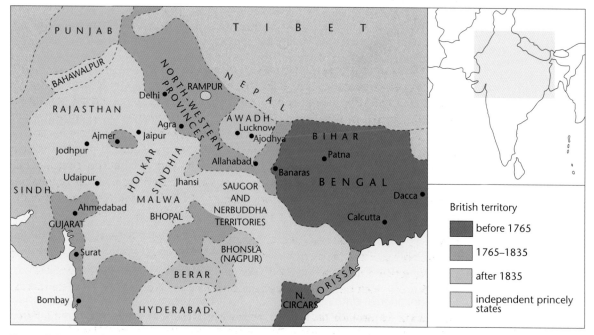

Figure 3.14 *British expansion in Northern India, 1750–1860. (Data from Bayly, C. A., 1988,* Indian Society and the Making of the British Empire, *Cambridge University Press, Cambridge)*

vast areas of India, such as Bengal, had been subordinated to Company rule. The Company's increasing administrative functions swelled the ranks of its bureaucracy, and its army grew to become one of the largest in the world.

Conflicts between the Company and various Indian polities, most notably the Marathas of Western India, caused great disruption and led to the spread of infectious diseases such as smallpox and cholera. Although there had been outbreaks of cholera outside Bengal — where the disease was endemic — these had been relatively isolated and confined to the Eastern and Western seaboards. However, in 1817, during operations against the Marathas and Pindaris (irregular cavalry formerly employed by the Marathas), the disease spread from Bengal to other parts of India and thence to many parts of the world. From 1817, cholera became a relatively common disease throughout the Indian subcontinent, killing millions of indigenous people. Whilst it is impossible to state with certainty the number of deaths from cholera, British figures suggest that on average some 80 000 died from the disease each year.

3.8.1 Medicine and military considerations

From the mid-eighteenth century, war in India placed a severe strain on the EIC's medical services. More surgeons had to be recruited from Britain and from other European countries, and all Company surgeons were required to serve at least two years with the *military* before becoming eligible for the *civil* medical service. In 1763, a permanent Medical Board was established to co-ordinate the civil and military branches of the medical service in Bengal, and similar organisations were set up in Bombay and Madras a few years later.

The conflicts of the mid-eighteenth century also highlighted the need for more hospital assistants and orderlies — posts which were often filled by Indians trained in the rudiments of Western medicine. The EIC increased its recruitment of Indians and organised them into a separate *Military Subordinate Medical Department*. By comparison with those in the 'superior' branch, which offered a serviceable if unremarkable income, these men were poorly paid and often complained bitterly of their position.

Military considerations were also dominant in the growth of institutionalised health care in eighteenth-century India. War against France provided the stimulus for the construction of the Royal Naval Hospital at Madras, and the British conquest of Bengal resulted in a hospital in Calcutta. In Bombay, by 1784, there were three large hospitals — two for British and one for Indian troops — whereas there had been only one before 1750. The need for such institutions was acutely felt, since mortality among British troops in India continued to be high throughout the eighteenth and nineteenth centuries.

● Look at Figure 3.15. In what ways might the conditions depicted in this barrack room be thought conducive to the spread of disease and the poor health of soldiers in India?

■ Ventilation is clearly a problem, as the rows of *punkahs* (fans) operated by a servant testify, despite the open windows. Sleeping, washing and recreation are all conducted in this confined area, with beds crowded close together.

Dragoon guards stationed in Britain, for example, suffered an average annual mortality of 14 per 1 000 in 1830–6, while British troops in the Bombay area suffered an annual mortality of over 47 per 1 000 between 1830 and 1849. The high mortality

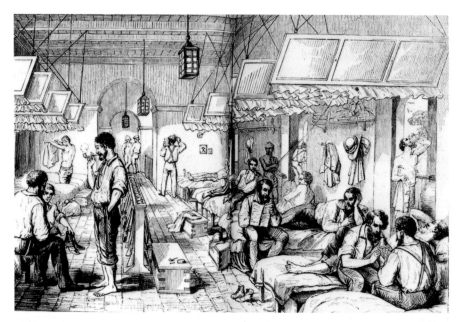

Figure 3.15 *From Florence Nightingale* Observations on the Sanitary Conditions of the British Army in India, *1863. (Source: British Library, London)*

among British soldiers in India at this time was partly a consequence of the spread of cholera throughout India following the British military conquests of the eighteenth and early nineteenth centuries, mentioned earlier. Anxieties about health, and the lower social prestige of the Indian medical/military services, deterred many Britons from seeking a career in India.

3.8.2 Medical practice in India

The EIC's increasing administrative commitments at the end of the eighteenth century presented both medical opportunities and medical problems. Company surgeons were quick to exploit the growing market for health care and many lucrative private practices were established in the three largest cities: Bombay, Madras, and Calcutta. As early as 1752, there were complaints in Madras that hospital surgeons paid more attention to their private practices than to their hospital patients.

However, as in Britain, *self*-treatment remained an important component of colonial health care until well into the nineteenth century. 'Self-help' manuals for Europeans were popular in India until the 1880s, some years after their appeal had waned in Britain. In the eighteenth century, and early years of the nineteenth century, it was not uncommon for these to be modelled on indigenous customs such as the avoidance of meat, alcohol and undue exercise. Translations of indigenous medical texts, by William Jones and other 'orientalist' scholars, had also enhanced European knowledge of Indian pharmacology.

3.8.3 The health of Indians

By comparison with the health care lavished on European civilians and troops, provisions for the indigenous population outside the armed forces remained meagre throughout this period. This apparent lack of concern with the health of Indians provides a point of contrast with the increasing interest taken in the 'political arithmetic' of health in Britain. There were, however, some notable exceptions. At the beginning of the nineteenth century, an 'Infirmary and Native Poor Asylum' was opened in Madras, under the auspices of a charitable fund raised by *subscription* among Europeans and wealthy Indians.

The EIC also played a role in institutional health care. In Bombay, for example, a 'native hospital' partly funded by the Company opened in 1809, and a dispensary some years later. By the middle of the nineteenth century, Indian gentlemen, like the Parsi philanthropist Sir Jamsetji Jejeebhai, were taking an active interest in Western medical care and funding the building of hospitals for the use of Indians. Charitable donations also supported the growth of the dispensary movement in India from the late 1830s — a movement that was to grow considerably in the second half of the nineteenth century, aided by the injection of funds from provincial governments and municipalities.

However, it is not easy to assess the level of demand for such institutions among Indians. The historian David Arnold has shown that considerable suspicion of hospitals remained into the late nineteenth century (Arnold, 1993). They were unable to escape their association with an alien and often oppressive regime, and the very concept of hospital treatment was foreign to the majority of Indians who were traditionally treated at home. But the dispensaries, or at least their out-patient clinics, proved far more popular, and became one of the principal outlets through which indigenous Indians encountered Western health care in the later nineteenth and twentieth centuries. Yet Indian women, bound by the Indian custom of *purdah* (the seclusion of women), continued to be ill-served by these dispensaries, which were only rarely supplied with female medical personnel.

3.8.4 Public health in India

The early nineteenth century also brought the first moves in the direction of public health in India. For the most part, sanitary reforms such as those begun in British cities from the 1830s were confined to military cantonments and to the European quarters of Indian cities. The vast majority of Indians remained untouched by these reforms until the twentieth century.

Vaccination against smallpox was the only exception to this rule. This began in India in 1802 and was performed on Indians at a relatively early stage. Like hospital provision, the vaccination of Indians was supposed to be read as a sign of the EIC's good intentions and of Western cultural superiority. Perhaps more important, however, was the concern with *economic efficiency*, which, as you will recall from earlier in this chapter, was a guiding principle of sanitary reform as espoused by Chadwick and other Benthamite reformers in Britain.

The extension of vaccination to rural areas of India in the 1820s and 1830s, similarly, occurred amidst reforms of India's administration, and was promoted by Benthamite administrators like Lord Elphinstone, Governor-General of Bombay. However, most of these vaccination programmes failed to meet their objectives. This was due to lack of financial support, and to resistance from the indigenous population, which had developed its own system of inoculation and which, in many cases, regarded arm-to-arm vaccination as ritually polluting, because people from whom the vaccine was transferred were usually Untouchables or low-caste Indians. It was not until the late nineteenth century that vaccination programmes began to reach substantial numbers of Indians — at about the same time as the anti-vaccination lobby was gaining ground in Britain (Figure 3.16).

3.8.5 Tropical hygiene

The other principal development in public health in nineteenth-century India was the changing nature and content of *tropical hygiene*. As a consequence of European political domination, reflected in the growing social distance of Europeans, Indian

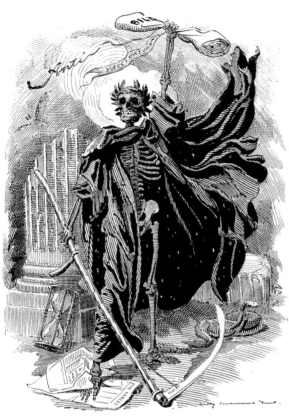

TRIUMPH OF DE-JENNER-ATION.
[The Bill for the encouragement of Small Pox was passed.]

Figure 3.16 *This* Punch *cartoon of 30 July 1898 refers to the passing of a 'Bill for the encouragement of Small Pox' — an Act of Parliament allowing parents in Britain to state their 'conscientious objections' as a valid reason for not having their children vaccinated. This prompted correspondents in India to write to medical journals at home inviting the objectors to come and see the effects of smallpox in the population there. (Source:* Punch, *July 1898)*

people, their dwellings, and their lifestyle, came to be viewed increasingly as 'reservoirs of dirt and disease'. Whereas Indians had once been consulted and, to some extent, emulated in order to facilitate European acclimatisation to the tropics, Indian culture and the Indian people came to be seen as part of the sanitary *problem* confronting Europeans. Increasingly, European medical texts began to recommend the separation of British from Indian settlements, and to view Indians as physically as well as culturally different. Only the 'martial races' of northern India, whose military traditions and physical stature endeared them to the British, continued to be viewed in a favourable light.

●   What similarities do you find between colonial attitudes towards the health of Indians, and the attitude of Benthamite reformers towards the health of the working class in Britain?

■   The 'fever nests' in working-class districts of Britain were viewed as threats to the health of the middle classes in the same way as Indian dwellings were to Europeans; the health of both groups was considered in terms of maintaining economic efficiency rather than as a moral responsibility.

This trend was accompanied by an increasing pessimism about the possibility of European acclimatisation to the tropical environment. In the eighteenth century, many doctors in India and the West Indies believed that, over time, and through the adoption of certain indigenous customs, they would become fully adapted to tropical climates. Some even believed they would acquire the physical characteristics of native peoples. But, in the nineteenth century, with the growing social separation of colonisers and colonised, such views became extremely rare.

The Company surgeon, James Johnson, writing in 1812, maintained that Europeans in India tended to 'droop', and, before long, to seek refuge in their native climate. The offspring of those who remained in India, he believed, would 'gradually degenerate', morally and physically (Johnson, 1812, p. 3). Johnson urged that much could still be done to make the existence of Europeans in India more comfortable but, in later texts, a more fatalistic attitude prevails, and is reflected in the growing interest in *medical topography* — the attempt to locate microclimates most suitable to Europeans.

This concern with medical topography led to two parallel developments: the gathering of medical and meteorological statistics from British military cantonments and towns from the 1830s, and the increasing resort to sanatoria and hill stations with more salubrious climates. At the same time, it became fashionable to send children back to Britain for their schooling. Ironically, with British influence approaching its zenith in India, Europeans had come to regard themselves as exotics, prone to wilt on foreign soil.

It was not until after 1858, with the assumption of government by the British Crown, and in the wake of the Indian Mutiny, that the British administration began to intervene more directly in public health in India, and then largely out of concern for the health of British troops. With the exception of smallpox vaccination and the establishment of a few charitable institutions in the larger cities, the EIC showed little concern for the health of the indigenous civilian population. Health-care provisions clearly reflected colonial, and especially military, priorities and, in the early nineteenth century, the increasing pessimism about European acclimatisation to the tropics. But, although belief in the possibility of bodily adaptation to tropical climates declined considerably in the years after 1830, the potential for transforming the tropical environment remained, and infused the rhetoric of the so-called pioneers of tropical medicine considered in Chapter 4.

OBJECTIVES FOR CHAPTER 3

When you have studied this chapter, you should be able to:

3.1 Define and use, or recognise definitions and applications of, each of the terms printed in **bold** in the text.

3.2 Identify the principal social and economic factors affecting health in Britain during the Industrial Revolution, where necessary relating the content of this chapter to relevant material in *World Health and Disease*, Chapters 5 and 6.

3.3 Indicate ways in which lay care and self-help changed — and did not change — in Britain in this period, as a result of industrialisation, urbanisation and Enlightenment ideas.

3.4 Comment on the degree to which different kinds of medical practitioner in Britain might have gained (or lost) by the growing professionalisation of medicine, associated with the trend towards formal qualifications.

3.5 Explain why pre-industrial mechanisms of public health were inadequate to deal with threats to the environment associated with industrialisation; and describe the ways in which the sanitarian movement addressed these threats.

3.6 Give examples that show how health-care systems in Britain and continental Europe in this period were influenced by attitudes towards the poor, including attitudes derived from religious belief.

3.7 Describe the origins of British medical intervention in India and explain its limitations.

QUESTIONS FOR CHAPTER 3

1   (*Objective 3.2*)

Here is Samuel Johnson again, in 1776, defending his birthplace, the cathedral city of Lichfield, against charges of idleness:

> We are a City of Philosophers: we work with our Heads, and make the Boobies of Birmingham work for us with their Hands... (Quoted in Corfield, 1989, p. 94)

This is a piece of evidence given to the Commission of 1842 enquiring into children's employment in mines:

> Mr Holroyd, solicitor, and Mr Brook, surgeon, practising in Stainland, were present, who confessed that, although living within a few miles, they could not have believed that such a system of unchristian cruelty could have existed. (Quoted in Thompson, 1975, p. 377)

What do these very different statements have in common? And what can they tell us about social conditions during industrialisation?

2   (*Objective 3.3*)

A local historian wrote in 1898 of the spa baths at Lockwood, near Huddersfield, created in the 1820s:

> The existence of mineral springs had suggested to the speculative mind dreams of an English Baden [Baden-Baden, in Germany, one of the most fashionable spas in Europe in the nineteenth century], or at least of another Harrogate [the spa resort in Yorkshire]. The river was spanned with a rustic bridge, grounds were laid, and a Bath Hotel opened its doors. (Quoted in Marland, 1987, p. 232)

The new baths were on the site of an old sulphur well. What points does the quotation illustrate about the connections between urbanisation and the search for health in this period?

3   (*Objective 3.4*)

A 'letter to the editor' written in 1827 and signed 'General Practitioner' read in part:

> I am not factious or querulous, but I fearlessly maintain, that the promised rights, which I naturally expected, as a member of the College and Hall, have no existence, and that those who have never been educated have had as many advantages, and much more, than those who qualified and received diplomas in surgery and pharmacy. As the profession is now constituted a man cannot select a worse mode of life than that of a general practitioner. (Quoted in Loudon, 1986, p. 181)

What kind of practitioner was this 'General Practitioner', and what grounds were there for his complaint?

4   (*Objectives 3.5 and 3.6*)

In 1839, Dr Southwood Smith reported as follows to the Poor Law Commissioners, who were looking for ways of reducing the 'rate-burden' arising from disease and destitution:

> While systematic efforts on a large scale have been made to widen the streets, to remove obstructions to the circulation...of air, to extend and perfect the drainage and sewerage, and to prevent the accumulation of putrefying vegetable and animal substances in the places in which the wealthier classes reside, nothing whatever has been done to improve the condition of the districts inhabited by the poor. These neglected places are out of view, and are not thought of...Yet in these pestilential places the industrious poor are obliged to take up their abode; they have no choice; they must live in what houses they can get nearest the places where they find employment. By no prudence or forethought on their part can they avoid the dreadful evils of this class to which they are thus exposed. (Quoted in Simon, 1897, p. 183)

What does this suggest about the obstacles to improving the living conditions of the poor?

5   (*Objective 3.6*)

What follows is part of a reply to objections made in the 1730s to the plan to found Winchester County Hospital — which, you may recall (see Figure 3.11) was the first English voluntary hospital outside London:

> It was objected that the poor dislike anything with the appearance of constraint or removal from their families. But any who desire it shall be considered and received as outpatients. Experience tells that whenever a hospital has been erected the poor have esteemed it a blessing and have flocked to it with eagerness; for there they get free air, wholesome and proper diet, clean and constant attendance, the best advice, and no more medicines than are necessary. (Quoted in Woodward, 1974, p. 13)

What does this suggest to you about the functions of the voluntary hospitals — and the attitudes and circumstances of their patients?

6   (*Objective 3.7*)

The following are extracts from the *Medical Topography of Calcutta*, written by the East India Company surgeon James Ranald Martin, and published in 1837.

> The Bengallee, unlike the Hindu of the North, is utterly devoid of pride, national and individual. His moral character is a matter of history...when we are looking forward with such well-founded hope to the improved results of European knowledge and example diffused among the natives....The natives have yet to learn that the sweet sensations connected with cleanly habits, and pure air, are some of the most precious gifts of civilization. (Martin, 1837, pp. 45, 24)

In what ways do these extracts illustrate the changes that were taking place in colonial medicine in India in the early nineteenth century?

CHAPTER 4

The era of public health, 1848 to 1918

4.1 From sanitarianism to personal responsibility 98

4.1.1 Darwinism and human society 98

4.1.2 Sanitarianism — success and failure 99

4.1.3 Imperialism and national deterioration 100

4.2 The erosion of lay care and lay control 101

4.2.1 Commercial growth 102

4.2.2 Lay care stretched beyond its limits 102

4.2.3 Institutionalisation and lay control 104

4.2.4 Inefficient mothers? 105

4.2.5 Lady visitors 106

4.3 Sanitarianism in action 106

4.3.1 The successes of propaganda 108

4.3.2 Medical Officers of Health 109

4.3.3 'Scientific' sanitarianism 110

4.3.4 The complex role of bacteriology 111

4.4 Different routes to professionalisation 112

4.4.1 Nursing: religion, gender and social class 112

4.4.2 Midwives: marginalisation to rehabilitation 116

4.4.3 The Medical Register: definition not prohibition 116

4.4.4 Changing definitions? Some challenges to the medical hierarchy 117

4.4.5 Medical power versus lay control 118

4.5 Institutions, insurances and the national interest 119

4.5.1 Asylums and hospitals 119

4.5.2 Financing health care 121

4.5.3 Impact of World War I 124

4.5.4 Mortality and medical progress 124

4.6 Medicine and imperialism: the 'scramble for Africa' 125

4.6.1 Tropical medicine 126

4.6.2 'The sick continent' 128

4.6.3 Missionary zeal 129

Objectives for Chapter 4 130

Questions for Chapter 4 131

Study notes for OU students

This chapter assumes a familiarity with the theory of evolution by natural selection (*World Health and Disease*, Open University Press, third edition 2001, Chapter 5, and *Human Biology and Health: an Evolutionary Approach*, Open University Press, third edition 2001, Chapter 3). It also refers to the 'bacteriological revolution' in the later part of the nineteenth century, when it was conclusively demonstrated that infectious diseases were caused by micro-organisms (*Medical Knowledge: Doubt and Certainty*, Open University Press, second edition 1994; colour-enhanced second edition 2001, Chapters 3 and 4). In this chapter, these developments in theoretical and practical biology are related to the social and political developments they helped to fuel.

Reference is also made to two articles in *Health and Disease: A Reader* (Open University Press, second edition 1995; third edition 2001) by Thomas McKeown and by Simon Szreter, which you read during *World Health and Disease*, Chapter 6. In Section 4.5.2 of this chapter, you will read an article in the Reader (second and third editions), by the historian Rosemary Stevens, entitled 'The evolution of health-care systems in the United States and the United Kingdom: similarities and differences'.

4.1 From sanitarianism to personal responsibility

The failed liberal revolutions of the 1840s in Western Europe were followed by decades of pragmatic politics, economic expansion and competition, the consolidation of nation states and, at the turn of the century, imperialism and World War I. Historians are increasingly finding links between major economic and social changes in this period, and rapidly developing areas of the human sciences, in particular evolutionary biology, sociology, anthropology and genetics. Here is the prominent sanitarian, William Farr, addressing the Statistical Society of London in 1872:

> Politics is no longer the art of Letting things alone, nor the game of audacious Revolution for the sake of change; so politics, like war, has to submit to the spirit of the age, and to call in the aid of science: for the art of government can only be practised with success when it is grounded on a knowledge of the people governed, derived from exact observation. (Quoted by Eyler, 1979, p. 28)

Major shifts in social policy, like sanitarianism, made overt reference to biological principles as applied to human populations — the effects on health and behaviour of crowding, for example. The interdependence of science and industrialisation was rationalised by the French philosopher Auguste Comte, in whose positivist account of human progress the most advanced stage was marked by the rise of the secular science of *sociology* and by successful *social engineering* based on scientific laws.[1]

4.1.1 Darwinism and human society

This inherently optimistic outlook was countered by more pessimistic trends as capitalism failed to ensure benefits for all. The principle, as put forward by Charles Darwin and Alfred Russel Wallace, of *evolution by natural selection* — the so-called 'survival of the fittest' — was in part a further development of *Malthusianism*,[2] and fostered continued adherence to economic individualism later in the nineteenth century. Unfettered competition, it seemed, was a 'law of nature', and not to be interfered with.

Natural selection, which depended upon another of Darwin's assumptions — the surplus production of offspring — encouraged speculation about 'fitness to survive' among human populations. Darwinism was readily deployed to discredit state intervention in the field of social welfare, to oppose feminism, and to defend imperialism and the subordination of 'inferior' races. So-called **social Darwinism**, reinforced by the new 'science' of **eugenics** (the devising of policies to improve the genetic quality of the human race, especially by selective breeding), provided a framework for exaggerated fears, contrasting the declining fertility of the middle classes with high fertility among 'degraded groups' in large industrial towns. This represented the dominant social philosophy among the Darwinists, but it was not the only legitimate construction. For instance, Wallace, co-founder of the theory of natural selection, supported socialism and women's rights. 'Neo-Malthusian' advocates of contraception, and social reformers, also looked to biology to reinforce their arguments.

---

[1] A discussion of positivism and the foundation of sociology can be found in *Studying Health and Disease* (Open University Press, 2nd edn 1994; colour-enhanced 2nd edn 2001), Chapter 2.

[2] The theories of Thomas Malthus (1766–1834) on the 'checks and balances' on population growth are discussed in *World Health and Disease* (Open University Press, 3rd edn 2001), Chapter 5.

4.1.2 Sanitarianism — success and failure

Sanitarianism instilled the conviction that epidemic disease acted indiscriminately, and did not in fact remove only the supposedly 'unfit'. Sanitary reform delivered considerable benefits in the course of this period, particularly with respect to water supply, sewage removal, and food production. Nonetheless, implementation was slow; the problem of inadequate housing was particularly intractable; and many reformers were disappointed to find, around the turn of the twentieth century, that some mortality rates remained obstinately high. This applied especially to infant mortality, and crude mortality rates in areas of high population density (as Figure 3.2 illustrated earlier).

● Can you think of one reason why both rates remained high?

■ The two were in fact related, in that an increasing proportion of most populations was urbanised — a higher proportion of babies was being born in poor conditions in densely populated areas.

Even now, there are difficulties in accounting for mortality trends in this period, since it appears that first adult and then infant mortality declined in most Western European countries at about the same time. A similar secular decline in fertility can also be detected.[3] Nonetheless, whatever the influences on overall rates, observers of the time were correct in discerning wide differentials of mortality between town and country, and between different social groups (see Figure 4.1).

TABLE XVIII.—**Deaths in 30 Large Town Districts** in the 10 Years 1851-60 ; and also the DEATHS which would have occurred in the 10 Years if the MORTALITY had been at the same Rate as prevailed in the 63 HEALTHY DISTRICTS (1849–53).

AGES.	DEATHS in 10 Years 1851-60.	DEATHS which would have occurred in the 10 Years at HEALTHY DISTRICT RATES.	EXCESS of ACTUAL DEATHS in 10 Years over DEATHS at HEALTHY DISTRICT RATES.
ALL AGES -	711,944	384,590	327,354
0— - -	338,990	135,470	203,520
5— - -	31,319	19,290	12,029
10— - -	14,240	11,020	3,220
15— - -	43,807	37,550	6,257
25— - -	48,625	36,150	12,475
35— - -	50,071	30,320	19,751
45— - -	49,638	26,680	22,958
55— - -	49,763	27,020	22,743
65— - -	47,445	31,510	15,935
75— - -	30,583	22,920	7,663
85 & upwards -	7,463	6,660	803

Figure 4.1 *This table, reproduced from William Farr's official report of 1865, illustrates the development of a standard of comparison for healthiness in terms of the rates of the so-called 'healthy districts'. Note also that Farr has corrected for differences in the age-structure of different localities (compare this with Table 3.1). (Source:* Supplement to the 25th Annual Report of the Registrar-General, *1865, p. xxvi)*

[3] Trends in birth and death rates in England during this period are described in detail in *World Health and Disease* (Open University Press, 3rd edn 2001), Chapter 6, which also examines the contribution of the decline in infectious diseases to these trends.

4.1.3 Imperialism and national deterioration

Towards the end of the nineteenth century, the balance of economic power was shifting away from Britain and towards Germany and the USA. Fears of economic decline at home, and loss of empire abroad, were sharpened by revelations of the physical state of the nation's manpower. Industrial supremacy required a fit labour force, and controlling the empire, an effective standing army: yet the examination of Boer War recruits, reinforced by many other surveys, produced a devastating picture of physical inadequacy (see Figure 4.2).

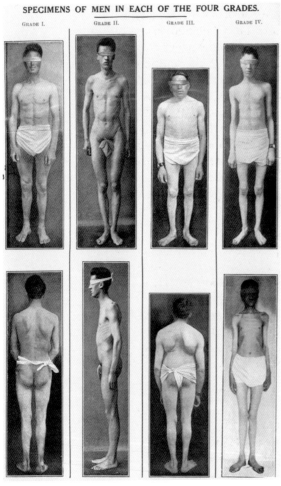

SPECIMENS OF MEN IN EACH OF THE FOUR GRADES.

GRADE I.   GRADE II.   GRADE III.   GRADE IV.

Figure 4.2 *Army recruits in World War I. These photographs underline the physical defects and class disparities in health that were revealed by the World War and previously by the Boer War. (Source: Ministry of National Service, 1919,* Report upon the Physical Examination of Men of Military Age by National Service Medical Boards from 1st November 1917 to 31st October 1918, *HMSO, London, Cmd 504)*

The evidence of these reports was discussed against the background of a changing climate of opinion about the causes of ill-health. Environmental solutions had been downgraded by the *bacteriological revolution,* and the establishment of the *germ theory of disease*[4] led to what the American historian Paul Starr has called a 'new concept of dirt' (Starr, 1982). Increasingly the focus was not the broad vision of nineteenth-century public health, but responsibility for health at the *individual* level, and especially at the level of individual *mothers.* A conviction that maternal inefficiency was a serious factor affecting working-class health prompted an armoury of devices aimed at delivering advice to mothers — although there was some realisation, as you will see, that 'efficiency' was severely constrained by housing conditions.

Even John Simon, whose crucial role in mid-nineteenth-century public health will be highlighted later in the chapter, could in later life share in the trend towards personal responsibility:

> Especially it would seem reasonable to connect the principle of Compulsory Insurance with the principle of Free Education; for surely, if the State is to provide gratuitous education for the masses of the people, it may reasonably require, as first-fruits from the receivers of such education, that they shall, as far as practicable, secure themselves against future pauperism, and thus guarantee the community against further costs on their behalf. (Simon, 1897, p. 462)

But services also expanded under the control of local authorities. In the first decade of the twentieth century a modest start was made, with child welfare and ante-natal clinics, the provision of school meals, and school medical inspection.

---

[4] Discussed in *Medical Knowledge: Doubt and Certainty* (Open University Press, 2nd edn 1994; colour-enhanced 2nd edn 2001), Chapters 3 and 4.

The national system of measures directed at mothers and children was part of a more general system of welfare benefits established under the threat of *national deterioration.* Legislation was passed for old age pensions in 1907, and National Health Insurance in 1911. This embryo *welfare state* was established not just out of humanitarianism, but through a desire to develop *national efficiency.* The sociologist Lesley Doyal has called the reforms an 'important element in the attempt to restructure British capitalism' (Doyal and Pennell, 1979, p. 160).

At another level, too, the focus was on individual responsibility. The downturn in infectious epidemic disease at the end of the century brought a shift in patterns of mortality and morbidity towards chronic diseases such as cancer, heart disease, and tuberculosis (TB). Alcoholism, sexually transmitted diseases (referred to as venereal diseases, VD, in this period), and mental 'deficiency' were perceived as major problems because of the threat of national deterioration through transmission and inheritance of these disorders of 'degeneration'. These 'diseases' were viewed within an individualistic, moralising framework. Concern about VD peaked during World War I and led to the establishment of venereal disease clinics, but not to other preventive measures. The wider impact of that war on health and health-care practice remains uncertain. Expectations were aroused that World War I would be followed by the creation of a national system of health services. The actual response fell far short of this goal.

4.2   The erosion of lay care and lay control

The legal boundaries between qualified and unqualified practice became clearer in this period, and some women carers began to be included in the professional hierarchy. On the ground, however, the informal sector remained strong, stretching from the paupers who continued to serve as nurses in workhouses, to the practitioners of homoeopathy and other 'alternative' systems who were increasingly presenting themselves as part of the formal sector. Examples such as the following show the persistence of the lay carer who was sanctioned by the community and paid in kind, rather than cash.

> **Praise of Sally Dunkirk, a lay practitioner from Slaithwaite, Yorkshire, around 1860**
>
> Any bad case of fever, or lunacy, of exceptional emergency, was a call for Sally's services. In such cases she became general, and house maid, doctor and nurse, friend and physician all in one ... A most useful woman was she for the times in which she lived ... If her treatment failed to restore the patient to normal health it was a case forthwith to be sent to a lunatic asylum. Her fees were never much more than a liberal supply of home-brewed beer, unrestricted stock of good 'bacca', and the indispensable long clay pipe, with a good 'table', and implicit obedience to her orders. (Quoted in Marland, 1987, p. 219)

4.2.1 Commercial growth

Lay care was also construed to be a matter of self-care and self-medication. Although earlier traditions of self-medication remained strong, a *commercial* tendency became increasingly apparent. A fall in the price of drugs was part of a general decline in the cost of raw materials in the 1870s and was accompanied by a rise in the real value of wages. The increased sale of patent medicines was a demonstration of greater prosperity among certain sectors of the working class (see Figure 4.3).

Newspaper advertising expanded; the advertising expenditure of pharmaceutical entrepreneurs like Thomas Holloway (see Figure 4.4) and Thomas Beecham reached unprecedented heights (Holloway's jumped from £5 000 a year in 1842 to £50 000 in 1883). Beecham promoted his Patent Liver Pills with the motto 'Worth a guinea a box', which became a famous catch-phrase for the best part of a century. Several of the leading proprietors and sellers of patent medicines, like Beecham himself, a herbalist, and Jesse Boot, who was expanding his chain of cash chemists in Nottingham in the 1870s, had strong connections with the earlier traditions of folk medicine and medical botany.

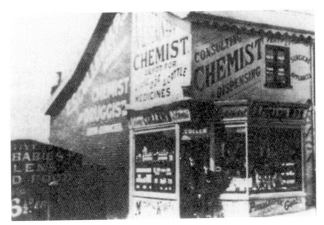

Figure 4.3 *Cullen's Drug Store, Norfolk, 1890s. The services and products offered include: 'Trusses [for rupture] a speciality'; photographic goods; teeth extraction; 'veterinary chemist'. (Source: Royal Pharmaceutical Society of Great Britain)*

Figure 4.4 *Royal Holloway College, opened in 1886 as a women's college of the University of London: modelled on a French château, and endowed by Thomas Holloway out of the proceeds of his patent medicine empire. (Source: Royal Holloway and Bedford New College, University of London)*

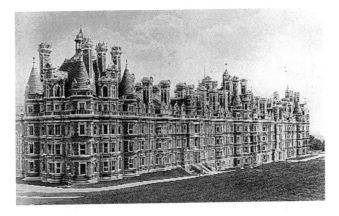

There were many abuses of patent medicine sale and advertisement (see Figure 4.5). Wild claims for efficacy were made, and leading public figures quoted as endorsing products they had probably never heard of. Pharmaceutical composition of remedies was variable. These abuses were attacked in a campaign promoted by the medical and pharmaceutical professions at the turn of the twentieth century.

4.2.2 Lay care stretched beyond its limits

In other respects, self-help systems were giving way under the strain. The Friendly Societies came under economic pressure from the effects both of 'unhealthy trades' and the changing demographic regime in which adults lived longer, but were not necessarily in better health (Figure 4.6). Lay care for the chronically sick was also affected by the absorption of married women into paid work.

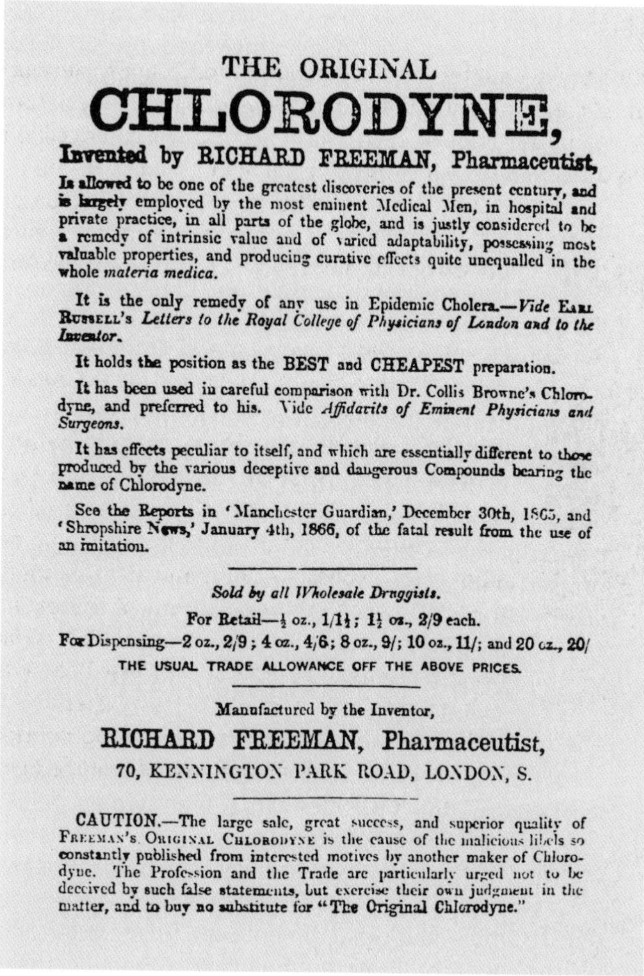

THE ORIGINAL
CHLORODYNE,
Invented by RICHARD FREEMAN, Pharmaceutist,
Is allowed to be one of the greatest discoveries of the present century, and is largely employed by the most eminent Medical Men, in hospital and private practice, in all parts of the globe, and is justly considered to be a remedy of intrinsic value and of varied adaptability, possessing most valuable properties, and producing curative effects quite unequalled in the whole materia medica.
It is the only remedy of any use in Epidemic Cholera.—Vide Earl Russell's Letters to the Royal College of Physicians of London and to the Inventor.
It holds the position as the BEST and CHEAPEST preparation.
It has been used in careful comparison with Dr. Collis Browne's Chlorodyne, and preferred to his. Vide Affidavits of Eminent Physicians and Surgeons.
It has effects peculiar to itself, and which are essentially different to those produced by the various deceptive and dangerous Compounds bearing the name of Chlorodyne.
See the Reports in 'Manchester Guardian,' December 30th, 1865, and 'Shropshire News,' January 4th, 1866, of the fatal result from the use of an imitation.
Sold by all Wholesale Druggists.
For Retail—½ oz., 1/1½; 1½ oz., 2/9 each.
For Dispensing—2 oz., 2/9; 4 oz., 4/6; 8 oz., 9/; 10 oz., 11/; and 20 oz., 20/
THE USUAL TRADE ALLOWANCE OFF THE ABOVE PRICES.
Manufactured by the Inventor,
RICHARD FREEMAN, Pharmaceutist,
70, KENNINGTON PARK ROAD, LONDON, S.
CAUTION.—The large sale, great success, and superior quality of Freeman's Original Chlorodyne is the cause of the malicious libels so constantly published from interested motives by another maker of Chlorodyne. The Profession and the Trade are particularly urged not to be deceived by such false statements, but exercise their own judgment in the matter, and to buy no substitute for "The Original Chlorodyne."

Figure 4.5 *Chlorodyne advertising, c. 1870. Rival inventors and distributors of chlorodyne (an opium-based patent medicine used in the treatment of diarrhoea and other ailments) attacked each other's products. This advertisement for Freeman's chlorodyne attacks Dr Collis Browne's remedy. (Source: Royal Pharmaceutical Society of Great Britain)*

INDEPENDENT ORDER
OF ODDFELLOWS
MANCHESTER UNITY
FRIENDLY SOCIETY
This is to Certify

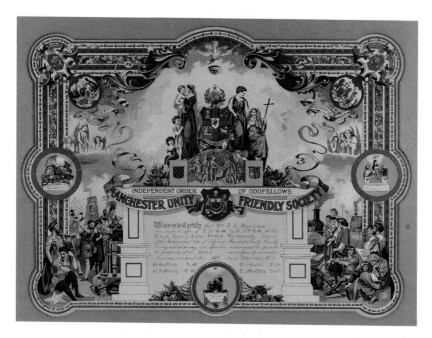

Figure 4.6 *This certificate was presented by the Manchester Unity Friendly Society to commemorate the services of members who acted as unpaid officers of its local Lodges. Nineteenth-century confidence in 'mutualism' and social progress is evident as the eye of God surveys the civilising work of engineers, artists, farmers, scientists, mathematicians, and the harmonious family of nations as well as individuals. But by the turn of the twentieth century, the drain on mutual funds to support members and their families in sickness, unemployment and retirement was becoming unsustainable. (Source: courtesy of the family of Thomas Leonard Harrison)*

The position of the elderly population had always been difficult, and was worsened by their longer survival. For all but a few groups (for example, army officers) there was no 'retirement age', and no age-related entitlement, for example to charity or poor relief, until state pensions were introduced in 1907.

Middle-class expectations of the poor were based partly on a hardening attitude to the division of responsibility between the family and the state, and partly on Victorian family ideals relevant only to the more prosperous. Poor households were unable to 'extend' to provide carers for older relatives, and even co-residence with relatives did not mean that the needs of the infirm elderly could be met. This became evident when, during the depression of the 1870s, strenuous attempts were made to force the care of parents on to their children, to avoid paying pensions from the poor rate. The end result of greater stringency was to increase the proportion of elderly people in the workhouses (see Figure 4.7).

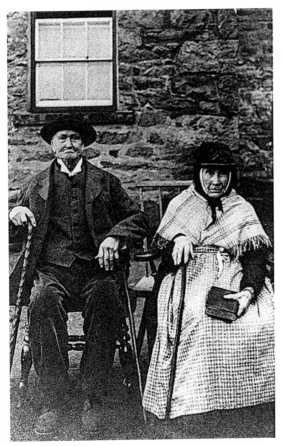

Figure 4.7 *Roland and Betsy Jones of Hen Hafod, Merioneth, in 1870. This self-respecting couple are known only by a Welsh inscription on the back of the original photograph: 'They entered the workhouse at Bala, but instead of separating them the Guardians permitted them to have a room to themselves'. (Source: Gwynedd Archives Service)*

4.2.3 Institutionalisation and lay control

The rate of institutionalisation also increased for the steeply rising numbers classified as mentally handicapped or insane. That medical men rather than laymen should control and inspect asylums was a well-established principle by the mid-nineteenth century, but as asylums grew to enormous size and ineffectiveness, this was at best an ambiguous development both for medicine and for the mentally ill. As the following pronouncement suggests, the boundaries between lay and formal care were considerably complicated by status and gender divisions:

The circumstance of a superintendent's wife acting as matron involves a sacrifice of social position injurious, if not fatal, to success. It is above all things indispensable that medical superintendents of asylums should be educated gentlemen; and if that is to be the case, their wives cannot be matrons. Indeed, it is inconceivable that a man of position and culture would allow his family to have any connection with an asylum. (J. M. Granville, 1877, quoted in Scull, 1979, p. 182)

With respect to lay control of other institutions of medical care, there was some shifting of boundaries. The Poor Law remained under lay control, as did much of the public-health administration evolving under the new structures of local government. Medical authority was increasing, but within, rather than in opposition to, existing lay hierarchies: examples are the army, asylums, and the voluntary hospitals, which we will look at later in this chapter.

4.2.4 Inefficient mothers?

The high, and even increasing, rate of *infant mortality* drew attention to the crucial importance of mothers as carers. Mary Scharlieb, a leading doctor, singled out the relationship between mothers' drinking and poor infant care. Her opinion was that:

> The high death rate amongst English babies is not dependent upon poverty alone … There is no doubt whatever that the drinking habits of the nation and especially of the women of the nation, are doing more harm to our financial and social position than is any depression in trade or other economic causes. (Scharlieb, 1907–8, p. 59)

● In what ways is Scharlieb's view of maternal responsibility characteristic of middle-class attitudes to the poor?

■ She was advancing an *individually* focused view of causes, which could instead be ascribed to poverty. Mothers were being blamed for the results of poor social and economic conditions.

Despite the emphasis on *maternal inefficiency*, few of the welfare benefits introduced at this time were available to individual working-class women. The aim of the welfare reforms was primarily economic, and women, even though more of them were at work, had little power in the market place.

This emphasis on motherhood did not lead to a rise in family size at any level of society. Exactly the opposite was the case. Middle-class women had been using *birth control* to limit the size of their families since the 1860s and, as you have seen, the birth rate was falling in the last quarter of the century. Immediately after World War I there was a brief increase in the birth rate, but the long-term trend was downward throughout Western Europe. This trend was assisted by the wider use of contraception which was spreading among working-class women by the turn of the century. The burden of unwanted births (see Figure 4.8) gradually began to lift.

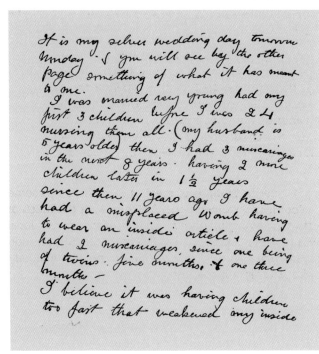

Figure 4.8 *A letter written to the Women's Co-operative Guild describes the burden of unwanted births and untreated health problems for women who did not have right of access to medical care. (Source: from Llewellyn Davies, M. (ed.), 1915,* Maternity: Letters from Working Women, *collected by the Women's Co-operative Guild, G. Bell & Sons, London; reprinted in 1978 by Virago, London)*

4.2.5 Lady visitors

Increased *outside* intervention in working-class homes and important shifts between lay and formal sectors of care both took place. Areas of lay care were taken out of the home by the institutional route — the removal of large numbers of elderly women into lunatic asylums is one example. *Volunteer visiting* of the poor had a long history, but this tendency also became more marked from the 1860s onwards. In 1862, the Ladies' Section of the Manchester and Salford Sanitary Association undertook to spread health information among the poor of the community. Visiting nurses moved rapidly into other areas of domestic responsibility, promoting the care and welfare of young children at home. In London, the work of the Charity Organisation Society from the 1870s was focused on 'close personal surveillance'.

The main development at the end of the nineteenth century was that these 'visitors' were more likely to have a professional, or at least a trained background. Formal health-visiting schemes expanded in the early years of the twentieth century, largely in response to growing concern over high levels of infant mortality. Encouraged by the Local Government Board, health visiting became one of the main growth areas of the work supervised by the Medical Officers of Health. The position of health visitors was ambiguous in that they were expected to befriend and gently influence, but also to monitor and report. Ultimately the focus of their work did not address the real needs of mothers and infants.

Evidence collected by the Women's Co-operative Guild (published in *Maternity*, 1915; see Figure 4.8) and other surveys, showed the impact of poor diet in pregnancy and the stretching of inadequate wages. Problems arising from living conditions and economic situation were on a far greater scale than any individual inadequacies. But the magnified role for health visiting also demonstrated how lay networks of care were increasingly giving way to outside intervention, initially on a voluntary basis and subsequently trained and professionalised.

4.3 Sanitarianism in action

The sanitarian movement reflected the best and the worst features of Victorian society. Against a neglect of the root causes of poverty must be set the energy and dedication which led to the transformation of the urban environment. The unbridled industrial activity which blighted the lives and health of a large proportion of the working population also produced the waterworks, embankments, and pumping stations which stand as monuments today (see Figure 4.9). Parsimony and obliviousness to the sufferings of others were matched by passionate concern and a strong sense of public duty.

The classic period of public-health reform is represented by four very different charismatic figures: Edwin Chadwick, the Benthamite lawyer, whom you met in Chapter 3 (Figure 3.6a, Table 3.1 and Table 3.2); William Farr of the Registrar-General's Office, the son of a Shropshire farm labourer (Figure 4.1); Florence Nightingale, the sickly upper-class woman, who spearheaded sanitary reform of the army and of hospitals (Figure 3.15); and John Simon, a surgeon of Huguenot descent, and creator, after the dismantling of Chadwick's General Board of Health, of a medical department of government which prefigured the Ministry of Health (Figure 4.10). These figures had in common the ability to deploy information to devastating effect, using the characteristic Victorian weapons of personal influence, 'bluebooks' (official government reports), the press, and the pulpit. All were long-lived, and their influence extended until the turn of the century.

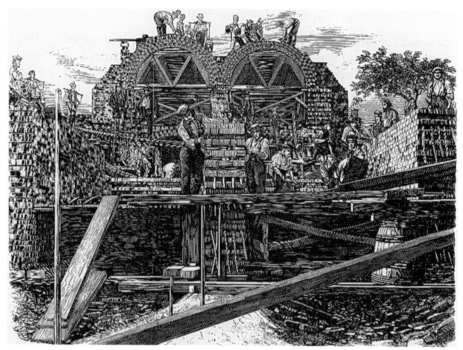

Figure 4.9   *6 000 men, directed by Sir Joseph Bazalgette, built London's main sewer system between 1858 and 1865: eighty miles of tunnel running north and south of the Thames with outfalls into the river at Barking and Crossness. 'The opening ceremonies at the southern outfall down the Thames were attended by the Prince of Wales, Prince Edward Saxe-Weimar, the Lord Mayor, the Archbishop of Canterbury, the Archbishop of York, and 500 guests, who dined on salmon while the city's excreta gushed forth into the Thames beneath them' (Wohl, 1983, p. 107). (Source:* Illustrated London News*)*

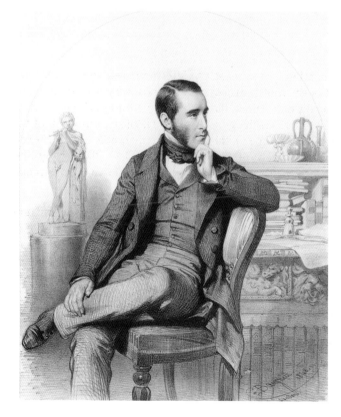

Figure 4.10   *John Simon, when Medical Officer of Health, City of London, from 1848 to 1855. This fine lithograph shows Simon as a young man of culture and elegance. His pose is one intended to convey masculine confidence, ease, and introspection. (Source: Wellcome Library, London)*

4.3.1 The successes of propaganda

The sanitary movement was very much a matter of effective propaganda and the creation of a responsive climate of opinion. Early sanitary legislation, from 1848 onwards, mainly facilitated the granting of powers to local agencies, and laid down administrative measures which had to be adopted only if local mortality rose to exceed a defined 'average' of 23 per thousand. Where powers did exist, the problems of enforcement were usually considerable. For the most part, early public-health administration consisted of talented and courageous use of duties to 'inquire and report'. The creation of *inspectorates* was central to sanitary campaigns. Much effort had to be devoted to the extraction and presentation of up-to-date data on changes in the level of mortality, since these constituted the basis on which action could be taken.

Victorian elites came to believe in quantification as a mode of reasoning, and *statistics* were central to the sanitary movement. However, medical certification of death was not compulsory until 1874; the notification of cases of certain infectious diseases, compulsory once adopted and providing information on morbidity, was not introduced nationally until 1889. In the meantime, William Farr, as Compiler of Abstracts, provided a running commentary on the broad generalisations issued in the Registrar-General's Reports, and constructed equations from the unpublished material which suggested natural laws of disease involving such factors as population density and height above sea-level. This was matched by independent inquiries conducted by individuals and local societies, like the Manchester Statistical Society (founded 1833) and the Epidemiological Society of London (founded 1850). The use of statistics by sanitarians is of course only one reflection of the development of the 'social sciences' — the sense that not only the natural world, but also human society, could be studied scientifically.

Early sanitarianism was dominated by water supply and drainage, along with a successful campaign to halt burials in crowded urban graveyards. Chadwick was chiefly responsible for the introduction of the smallbore sewer pipe, an innovation which his successor Simon could hardly praise sufficiently:

> The adaptation of glazed earthenware pipes to serve as domestic
> and urban drains was the most valuable sanitary contrivance which
> had been introduced since Roman times. (Simon, 1897, p. 226)

Chadwick envisaged, but could not implement, a perfect, cyclic system in which flowing water scoured the sewers and the sewage was transported to enrich agricultural land. This system presupposed central, single-authority control. Chadwick's Board was axed by government in 1854 (a cholera year), and health responsibilities were transferred to the Privy Council. Simon, having attracted much attention as Medical Officer of Health to the City of London, moved to become 'Medical Officer of the Committee of Council on Health'.

Simon initially avoided the Benthamite emphasis on direct central administration, and was only gradually converted to it because of the unreformed structure of local government. From the outset, however, he advocated a Ministry of Health, and defined areas requiring legislative intervention, including:

> The uncontrolled letting of houses unfit for human habitation; the
> unregulated industries of sorts endangering the health of persons
> employed in them; the unregulated nuisance-making businesses;
> the unchecked adulterations of food [see Figure 4.11]; the

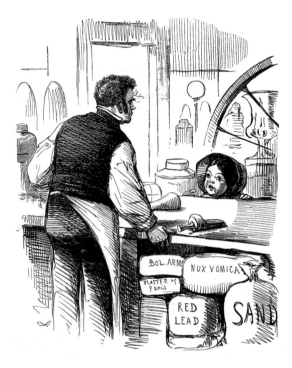

Figure 4.11 *Urbanisation and industrialisation increased the scale and severity of food and drug adulteration. In spite of spirited press campaigns, and legislation from 1860 onwards, effective and widespread testing was not established before the twentieth century. The little girl says: 'If you please, sir, Mother says, will you let her have a quarter of a pound of your best tea to kill the rats with, and a ounce of chocolate as would get rid of the black beadles!'* (*Source:* Punch, *4 August 1855*)

> unchecked falsification of drugs; the unregulated promiscuous sale of poisons; and the absence of legal distinction between qualified and unqualified medical practitioners. (Simon, 1897, p. 255)

These were not new issues, but ones in which sanitarianism reasserted the moral duty of interference between buyer and seller.

4.3.2 Medical Officers of Health

Simon did however represent a shift of emphasis in sanitarianism which occurred as medical involvement increased. **Medical Officers of Health** (MOHs), at first attached to temporary Boards of Health in periods of epidemic crisis, became compulsory in London districts in 1855, in all local government areas in England and Wales in 1872, and in Scotland in 1889.

For some practitioners, a Medical Officership was a routine part-time local appointment, somewhat better paid and higher in status than a Poor Law surgeoncy. Some MOHs were able and dedicated innovators with well-developed research interests. However, the reforming MOH was often unpopular, as in Darlington in 1851:

> The indiscriminate publication at length of the report...of the Officer of Health having been considered by the Board, it is resolved that indiscriminate publication is calculated to be injurious to the town. (Quoted by Brockington, 1965, p. 159)

● The origin of the MOH can be traced to Chadwick, who had stressed the need for health officers to be full-time, salaried public employees. Can you suggest reasons for this requirement?

■ Conscientious MOHs were very often in difficulties because the insecure, low-paid, part-time nature of their employment left them dependent on continuing in private practice among the very people whose local interests they were seen as attacking.

The basic sanitary truths about filth and disease became enshrined in the public mind, and were reiterated for the whole of the period. Reiteration was often necessary, as the Rev. Joseph Dare of Leicester found in 1852:

> The completion of the Water Works will be a great blessing to the town...From the far villas on the London-road, to the extremities of 'the North' and the Belgrave-gate, fever and diarrhoea have spread their desolating blight. From these and other causes vast numbers of the poor are always in a low state of health. This is no doubt the reason why they are perpetually seeking after the nostrums of quackery. Of course, I have heard of the 'Wise Woman of Wing'. The London Board, by its dilatoriness and needless objections to the proposed Drainage Scheme, has been the best patron she has had in this neighbourhood. (Quoted in Haynes, 1991, pp. 43–4)

Moreover, it was not only the poor whose habits had to be changed, as Simon later recalled about his successes as MOH for the City of London:

> The abomination of cesspools had come to an end. At a time when cesspools were still almost universal in the metropolis, and while, in the mansions of the west-end, they were regarded as equally sacred with the wine-cellars, they had been abolished, for rich and poor, throughout all the square mile of the City. (Simon, 1897, p. 252)

4.3.3 'Scientific' sanitarianism

Little legislation on public health was added to the statute book after the great legal codifications of the 1870s; the gap between legislation and its effective implementation is illustrated by the following extract from the 'New Closet Regulations' of Hartlepool Engine Works, notified to workers in November 1880:

> The Middleton Local Board finding it impracticable, owing to the tidal action, to keep the drains in working order, have passed a resolution that the drain connected with the Hartlepool Engine Works be cut off. It has therefore been necessary to adopt a Closet on the Dry-earth System adjoining the Gatehouse. There is, however, so much trouble and difficulty in keeping such Closets in a proper sanitary condition, that whilst providing such a convenience, it is strongly recommended to the workmen to use instead their own conveniences at home. (Quoted in Shellard, P., 1970, *Factory Life 1774–1885*, Evans Bros., London)

By the 1920s, public-health agencies had built up a formidable system of controls, expanding into food production, workplaces, shops, housing, schools, hospitals and clinics (see Figure 4.12).

However, the 'scientising' of public health from about 1860 meant a shift *away* from focusing on the environment *towards* the control of particular diseases and their causes — a move away from the 'filth diseases' like cholera, typhoid and dysentery, towards diseases spread by person-to-person contact and the behaviour of the infected individual.

The more refined epidemiology of Simon and his department was partly a political strategy, and partly a reflection of Simon's awareness of scientific developments in mainland Europe. Simon was able to capitalise on his contemporaries' belief that

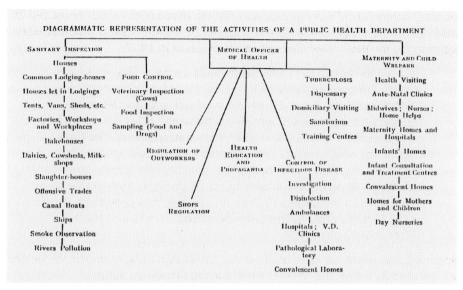

Figure 4.12   *This textbook diagram outlines the pyramid of responsibilities which had accumulated under the Medical Officer of Health by the late 1920s (Source: Bannington, B. G., 1929,* English Public Health Administration, *P. S. King & Son Ltd, London, frontispiece from 2nd edition). The chief difference noted by the author since the first edition of 1915 was the growth of maternity and child welfare.*

science was ultimately the means ordained for ordering the chaos with which many Victorians felt themselves to be surrounded. This is not to say that science in the public domain went unquestioned. The anti-vivisection agitation of the 1870s is the most obvious example of this.

Moreover, the scientifically informed campaign against the infected individual had a strong tendency to bear hardest upon the most disadvantaged. *Vaccination* against smallpox, compulsory for infants since 1853, was closely associated with the Poor Law, and often poorly administered, and consequently had bred popular resistance from its inception (look back at Figure 3.16). The later phases of this resistance stored up opposition to subsequent immunisation programmes.

In the 1860s, inequity in public-health policy was taken to an extreme by the Contagious Diseases Acts, which sought to control sexually transmitted disease by allowing, in garrison towns, the *compulsory* medical treatment of those suspected of prostitution. Many sanitarians advocated the extension of this legislation to the civilian population; the controversy went on even after repeal of the Acts in the 1880s. All policies of disease notification, disinfection, and segregation were more readily evaded by the better-off than by the poor, who were also more disadvantaged by loss of earnings or property.

4.3.4 The complex role of bacteriology

Public-health medicine gained new scientific credibility from the rise of the 'germ theory' which began in the 1860s. However, **bacteriology** — the scientific study of micro-organisms[5] — had wider implications. The speed with which Louis Pasteur's discovery of living micro-organisms was taken up by conservative politicians and the medical establishment reveals their reluctance to acknowledge social and

[5] The revolution in the scientific understanding of bacteria as the causes of many infectious diseases, from the 1860s onwards, is described in *Medical Knowledge: Doubt and Certainty* (Open University Press, colour-enhanced 2nd edn 2001), Chapters 3 and 4.

material explanations for infectious diseases. For some, bacteriology encouraged a sense of fatalism, or of alienation; it appeared to suggest the impracticability of modern urban society — that God, or nature, had ordained that human beings could not live together without danger.

The undoubted successes of bacteriology instilled both a 'single-factor' style of explanation for disease, in which all the emphasis was placed on the invading organism, and an expectation of equally single-factor solutions — 'magic bullets', like the drug salvarsan, the specific remedy for syphilis discovered in 1907 — which in practice were rarely forthcoming. Bacteriology gave medicine an almost unprecedented reputation for effectiveness; but, because it shifted the centre of gravity of medical legitimation *away* from the hospital and the private patient and *towards* the laboratory, bacteriology also drove a wedge — especially in Britain — between the clinician and the laboratory scientist.

However, the focus on *single-factor* explanations was never absolute. Public-health doctors continued to advocate *environmentalist* views in the early twentieth century, with an updated emphasis on persistent re-infection among crowded populations. The environmentalists also turned to collectivist social remedies against infectious disease, demanding improved housing and diet, and town planning, in order to promote bodily resistance to infection. Medicine in general was deeply reluctant to relinquish its emphasis on the *constitution* of the individual (which by now had been given eugenic connotations). Doctors favoured a multifactorial, rather than a single-factor, approach even to infectious disease. Thus, even in a post-bacteriological era, many who would otherwise be opponents, could agree on the virtues of therapies such as open air and sunlight.

Overall, however, the end of the period saw a gradual shift away from collective, environmental approaches, towards an emphasis on individual responsibility and individual liability to disease. Public health had also moved somewhat away from concern with the acute infectious diseases, to consider conditions like cancer, TB, sexually transmitted diseases, and alcoholism.

4.4   Different routes to professionalisation

Medical practice continued to professionalise in this period, both to meet middle-class demand and to answer the requirements of an increasingly bureaucratic society. Nonetheless, both training and the rewards of practice remained very far from uniform, and the search for recognised qualifications was in part a response to pressures within an 'overstocked' profession.

Medical men (not women as yet) were also struggling to remain at the top of pyramids of public administration which were growing in areas like public health and education. The supervision of other health workers, such as nurses and midwives, formed part of this struggle and, as in earlier periods, could lead to medical sponsorship of the professionalisation of these groups. It would be wrong, however, to see factors related to professionalisation as the only cause of these changes. *Nursing* is an excellent example of this.

4.4.1 Nursing: religion, gender and social class

Because of the dominance of the Nightingale story, and because nurses are easier to detect in hospitals than elsewhere, the myth by which the down-at-heel, drunken, middle-aged 'Sairey Gamp' (immortalised by Dickens in *Martin Chuzzlewit*) was

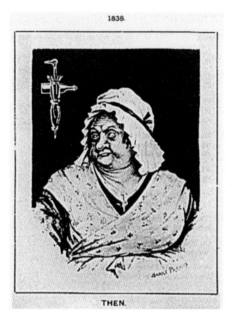
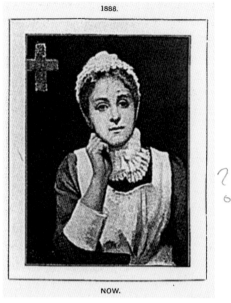

Figure 4.13   *These 'then and now' images should be seen as loaded with the biases of the later nineteenth-century campaigns for nursing 'sisterhoods'. Note the resemblance of the young nurse's uniform to a religious habit, and the cross behind her; the older nurse, on the other hand, has been given as her device a bottle of drink and an umbrella (or 'gamp'). Note too the element of prejudice against the mature woman, who is likely to have worked independently, on a self-employed basis. (Source:* Supplement to the Nursing Record, *20 December 1888)*

transformed into the young, pure, vocational nurse (see Figure 4.13) has been placed firmly in the context of the *reform of hospitals*, military and civilian.

However, this is to overlook other important factors that shaped nursing. The historian Anne Summers has stressed the need to see nursing history as a subplot to the history of Victorian Christianity (Summers, 2000). Earlier in the century, the churches had seen the pressures of industrialisation undermine the traditional practice of visiting the sick poor to advise on the health of body and soul. 'District Visiting Societies' emerged, which were successful enough to preserve the term *district nurse* for later use. The 'sisterhoods' of domiciliary nurses trained by some of these religious societies attended the poor without charge, but were in increasing demand in better-off households and in hospitals. Summers argues that hospital patients benefited from the higher standards of care imported by these nurses from their upper-class employments.

These developments precede the well-known story of Florence Nightingale's experience in the Crimean War (1854–56), shortly after which St Thomas's Hospital became home to the Nightingale School, established to implement her ideas on nurse education (Figure 4.14 overleaf). They also look forward to the marked trend at the end of the century towards home visiting, which we discussed earlier. We should also note that, although nursing was being recognised as an occupation, this was in the context of nurses being supervised by, and accountable to, their social superiors, whether these were male medical practitioners, or women philanthropists.

This social division was of importance in the struggle to organise nursing more formally as an occupation. The actual social background of recruits had changed much less by 1918 than might have been imagined. A handful of well-born women had become matrons or lady superintendents, but the majority of nurses still came from relatively humble backgrounds.

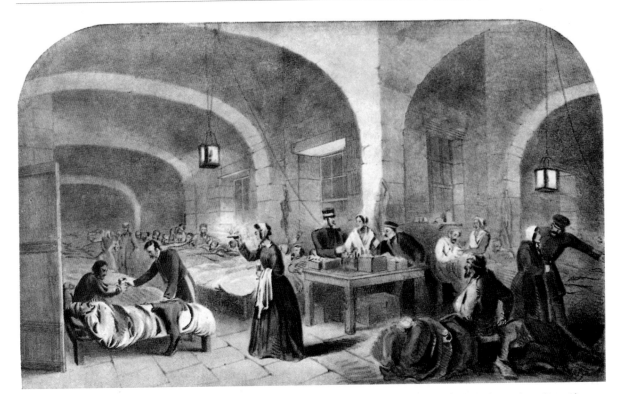

Figure 4.14   *Florence Nightingale's nursing work at the hospital at Scutari (depicted here), filtered into the reform of nursing practice. But it would be a mistake to suppose that this applied to the whole of English nursing, which remained divided according to class of nurse and the type of health care offered. (Source: lithograph by J. A. Bonwell, from Graves, C., 1947,* The story of St. Thomas's 1106–1947, *Faber and Faber, London)*

Table 4.1   Distribution of previous work experiences of recruits to nurse training, 1881–1921 (shown as percentages).

Previous work experience	Manchester Royal Infirmary (1881–1921)	The London Hospital (1881–1921)	Leeds Poor Law Infirmary (1895–1921)
actual number of recruits	1 696	4 454	370
	%	%	%
nil	28	28	28
nursing	39	26	35
domestic service	21	29	22
clerical and commercial	4	5	3
clothing and textiles	1	2	5
shop work	2	2	4
education	5	5	2
war work and miscellaneous	1	3	1

Data from Maggs, C. J. (1983) *The Origins of General Nursing*, Croom Helm, Beckenham, Table 2.2, p. 67.

● What can you infer from Table 4.1 about the social background of nursing recruits and the social status of nursing?

■ Nurses were mostly from a working-class background and nursing shared a similar social status with domestic service and other manual occupations.

This division created tensions in establishing the status of nursing which have continued to the present day.[6] Was nursing to be a 'new profession for women'; or was it a form of refined domestic service, assigned a subordinate position in the hospital?

To this division was added that between the *general nurses* of the voluntary hospitals, and those engaged in *Poor Law nursing* which, despite its numerical significance, was seen as very much the poor relation. Following a professional pattern, general nurses stressed vocation, selflessness and dedication. They formed the dominant element in the College of Nursing established in 1916. This steadily grew in influence and was granted its royal charter in 1939. Asylum and Poor Law nurses, on the other hand, tended to join the trades union movement.

The principal arena for contests over the resolution of these complex divisions was the struggle for *nurse registration*, which began in the 1880s. For the next thirty years a 'nursing war' took place against a background of changed and widening employment opportunities for women of all classes. At the same time the number of hospitals increased and so did the demand for nurses.

The question of the *nursing shortage* (another parallel with present-day nursing issues) was an added and continuing complication in the debates around how nursing status could be established. In 1909, the Red Cross devised Voluntary Aid Detachments (VADs) as a means to ease the shortage of nurses and related staff during military emergencies. VAD nursing staff became particularly important during World War I (Figure 4.15). Because these women were given only minimal and non-standardised training, there was fear among professional nurses that VADs would become a vehicle for diluting the civilian nursing profession.

Registration of nurses was finally secured after the war in 1919 and established a standard system of accreditation; but it did not eliminate the tensions within nursing, between 'aristocratic' and 'democratic' conceptions of its role and status.

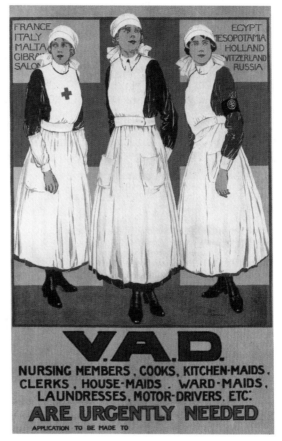

Figure 4.15 *A World War I recruiting poster for the Voluntary Aid Detachment. During the war some thirty thousand women were trained as VAD nurses and around twelve thousand served in other capacities, such as laboratory assistants, telephonists, cooks, cleaners and ambulance drivers. The VAD movement was attractive to the government because it released men for combatant duties. (Source: Imperial War Museum, London)*

---

[6] For detailed discussion of present-day issues affecting the status of nursing, see another book in this series, *Dilemmas in UK Health Care* (Open University Press, 3rd edn 2001), Chapter 5.

4.4.2 Midwives: marginalisation to rehabilitation

Issues of internal stratification and of gender also affected the status and development of *midwifery* in this period. As you will recall from Chapter 2, in the seventeenth century nearly all babies had been delivered by women. But in the eighteenth century more men had entered this area, aided by technological innovation. Soon the stereotype of 'ignorant midwives' was commonplace, much as the image of drunken old hags had tainted untrained nurses. By the middle of the nineteenth century, midwives had been virtually confined to attendance on the poor, combining help at childbirth with general work such as washing and cleaning.

But moves by women of 'professional' status to enter medicine had their impact on midwifery, as much as on medicine and nursing. The emergence of a class of highly educated and vocal midwives as a professionalising pressure group led to efforts over the last three decades of the nineteenth century to bring about training and control. The battle was between medical pressure groups seeking legislation to control midwives in their own interests, and the middle-class section of midwifery seeking independent professional status.

The Midwives Act 1902 was to a great degree a compromise. It prohibited unqualified practice, but it placed midwifery in a disadvantaged professional position in the sexual division of health labour. The Central Midwives Board had a *medical* majority and local supervision was by the MOH. Moreover, the Act's immediate impact on unqualified practice was muted. By 1914 many such women continued to practise, for the Act allowed women in 'bona fide' practice to continue to work. The proportion of trained women had risen considerably by the early 1920s (see Table 4.2).

Table 4.2   Percentage of trained midwives in three cities, 1911–35.

	1911	1915	1920	1925	1930	1935
Birmingham	n.d.	31.5	53.3	76.4	90	97.6
Hull	30	43	38.9	83	91	96
Liverpool	88	86	100	100	100	100

n.d. = no data. Data from the annual reports of the Medical Officers of Health for Birmingham, Liverpool and Hull, cited in Lewis, J. (1980) *The Politics of Motherhood*, Croom Helm, Beckenham, p. 143.

4.4.3 The Medical Register: definition not prohibition

The modern definition of medicine as a *profession* is commonly dated to the Medical Act 1858, which created the General Medical Council (GMC) and gave it responsibilities for medical education, registration and discipline. The qualifications it defined were valid throughout the British Empire. The 1858 legislation placed regulation almost completely in the hands of the doctors themselves. As the historian Anne Digby has pointed out, the GMC acted as a convenient forum for settling professional wrangles 'away from the public gaze', which protected the image of the medical profession. Digby also adds: 'how effectively the profession safeguarded the public interest is doubtful, given the tiny numbers of those whom the GMC found unfit to practise' (Digby, 1994, p. 60). As you will see in Chapter 7, it was only in the 1990s that the full gravity of this flaw in the character of professional regulation was brought home to the public.

Thus, the 1858 Medical Act was a limited achievement. It did not outlaw unqualified practice, but merely laid down what the law would recognise as a qualification.

Homoeopaths and others were little hindered until *employment* was restricted to registered practitioners, as for example under the National Health Insurance scheme begun in 1911 (as discussed later in this chapter).

Moreover, the medical organisations were unable to agree on a 'single-portal' system involving only one set of national examinations. Consequently a wide range of qualifications were given legal status, and the numerous qualifying bodies could continue to set standards independently of each other. A *minimal* qualification was enough to ensure eligibility for the public service; and any *one* qualification legally entitled the practitioner to practise *all* parts of medicine, surgery and midwifery — even though his training may not have been of this general kind. As in earlier periods, the major call from patients was for general, not specialised practice.

●   You have seen that midwifery had low status; it was unremunerative and time-consuming. Yet many *male* GPs engaged in it. Can you suggest reasons for this?

■   Midwifery was in demand, and competition among practitioners meant that many could not pick and choose what services they offered. Practitioners offered midwifery services in the hope of securing the custom of the whole family.

Similarly, there was an incentive for doctors to sell drugs, however demeaning this was thought to be, because it was lucrative. Not surprisingly, medical practitioners pressed for regulation of their rivals in this area, the chemists and druggists.

4.4.4 Changing definitions? Some challenges to the medical hierarchy

Owing to the 'dreary and thankless task of learning the intricacies and jealousies of medico-professional politics' (Simon, 1897, p. 308), the necessary government interest in the defects of the 1858 Medical Act was slow to develop; effective action was delayed until 1886. By the 1870s the clinical ideal of *training by example*, on the basis of a gentlemanly background in natural philosophy, was being challenged by a stress on *scientific laboratory-based training* which derived from the research institutes developed in continental Europe. In this field, Britain was far behind developments in Germany and the USA.

The medical academic scene in Germany had been an important influence on the Johns Hopkins School of Medicine in the USA, founded in 1889. In Germany, *research* became an essential component of medicine and a strong biomedical scientific influence was brought to bear on clinical medicine. The 1910 Flexner Report (produced by a layman, Abraham Flexner, working for the Carnegie Foundation) proposed that all American medical education should be based on the German model. In Britain there was reluctance to embrace this emphasis on research, and full-time academic appointments, which could confer independence from private practice, did not develop in the London medical schools until after World War I.

Professional success in medical practice continued to be closely linked to social status and family connections, partly because of the relevance of family circumstances to the kind of education which could be afforded. Social status underpinned the distinction between consultants in metropolitan hospitals and GPs, which as yet had little to do with specialisation within medical practice (although specialties, for example in gynaecology, ophthalmology, neurology and psychological medicine, certainly existed).

The different grades of medical practitioner earned very different levels of income. For most, profitable private practice with a prestigious hospital connection was a remote ideal. The reality consisted of competing for appointments in insurance companies, prisons, the army, the police, Friendly Societies, factories, mining companies, railway companies and Poor Law Unions.

You may have been wondering what part *women* doctors had in these events. Qualified medical practice remained a male preserve until the 1860s, and the first women entrants in Britain and the USA had to follow a policy of 'separate development', in separate medical schools and even hospitals. Integrated training did not necessarily prove advantageous: later, women practitioners tended to be concentrated in specialties relating to women and children, or in lower-status options such as the School Medical Service (see Figure 4.16).

Figure 4.16 *The School Medical Service. Basic medical inspection (not treatment) of school children became the norm after the institution of this service in 1907 and served further to reveal social inequalities in health. (Source: London Metropolitan Archives)*

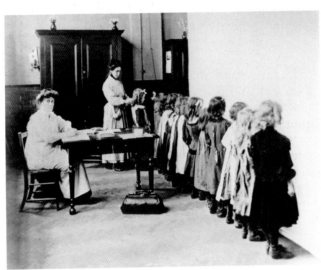

4.4.5 Medical power versus lay control

The external power relationships of medicine were also fluid. Although much of medical practice remained under lay control at the end of the century — as for example where doctors were employed by Friendly Societies and 'sick clubs' — the balance of power was beginning to alter. The shifting pattern of authority within hospitals in this period shows a move from lay to medical control. Increasingly, lay trustees exercised control *indirectly* through bureaucratic channels symbolised by the appointment of house committees and senior lay administrators like hospital secretaries. Doctors, on the other hand, formed themselves into medical committees to ensure that their interests were represented in hospital management.

By the 1860s, a general pattern was for lay and medical committees to work in tandem, with responsibility for their own areas. In the latter part of the century, the balance of power shifted still further to the medical sector as the hospital moved towards becoming a more specialist scientific and research-based institution.

In the USA, doctors were less dominant in hospital management, and health managers and administrators were a more powerful group. In Britain, as you will see in Chapter 7, the development of *health management* as a challenge to medical power came only in the 1980s.[7] In some respects, this tension has echoes of the nineteenth century. The struggle between, first, lay-and-voluntary and, subsequently, lay-and-bureaucratic forms of control, and medical dominance, is a theme which can be traced through from the eighteenth to the late twentieth centuries.

4.5   Institutions, insurances and the national interest

As you have seen earlier in this chapter, the latter half of the nineteenth century saw an expansion of institutional care; and, increasingly, in the first two decades of the twentieth century, publicly funded and centrally regulated health care developed as an outgrowth of the concern for national efficiency.

4.5.1   Asylums and hospitals

The asylum continued its inexorable growth.

● What does Table 4.3 show about changes in the institutional system for the treatment of insanity in the second half of the nineteenth century?

■ It demonstrates two developments: the increased number of institutional places available; and the rise in importance of the publicly funded County and Borough asylums. In fifteen years the numbers in these asylums had quadrupled. (Note also that large — perhaps greater — numbers of the 'insane' were kept in Poor Law institutions, notably the workhouses (see Figure 4.17), which are *not* included in the table.

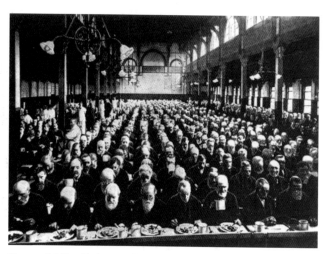

Figure 4.17   *Christmas dinner, Marylebone Workhouse, c. 1900. (Source: Mary Evans Picture Library)*

Table 4.3   Mid-nineteenth-century asylum statistics, England.

| | Patients in asylums (in year) | | | | | |
| | 1844 | | 1860 | | 1870 | |
Institutions	No.	%	No.	%	No.	%
provincial licensed houses	3 346	30	2 356	10	2 204	6
metropolitan licensed houses	1 827	16	1 944	8	2 700	8
County and Borough asylums	4 489	40	17 432	73	27 890	79
others	1 610	14	1 985	8	2 369	7
total	11 272	100	23 717	100	35 163	100

Data (rounded to nearest whole number) based on Scull, A. (1993) *The Most Solitary of Afflictions: Madness and Society in Britain 1700–1900*, Yale University Press, New Haven, Connecticut.

[7] Shifts in the balance of power between health service managers, doctors and groups representing patients' interests in the 1990s, following the re-organisation of the National Health Service, are also referred to in several chapters of *Dilemmas in UK Health Care* (Open University Press, 3rd edn 2001).

● In the years between 1807 and 1890, the numbers of persons officially identified as insane (including those in workhouses and the community) in England and Wales rose from about 2 per 10 000 population to almost 30 per 10 000. What different explanations can you think of for the steep rise?

■ There are three possible explanations:

  1 that this represented a real growth in the extent of insanity in the population;

  2 that it was an artefact (the collection of statistics was poor in the first half of the nineteenth century and medical diagnosis was less developed);

  3 that the increase represented a major reduction in the community's ability or willingness to contain and tolerate disturbed behaviour.

The American historical sociologist, Andrew Scull, has argued in favour of the last explanation (Scull, 1979, 1993). The growth of the asylum and the rise in the number of its inmates, in his view, were outgrowths of a rapidly urbanising society in which families were no longer able to support unproductive relatives. By the end of the nineteenth century, the pauper insane formed 90 per cent of the asylum population.

The *function* of the asylum also changed. The reformers who had supported its expansion had seen the asylum as a welcoming refuge, modelled on the pioneering Retreat at York. But the reality turned out to be very different.

> It is a vast and straggling building, in which the characteristics of a prison, a self-advertising charitable institution, and some ambitious piece of Poor Law architecture struggle for prominence. The gates are kept by an official who is attired in a garb as nearly as possible like that of a gaoler. All the male attendants are made to display the same forbidding uniform. (Mortimer Granville on Hanwell Asylum, London, 1877, quoted in Scull, 1979, p. 195)

● What does this suggest to you about the function of the asylum?

■ By the end of the century the asylum was custodial, a prison for those classified as insane.

The *hospital system* also expanded in the late nineteenth century. This was not simply a matter of the growth of specialisms. To the voluntary hospitals were added the Poor Law infirmaries which expanded in London after a major onslaught on workhouse infirmary conditions by *The Lancet* and medical groups in the 1860s.

The Metropolitan Poor Act 1867 was a means by which finance could be raised for building large infirmaries. The Metropolitan Asylums Board, also established in 1867, developed one of the largest hospital systems in the world (note that the term 'asylum' was here being used in its general sense of 'place of refuge'). The Board's infectious diseases hospitals were originally intended only for use by paupers, but during epidemics they were used by all classes. In this way the principle of entitlement to free treatment was established. By 1908, over 18 per cent of all deaths in England and Wales occurred in public institutions, a figure which had doubled over the previous thirty years.

● Table 4.4 shows some basic statistics about the growth of hospital provision in England from 1861 onward. What developments do you notice?

- (The numbers of beds in both voluntary and public hospitals had increased proportionately to population in this period. But the public hospital sector was far larger and continued to grow at a higher rate.)

Table 4.4   Growth of hospital provision (numbers of beds) in England after 1861.

Year	Public hospitals		Voluntary hospitals		Total	
	Beds	Per 1 000 population	Beds	Per 1 000 population	Beds	Per 1 000 population
1861	50 000	2.6	11 000	0.6	61 000	3.2
1891	83 000	2.9	29 000	1.0	113 000	3.9
1911	154 000	4.3	43 000	1.2	197 000	5.5
1921	172 000	4.6	57 000	1.5	229 000	6.1
1938	176 000	4.3	87 000	2.1	263 000	6.4

Data (rounded to the nearest thousand) based on Abel-Smith, B. (1964) *The Hospitals, 1800–1948*, Heinemann, London, pp. 46, 152, 200, 353, 382–5.

(These developments brought changes in the role of patients and the relationship between doctors in and outside the hospital. One change was that out-patient numbers increased dramatically at the end of the century. Hospital out-patient departments, especially in London, provided primary health care for the entire local population. Indeed, before the National Insurance Act 1911 (described in Section 4.5.2) 'going to the doctor' in his surgery was unusual for most of the British population.)

The historian Rosemary Stevens has compared the evolution of the health-care system in the USA with that in the United Kingdom in this period.[8]

- According to Stevens, how did the expansion of the hospital system which took place on both sides of the Atlantic, have different effects in the USA and Britain on the relationship between doctors inside and outside hospital medicine?

- Stevens argues that in the USA the use of out-patient departments, and the rise of special hospitals in the last quarter of the nineteenth century, threatened the position of the GP; general practice was largely moribund by World War I. But in Britain, the relationship between the hospital specialist and the GP was settled to accommodate a continuing role for the GP (as you will see in greater detail in the next three chapters).

4.5.2 Financing health care

(The expansion in hospital usage brought particular problems for the *voluntary hospitals*. The proportion of beds they provided grew, but this led to financial crisis. Higher levels of success, with more patients surviving, brought increases in costs of nursing and medical care. The voluntary hospitals provided almost all the *acute*

[8] An edited version of her 1976 article, 'The evolution of health-care systems in the United States and the United Kingdom: similarities and differences', appears in *Health and Disease: A Reader* (Open University Press, 2nd edn 1995; 3rd edn 2001). Open University students should read it now, and then answer the question above.

beds (i.e. those dedicated to short-stay patients in acute need of care); costs escalated owing to medical advances such as antiseptic and then aseptic surgery. Acute-care patients need more intensive nursing, and consequently running costs were also higher.

Money was raised through private charity and the introduction of *pay beds*. The charitable Hospital Sunday and Hospital Saturday Funds (which organised flag days and fund-raising) were established as sources of hospital finance in the 1870s. Hospitals, which had previously had a solely working-class clientele, began charging any patients judged capable of paying, and also established private blocks, thus instituting first- and second-class forms of treatment.

Sickness insurance in Germany

There were moves to establish a broader entitlement to health care in Britain. The National Insurance Act 1911 was a significant step in this direction (see below), but Britain was slower to introduce a state insurance-based sickness system than many European countries.

Compulsory sickness insurance was introduced by the German Chancellor, Otto von Bismarck, in 1883. This superseded earlier voluntary and co-operative sickness funds, which had appealed to the better-educated workers in relatively stable occupations. The motives were both economic and political. Bismarck had introduced anti-socialist legislation between 1878 and 1891. Threats of opposition were defused by making sickness insurance funds *(Krankenkassen)* available only to certain wage bands of urban workers who were the main supporters of socialism. Yet the insurance funds were autonomous, with worker and employer representation on a 2:1 basis. Ironically, from the 1890s, a number of leading socialists had careers in sickness insurance fund administration, and they were keen to extend benefits to family dependants, to emulate French schemes for maternity benefits (these were discretionary in Germany), and to include certain categories of disease (like sexually transmitted diseases), initially excluded from the scheme as attributable to personal moral failings.

In the longer term, sickness insurance was extended by state legislation, so that by 1913 it covered 25 per cent of the German population (including, from 1911, such groups as domestic servants and agricultural workers), half of this proportion having family dependants. In contrast to the British scheme, German workers contributed on a graduated scale in proportion to their earnings. The market for medical care was greatly extended, bringing new social sectors into regular contact with university-educated physicians. The prospect of a steady income from insurance fees stimulated a doubling in numbers of the German medical profession between 1889 and 1898.

German socialist criticisms of unhealthy social conditions, and of the poor law as depriving recipients of civil rights, prompted the Prussian ruling elite in 1895 to launch an association for providing *sanatoria* for patients with TB. Once these were opened, patients' costs could be covered by sickness insurance schemes, and by 1911 Germany had more public sanatoria *(Volksheilstätten)* than any other country.

As the cost of such sanatoria was high, welfare clinics and home-visiting schemes were devised, using pioneer French dispensary clinics as models. Whereas the French clinics provided treatment, pressure from the German medical profession limited the role of the German equivalents to diagnosis and the provision of welfare benefits. Dispensary clinics were organised for infant welfare, for alcoholism and, by 1914, for sexually transmitted diseases. Networks of urban 'polyclinics' supplemented the French and German municipal hospital systems which were being extended and modernised from the 1880s. Improvements in hospital design and new therapies meant that by the turn of the century a broader social spectrum was making use of new children's hospitals.

Sickness insurance in Britain

The German system of social insurance became an influential international model. But the British system, although influenced by German example, was significantly different in several respects. The 1911 *National Health Insurance* (NHI) scheme limited benefits to the contributor alone, below a certain level of income, and did not include dependants (see Figure 4.18). However, a modest maternity benefit was available to insured working women and to the wives of working men.

Contributions were not graduated according to income, but were paid at a flat rate, approximately half by the employee and half by the employer. The state played a background role, mainly serving to regulate the system, which was largely self-financing. Cash benefits for sickness, accident and disability were paid at a fixed amount regardless of severity, and continued to be distributed through familiar insurance companies, the so-called *approved societies*. Insured contributors had the right to free but limited care from a doctor on a local list or *panel* and the doctor received a **capitation fee** — a standard payment for each panel patient. Hospital treatment was available only to patients with TB.

The historian Bentley Gilbert has commented that:

> The aim of national insurance was to replace lost income, not to cure sickness. (Gilbert, 1966, p. 318)

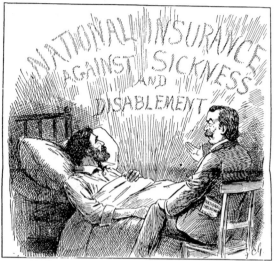

THE DAWN OF HOPE.

Mr. LLOYD GEORGE'S National Health Insurance Bill provides for the insurance of the Worker in case of Sickness.

Support the Liberal Government
in their policy of
SOCIAL REFORM.

Figure 4.18 *The National Insurance Act 1911 established for the first time in Britain the concept of benefits as a right, based on records of contributions. (Source: Hulton Getty Picture Collection)*

The avoidance of pauperism was the main incentive: Lloyd George's intention was that sickness insurance, despite its limited coverage, should supersede the Poor Law. Yet even this limited scheme did not become law without a struggle. Doctors, via the British Medical Association, fought hard to secure realistic capitation fees, to prevent interference by the approved societies, and generally to protect their independence of professional action. The government largely acceded to their demands, with the result that GPs ultimately clamoured to be admitted to the panels, which offered many a larger and steadier income than ever before. As a result of the panels, a GP service became available to manual workers, which resolved the conflict over hospital out-patients and brought clarification of the division between the GP/primary level of health care and the secondary/tertiary level of acute and specialist hospital care — a crucial development in British health policy.

One significant offshoot of the National Health Insurance system was the establishment of the Medical Research Committee in 1913, funded from the proceeds of the National Insurance Act and originally intended to develop research into TB. Renamed the *Medical Research Council* after World War I, it financed a wide-ranging programme of medical research, focusing on the pre-clinical sciences.

4.5.3 Impact of World War I

In Germany, the war had a considerable impact on health services. The various state sickness insurance and voluntary medical measures were subject to increasing control by the central state (or *Reich*). The state began to acknowledge its responsibility to maintain the health of the population in the context of total war, and health innovations were accompanied by pronatalist propaganda in favour of 'child-rich' families. Legislation was introduced for maternity allowances, schemes were instituted to improve midwifery services on a domiciliary basis, district health and welfare centres were opened, and condoms as a barrier to sexually transmitted infections were officially sanctioned.

In Britain, developments were on a smaller scale. The pre-existing concerns for the health of mothers and babies rose to a new height during the war. The argument that it was more dangerous to be a baby than a soldier was well publicised. Infant mortality had, in fact, been in decline since the early years of the twentieth century and continued to fall during the war. The number of clinics and health visitors expanded, and the Maternity and Child Welfare Act 1918 imposed an obligation on local authorities to provide services in this area. However, the historian Jay Winter has concluded that rising incomes, and consequent better nutrition, had a more significant effect on the health of mothers and children than the patchy local provision of health services (Winter, 1986).

Somewhat surprisingly, civilian mortality rates also improved; even though 14 000 doctors were diverted to military service during the war, lack of medical attention did not prevent an overall increase in life expectancy.

Against this generally 'optimistic' picture must be set the increased death rate from TB (primarily a young person's disease), possibly because of cross-infection from troops and deteriorating housing; and higher death rates among the elderly, who were removed from hospitals and institutions to make way for the wounded. *Sexually transmitted diseases* ('venereal diseases' or VD) also spread rapidly in war-time conditions.

Government action was forthcoming in the cases of TB and sexually transmitted diseases. The government had made free treatment for TB (including sanatoria) available to insured workers and their dependants in 1911 under the National Insurance Act; an Act in 1921 extended local-authority responsibility for the treatment of TB; and an Act of 1917 established a network of local-authority VD clinics where treatment was free and confidential. Arguments about condoning or encouraging immorality (paralleled by the arguments in the 1980s around the promotion of 'safe sex' and condom use against AIDS), prevented distribution to the troops of prophylactics against VD. Thus, World War I had some impact on health-care provision, but little of the generalised effect of World War II (as you will see in Chapter 5); rather, there was a patchwork of services for special groups.

4.5.4 Mortality and medical progress

The latter half of the nineteenth century and the beginning of the twentieth was a time of *innovation* in hospital-based procedures and therapies in Britain and continental Europe.[9] Two crucial questions arising from these developments are: what *relevance* did they have for the general population; and what *impact* did they

---

[9] Discussed in *Medical Knowledge: Doubt and Certainty* (Open University Press, 2nd edn 1994; colour-enhanced 2nd edn 2001), Chapter 4, particularly in relation to the treatment and prevention of TB.

have on mortality and morbidity rates in this period? The debate about the impact of medical care is typified by two articles by Thomas McKeown and Simon Szreter.[10]

● Can you recall the main thrust, first of McKeown's argument, and then of what Szreter has added to McKeown?

■ McKeown's interpretation downgraded the role of medical treatment and immunisation against infectious disease as the main contributors to the decline prior to World War I, in favour of a greater role for improved nutrition. Szreter revised the McKeown account and emphasised the role of public-health measures in the rapidly falling mortality and morbidity from infectious diseases.

The general thrust of the McKeown argument still holds good. It makes the important point that scientific, high-technology medicine is often of limited impact by comparison with general improvements in living standards and the overall nutritional status of the population. These types of argument were important in later moves to reduce hospital dominance in the British health system and to upgrade the status of primary health care.

However, as you will see in Chapter 5, medicine's claims to effectiveness increase considerably *after* this period, on the basis of (for example) a wider range of immunisations, blood transfusion, vitamins, improved understanding of vector-borne diseases like malaria, and more potent drugs such as the sulphonamides.

4.6 Medicine and imperialism: the 'scramble for Africa'

The most important aspect of European expansion overseas in this period was the so-called 'scramble for Africa', beginning in the 1880s, in which Britain, France, Germany, and other European countries began to carve up the continent into colonies and 'protectorates' (see Figures 4.19 and 4.20 overleaf). No single theory can explain why this development occurred, but behind imperial rivalry was increasing political and economic competition between Britain, France and the new German state. As you saw earlier in this chapter, these changes were bound up with the rise of industrial capitalism, the social consequences of which led to new forms of medical intervention, particularly in the field of public health. In much the same way, imperial expansion created or exacerbated a whole range of medical and social problems in the colonies, which posed a threat not only to the health of indigenous peoples, but also to the durability and profitability of the colonial enterprise.

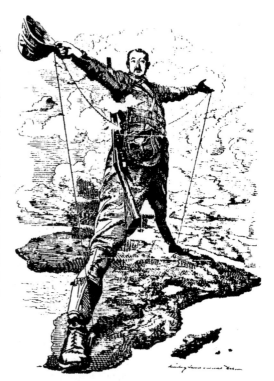

Figure 4.19 *British-born South African statesman Cecil Rhodes, shown by* Punch *as a colossus straddling the continent of Africa, was instrumental in expanding British territories. (Source:* Punch, *4 August, 1895)*

[10] The articles in question are 'The medical contribution' by Thomas McKeown (1976) and 'The importance of social intervention in Britain's mortality decline, *c.*1850–1914' by Simon Szreter (1988), in *Health and Disease: A Reader* (Open University Press, 2nd edn 1995; 3rd edn 2001). Both were set reading for Open University students studying another book in this series: *World Health and Disease* (Open University Press, 3rd edn 2001), Chapter 6.

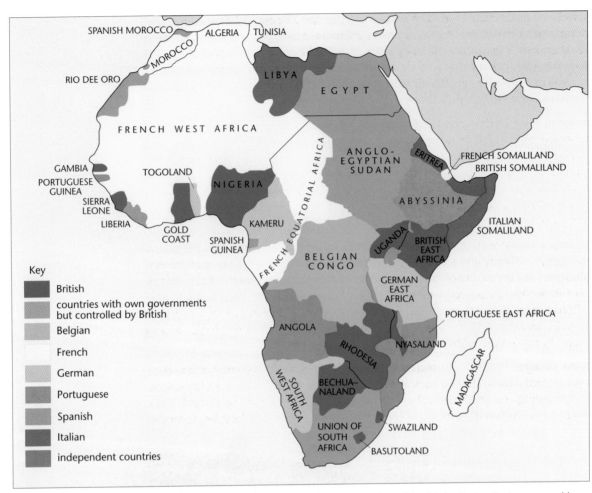

Figure 4.20   *The European partition of Africa, 1914. Medical provision varied considerably in the territories annexed by the European powers. Generally, medical services were focused on the needs of Europeans themselves, although in some colonies public-health measures were coercive. In Portuguese Angola and the Belgian Congo, for instance, colonial medicine was a powerful instrument of social control, constraining the movement of the indigenous population, or providing a pretext for their forcible relocation.*

Problems of imperial efficiency had a profound effect on the development of medicine in Europe, particularly on the new sciences of bacteriology and parasitology, which formed the basis of a new discipline — **tropical medicine**. But the indigenous inhabitants of Africa benefited little from these advances in medical knowledge, or from the sanitary reforms that were transforming the urban environment in Europe. More often than not, if they encountered Western medicine, it was in the form of a coercive power, or was conditional upon the acceptance of European norms and values.

4.6.1 Tropical medicine

As you saw in Chapters 2 and 3, Europeans had begun to acquire a knowledge of the diseases of 'warm climates', based on a mixture of European and indigenous medical knowledge, and observations of the tropical disease environment. With few exceptions, however, this specialised knowledge had not been institutionalised; but from the 1880s, with the rise of a popular and political culture of imperialism, this began to change.

As well as being transformed internally by the specialisms of bacteriology and parasitology, tropical medicine was being shaped externally by a growing concern over economic and military efficiency in the colonies. The Liverpool School of Tropical Medicine founded in 1898, and the London School of Tropical Medicine founded in 1899 (Figure 4.21), owed their existence to financial contributions from colonial merchants and the Colonial Office respectively.

However, the Liverpool and London schools embodied the professional aspirations of medical men as much as the economic objectives of European businessmen and politicians. In the last two decades of the nineteenth century, medical men in the colonies had made a number of discoveries that would eventually revolutionise the prevention and treatment of disease in the tropics. The micro-organisms causing malaria, cholera, brucellosis, sleeping sickness, bubonic plague and leishmaniasis were all discovered in the years between 1880 and 1918.

But until 1900, at least, those engaged in medical research in the colonies received little support from either their respective governments or their professional colleagues in Europe, many of whom were suspicious or ignorant of bacteriology and microscopical research. In the 1890s, professional journals, such as the *Journal of Tropical Medicine*, began to appear with the object of uniting those working in the field, and medical men began to lobby governments in the colonies and in Europe to make better provisions for laboratory research.

Those engaged in medical research in the tropics frequently presented themselves as heroic individuals, striving against official indifference and indigenous ignorance. For 'crusading' colonial medical officers like Ronald Ross (later, Sir Ronald Ross), who became the first director of the Liverpool School of Tropical Medicine, European

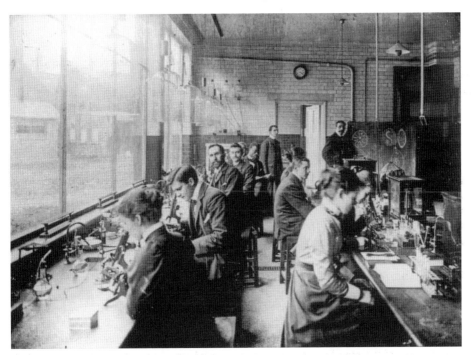

Figure 4.21   *The first class at work at the London School of Tropical Medicine in its foundation year, 1899. At the blackboard, Dr D. C. Rees is demonstrating the life-cycle of one of the species of* Plasmodium, *the parasites that cause malaria. (Source: Courtesy of the London School of Hygiene and Tropical Medicine)*

imperialism was first and foremost a civilising force, capable of bestowing immense benefits upon indigenous peoples. According to Ross, Europeans were:

> ... superior to subject peoples in natural ability, integrity and science ... They [had] introduced honesty, law, justice, order, roads, posts, railways, irrigation, hospitals ... and what was necessary for civilization, a final superior authority. (Ross, 1923, p. 17)

This paternalistic, if not racist, rationalisation of European domination was to set the tone for much of the propaganda surrounding tropical medicine until after World War II.

In reality, it was far from clear, at least before 1918, that tropical medicine had bestowed any substantial benefits upon the populations of European colonies. Research institutions established in the colonies before 1918, such as the French Pasteur Institutes and the Central Research Institute which opened in India in 1907, were little more than icons of Western scientific progress, whose research had direct benefit for only a small proportion of the indigenous population. The majority of medical research conducted in the colonies in this period was directed at health problems impairing military and economic efficiency.

This was clearly the case with the early work of the Liverpool School of Tropical Medicine in Africa. Its research and disease-prevention programmes were, in the words of the historian Michael Worboys, 'entrepreneurial activities', funded by subscriptions from among Liverpool merchants, which had the ultimate aim of improving labour efficiency in the colonies (Worboys, 1988b).

Most prominent among the school's early activities were *anti-malarial programmes* which attempted to control the disease by the eradication of its vector, the *Anopheles* mosquito (identified by the school's director, Ronald Ross). These early, isolated, attempts at mosquito eradication in Africa appear to have met with little success — not surprisingly, since they were rarely followed up by colonial governments.

4.6.2 'The sick continent'

Disease in African society was a social metaphor as well as a biological fact. For Europeans, 'African' diseases came to symbolise everything they considered degenerate or threatening about African society. *Sleeping sickness* became a metaphor for the 'laziness' of the black African, while *plague*, which was introduced into Africa in the late 1890s, came to represent all that was considered unclean or dangerous about the indigenous population. In the French North African port of Dakar, as in many other cities throughout the European colonies, plague provided a medical rationalisation for racial segregation. The Dakar Sanitary Commission demanded:

> ... the transfer of the native population which takes pleasure in a deep-rooted and incurable filthiness, to a place far from the city, and the destruction or demolition of all shacks and huts, as the only measure able to stop the spread of the current epidemic. (Quoted by Headrick, 1988, p. 163)

● Are there any similarities between this statement and the extract from Sir Ronald Ross's memoirs, cited above?

■ Ross stresses Europe's 'civilising mission' whereas the Commission seeks only to protect Europeans, but both view native peoples as culturally inferior to Europeans, and both are extremely authoritarian.

The high incidence of *malarial infection* among African children also led to attempts to segregate Europeans from native peoples. In Cameroon (Kameru in Figure 4.20), in 1910, German administrators began a scheme to relocate the entire black population of the harbour city Duala to a fenced-off area inland. Although not fully completed before Germany lost the colony after World War I, the legacy of segregated housing and poor sanitation was upheld by the colony's new masters, the French.

4.6.3 Missionary zeal

In most areas of colonial Africa before 1918, and in many cases until the 1930s, indigenous peoples were most likely to experience Western health care in the form of **medical missions**. It was the medical missions which first introduced rural health care in Africa and which began to train Africans in midwifery and rural health work.

But while mission medicine employed the same medical technologies as the secular colonial state, its mode of operation was substantially different. An emphasis on spiritual salvation and on the Christian tradition of healing frequently obscured the humanitarian objectives of medical missions. Indeed, medical work was generally subordinated to the more urgent task of saving souls. Long-term care of the sick in leper asylums and mission hospitals presented missionaries with the best opportunities for evangelisation (see Figure 4.22), and *leprosy*, with its biblical connotations, became their *cause célèbre*.

The extent to which indigenous peoples availed themselves of the opportunities provided by the missions is far from clear, yet it seems that mission dispensaries offering Western therapies and vaccination against smallpox had become quite popular in some areas of Africa by 1918. Certain forms of surgery such as the removal of cataracts also quickly gained the confidence of Africans. The results of cataract operations were fairly immediate and often impressive, and not unlike the biblical miracles preached by the missionaries.

Indeed, in Africa especially, the missions did succeed in converting a substantial number of their patients, many of whom went on to train as nurses and midwives. Generally, though, Africans were selective and incorporated only certain aspects of Western medicine and Christianity into their traditional systems. Missionaries viewed this tendency with some alarm, since African society was seen by them not only as heathen but as, itself, fundamentally sick.

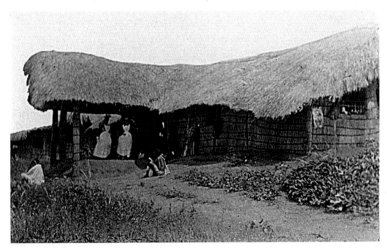

Figure 4.22 *Mengo missionary hospital, Uganda, 1898, from Foster, W. D. (1978) Sir Albert Cook: A Missionary Doctor in Uganda, Newhaven Press, Newhaven, Sussex. (Source: Church Missionary Society) Elsewhere in a missionary journal Cook commented: 'It is not our job, nor have we the power, to convert the souls of men, yet we do see again and again death beds irradiated by the smile of hope and peace given from on high'. (Mercy and Truth, 1904, 95, p. 338)*

Figure 4.23 'A Congo Child's Appeal', from Medical Missionary, 1909, 8. (Source: Bodleian Library, Oxford)

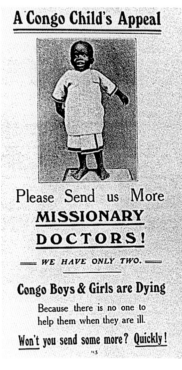

- What does Figure 4.23 suggest to you concerning the way in which Africans were portrayed by missionaries?

■ The appeal depicts Africans as sick, vulnerable, and unable to survive without Western medical aid.

The peoples of colonial Africa, like the inhabitants of India considered in Chapter 3, benefited little from the advances made in tropical medicine or from other 'fruits' of Western civilisation. Tropical medicine was not developed for the benefit of colonial peoples, but to improve colonial *productivity* and to safeguard the health of Europeans in the 'white man's grave'. Further, when Africans encountered Western medicine, it was often in the form of coercive public-health measures or missionary medicine, in which the task of healing the sick was perceived as less important than the saving of souls.

More generally, by representing African society as diseased, Western medicine was instrumental in creating a negative image of black Africans which has persisted in Western culture even to the present, reinforced by AIDS, which is considered in Chapter 8.

OBJECTIVES FOR CHAPTER 4

When you have studied this chapter, you should be able to:

4.1 Define and use, or recognise definitions and applications of, each of the terms printed in **bold** in the text.

4.2 Explain the shift from the ascendancy of the sanitarian movement and its representative, the MOH, to the deepening crisis of confidence over the state of health and health care, culminating in the concern over threats to 'national efficiency'.

4.3 Describe the ways in which the role of the family and the community in health care was eroded by professional, institutional and commercial developments.

4.4 Describe the moves towards professionalisation of nursing and other health-care occupations, noting the trend in control from lay to medical authorities.

4.5 Outline the moves in Europe towards social welfare systems providing health insurance and the way in which this trend was manifested in Britain.

4.6 Explain the ways in which European medicine was affected by colonial expansion and how European priorities dominated the provision of health care in colonial Africa.

QUESTIONS FOR CHAPTER 4

1 (*Objective 4.2*)

The Rev. Joseph Dare of Leicester, long an ardent sanitarian, reported in 1875:

> In view of the excessive mortality of the 'little ones' that has so long distressed the town, and which must show that its causes are not yet well understood, a medical gentleman recently inquired of me, 'whether married female labour had not lately much increased?' I have made many inquiries amongst different branches of labour, and the general impression seems to be that it has much increased of late years. (Quoted in Haynes, 1991, p. 49)

What change of view about the causes of major health problems does Dare (and the 'medical gentleman') represent?

2 (*Objective 4.3*)

Read the following extract from an article published in 1906 in the *British Medical Journal*:

> The health visitors…must carry with them the carbolic powder, explain its use, and leave it where it is accepted; direct the attention of those they visit to the evils of bad smells, want of fresh air, impurities of all kinds; give hints to mothers on feeding and clothing their children — where they find sickness assist in promoting the comfort of the invalid by personal help, and report such cases…they must urge the importance of cleanliness, thrift, and temperance on all possible occasions. They are desired to get as many as possible to join the mothers' meetings of their districts, to use all their influence to induce those they visit to attend regularly at their respective places of worship, and to send their children to school. ('A Model Ladies Health Society', *British Medical Journal*, 1906, **i**, p. 152, quoted in Davies, 1988, p. 43)

What changes in patterns of family care does this advice to health visitors represent?

3 (*Objective 4.4*)

In 1898, just before the (second) Boer war, a Miss Phipps wrote to a well-placed friend to ask:

> …how I, an amateur nurse, can get into the Red Cross Society — tell him [Lord Wantage, head of the National Aid Society] that I have done good work under St John Ambulance for which I got a Jubilee Medal and have worked as a nurse in a surgery in Rome — and all my life practised on our farm people — how brutal that sounds!…I *would* like to have the chance of being a R.C. [sic] nurse in case of war. (Quoted in Summers, 1988, p. 194)

How typical was this eager volunteer? And what does her background tell us about the state of nurse training at this time?

4   (*Objective 4.5*)

To what extent did the sickness insurance scheme introduced by Lloyd George improve upon defects in German sickness insurance provisions, and what were the limitations of Lloyd George's scheme?

5   (*Objective 4.6*)

What does the pattern of health care in colonial Africa tell us about the nature and objectives of colonial medicine in this period?

CHAPTER 5

The impact of war and depression, 1918 to 1948

5.1   **Europe between the wars   134**
        5.1.1 Financing health care in Britain   135
        5.1.2 The advance of social welfare   136

5.2   **The health-care system: chaos and change   137**
        5.2.1 A ramshackle system   137
        5.2.2 Hospitals in crisis   138
        5.2.3 Health-care finance in crisis   140
        5.2.4 Pressure for change   140
        5.2.5 The birth of the NHS   141

5.3   **Lay care and boundaries with formal care: tipping the balance   144**
        5.3.1 Establishing the boundaries   145
        5.3.2 Rising aspirations   148
        5.3.3 Birth control and maternity services   148

5.4   **Public-health services: in search of an identity   150**
        5.4.1 The neglect of social causes of ill-health   151
        5.4.2 Housing and health   153

5.5   **Formal health-care occupations: disputed boundaries   154**
        5.5.1 Regulating the 'para-medical' professions   154
        5.5.2 The role of the general practitioner   155
        5.5.3 The crisis in nursing   157

5.6   **Empires and exchanges: the limits of paternalism   159**
        5.6.1 India: devolution and diversity   159
        5.6.2 Africa: the 'great campaigns'   161
        5.6.3 Colonial medicine in transition   162
        5.6.4 Malnutrition in the colonies   163

Objectives for Chapter 5   165
Questions for Chapter 5   165

Study notes for OU students

Chapters 2 to 5 generally deal with events in Britain, meaning England, Scotland, Wales and Ireland. After the independence of the southern part of Ireland in 1922, links between the British mainland and Northern Ireland became closer. Consequently, later chapters of this book generally refer to the United Kingdom (UK) as a whole, meaning England, Scotland, Wales and Northern Ireland. The social welfare system which emerged in Britain during this period included a focus on the effects on health of poor housing and nutrition, especially among mothers and children. Data on the epidemiological associations of certain diseases with housing quality and nutrition were discussed in *World Health and Disease* (Open University Press, third edition 2001), Chapters 10 and 11. During this chapter, we will refer again to the article by Rosemary Stevens, which you read in Chapter 4; it is in *Health and Disease: A Reader* (Open University Press, second edition 1995; third edition 2001).

5.1   Europe between the wars

The period covered by this chapter begins and ends with a world war. War, and in particular 'total war' of the type experienced in 1914–18 and 1939–45, has been said by historians to lead to significant social change. This was more the case for World War II than for World War I (although in the rest of Europe, the first war did lead to the establishment of welfare systems for the civilian population). World War II led to the establishment of the National Health Service (NHS) in Britain, the first comprehensive state-funded system of health care in the West. The impact of World War I on health care has been more controversial, as we noted in the last chapter. The aftermath of World War I did not lead to the sort of reconstruction associated with World War II (see Figure 5.1). There was no mood for radical change among the ruling elite; that section of society instead believed that the war had been fought to restore the world as they knew it before 1914.

The period following World War I remained one of ebbs and flows in entitlement to health care in its widest sense, including social welfare. Post-war reconstruction was more limited than that after World War II, but did point towards greater collectivism. Bureaucracies were now assuming that they could intervene in complex socio-economic affairs. Ministries of Health were established all over Europe and elaborate insurance-based health-care systems were enacted. In England, the Ministry of Health was established in 1919, as a partial realisation of the earlier aims of John Simon and other public-health reformers (as described in Chapter 4). Autonomous and semi-autonomous health departments in Scotland and Wales respectively also date from this period. (Later in the chapter, Figure 5.6 shows how the new NHS specifically affected the Scottish health system.)

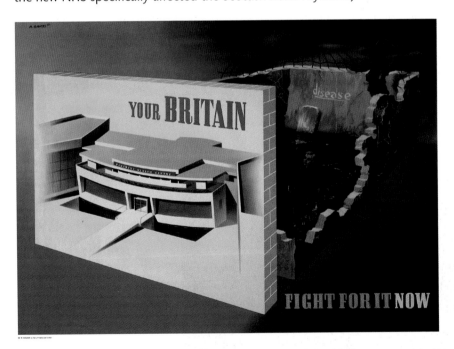

Figure 5.1   *This poster from World War II shows the Finsbury Health Centre, completed in 1938 (see Figure 5.11). It was part of a series intended to persuade the armed forces to fight for a better Britain, but was banned by Churchill, who disliked its portrayal of conditions prevailing in Britain before the war; (note, the depiction includes a child with the characteristic bowed legs of rickets). The poster nevertheless represents the emergent wartime optimism about the possibilities of post-war reconstruction — a positive mood which was strikingly absent after World War I. (Source: The Estate of Abram Games, by kind permission)*

The war also led to the beginnings of *international standard-setting*, not only for medicines but also for health care. The newly established League of Nations set optimal standards for *nutrition* which made it possible to begin to evaluate deficiencies at a national level. The Rockefeller Foundation's global policies promoted medicine on a collectivist and scientific basis, policies that were controversial because of their stress on training new elite specialists in public health.

The inter-war years are, nevertheless, with good reason generally portrayed as a time of depression. In Britain, the period was dominated by rising unemployment, which never fell below a million, and rose at its peak to more than three million. (This represented a far graver recession than the 'slumps' of the early 1980s and early 1990s because a larger proportion of the 'working' population was unemployed.) The collapse of the Western economies in 1929 meant that developments in health care must be seen against a background of national crisis.

There were also continuing *crises of subsistence* and of *disease*. The 1919 'flu pandemic brought a huge number of deaths in its train (perhaps 200 000 in Britain alone). There were epidemics of typhus and of cholera associated with a severe famine in Eastern Europe in 1920–2, causing the deaths of many millions.

5.1.1 Financing health care in Britain

In Britain, the inter-war years were also a time of *financial conservatism*. The Treasury fulfilled its traditional role of cutting short any reform involving significant public expenditure. The coverage of health and unemployment insurance was extended, but benefits were denied to the families of wage earners covered by the scheme. Despite this major shortcoming, there was no attempt at a wide-ranging reorganisation of health services nor any attempt to bring order into the funding of them.

There were a number of possible options facing policy makers in the inter-war years. These included the extension of the National Health Insurance (NHI) system (Figure 5.2), or basing health services firmly on the local authorities. The National Insurance Act 1911 and its subsequent revisions, as we have noted in Chapter 4, made only

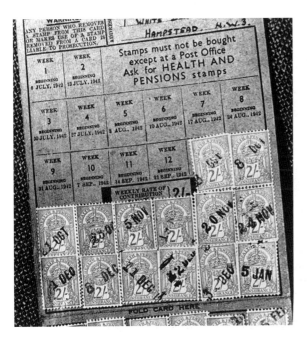

Figure 5.2 *The basis of National Health Insurance in Britain — a stamped up card for 1942. (Source: G. A. Paddon/ The Pilot Press)*

lower wage-earners eligible for state-subsidised insurance. But there were also other fundamental shortcomings in the insurance system. The system gave imperfect access to specialist services and many of those services, as you will see in the next section, were in a state of crisis — the voluntary hospitals in particular.

Other aspects of health administration were mostly left to local authorities, but here again there were problems, especially as the system of local taxation (rates) tended to result in the poorest services in the poorest areas. The downward trend of infant mortality and the decline in the major infectious diseases encouraged complacency and government economy. Exchequer contributions to the National Health Insurance fund fell in the 1920s and the government refused to finance any extra burden of access to health care out of taxation. Government was determined to retrench and refused to extend health insurance further.

5.1.2 The advance of social welfare

Social welfare systems were established in all Western European countries in this period, in spite of their contrasting political systems. Totalitarian regimes established in Italy and Germany produced their own solutions. Fascism, like its socialist antitheses, stressed the nation's health as was shown by Italian innovations in setting up a single (but inadequately financed) authority for maternal and child welfare, promulgating pronatalism geared to Mussolini's schemes for military conquest. At the same time, as part of the racial machinery of the Nazi state, there were efforts to promote a centralised welfare state by co-ordinating the hitherto autonomous sickness insurance funds, ending municipal autonomy by unifying state and municipal public health, and taking control of the Red Cross and other hitherto voluntary agencies.

Social welfare systems involving health care were also established elsewhere. The *New Deal* introduced under F. D. Roosevelt's Presidency in the 1930s included maternity and child health and child welfare services, all of them restricted to lower-income groups. The 'New Deal' was a kind of 'half-way house'; and when production began to recover in 1937, all government spending was cut back. Social democracies in Europe, most notably Sweden in the 1930s, introduced major programmes of social insurance and social reform — although *health* was not included in the minimum universal provision made in the decade after World War II for eradicating most of the major causes of poverty.

New directions for health care were apparent also in the post-revolutionary Soviet system. By the 1930s the Soviets could claim that the 1917 October Revolution had produced a radical change in the health position in the country and that they had successfully built the first mass national health service in the world. Western social and health reformers of the time were enthusiastic but often naive in their reports of Soviet achievements.

Various models of health care developed in Europe in the inter-war years; in the colonies, as you will see later in this chapter, a paternalistic model of health care prevailed.

It was not until after World War II in Britain that comprehensive reconstruction of health services was attempted. The election of a Labour government in 1945 was partly in reaction to the financial stringency of the National government in the 1930s. Radical reconstruction was achieved, as it had not been after World War I. The Labour government succeeded in establishing a system of comprehensive health care for the first time in Britain but, as you will see shortly, its organisation and funding were rather different to what might have been expected from looking at the inter-war health services. Neither of the apparent options facing policy makers after World War I — extension of National Health Insurance or increasing access to local-authority-based services — were in the event adopted.

5.2   The health-care system: chaos and change

Two questions concern us in this section: what was the state of the health-care system in Britain between the wars? and what led to the establishment of the post-war National Health Service?

5.2.1   A ramshackle system

Health-care provision after World War I was a patchwork of ramshackle and uncoordinated services. The health-care system in Britain proved increasingly chaotic in its funding, operation and with respect to access: the *voluntary hospitals* often limited their admissions to specialised cases; the *workhouse infirmaries* coped with the mentally handicapped, senile, 'venereal' and chronic and elderly patients; *local-authority ante-natal clinics* and *GP panel services* under the NHI Commission catered for a minority of the population. There was poor coordination between services and relations were often openly hostile, leading to criticism of clinical standards. Any attempts at wide-ranging rationalisation or reform of the system were prevented by the stance of governments in the inter-war period towards economic problems, which were concerned with financial retrenchment rather than investment.

The *Dawson Report* of 1920 provided an ambitious blueprint for the integration and coordination of preventive and curative services. Its recommendation of a two-tier network of GP and specialist **health centres**, in which services would be concentrated and coordinated, stressed planning of local GP-based services and the accessibility of specialist care. But, as Sir George Godber, later the Chief Medical Officer in the Department of Health, subsequently pointed out in the 1980s:

> The British did not really believe in the capacity of government at
> any level to run such human services in 1920. (Godber, 1983, p. 4)

The Dawson Committee's recommendations remained unimplemented in the inter-war years. As you will see in Chapter 6, health centres only became a reality in the 1960s and then in rather a different form. Models of health-care provision were discussed in the 1920s, but little was achieved in the inter-war years to rationalise a hotch-potch provision of overlapping and 'special interest' services, dealing with conditions such as tuberculosis or sexually transmitted disease.

More was achieved in other Western European countries. During the 1920s, socialist municipalities in cities like Berlin and Vienna promoted innovative schemes in social medicine[1] with health centres and model housing schemes. Soviet social medicine placed a high priority on preventive medicine, and medical services were shaped by theories that diseases were socially caused. *Preventive* health care became linked with the promotion of *positive health*. There were innovative experiments with birth-control clinics, child-guidance clinics (incorporating psychoanalysis) and cosmetic services for sufferers from facial cancers and other disfiguring illnesses. Feminists praised the liberality of Soviet abortion legislation (overlooking the fact that abortion was subject to medical decisions by a physician).

---

[1] Variations in the construction of what constituted 'social medicine' in different countries and in different periods were noted in Chapter 3.

In Britain, the recommendations of other committees of enquiry — for example, the 1918 Maclean Committee, or the 1926 Royal Commission on National Health Insurance, which attacked the hotch-potch of benefits and provision offered by the existing NHI scheme — all foundered in the face of government economy measures. The Economy Act 1926 incorporated a wide range of cuts, including the government contribution to the health insurance scheme which was reduced from two-ninths to one-seventh. Further cuts followed the world financial crisis of 1931; cuts in benefit to married women were made in 1932.

5.2.2 Hospitals in crisis

A significant weakness of the NHI scheme (in addition to the exclusion of dependants from medical treatment) was the *lack of hospital treatment*. But the hospital services in the inter-war period were a chaotic mixture: they were unevenly distributed and especially limited in rural areas (Figure 5.3). The voluntary hospitals were in a state of crisis: they provided 25 per cent of all beds and had increasing financial problems. In 1921, a Committee headed by Viscount Cave pointed out that they were suffering from rising costs and recommended a £1 million subvention from the state. The government provided only half the amount and refused any permanent commitment.

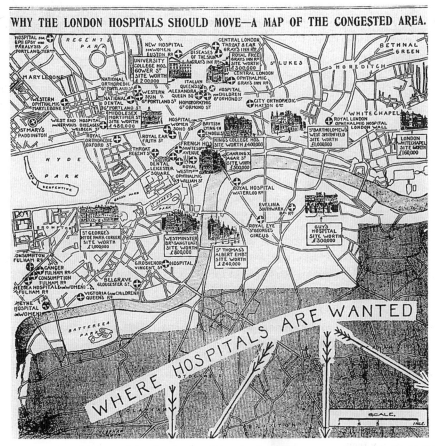

Figure 5.3 *This map of the distribution of London hospitals appeared in the* Daily Mail *in 1902, and graphically illustrates the mismatch between hospital location to the North of the Thames and the needs of the population living South of the river. (Source: Prochaska, F. K., 1992,* Philanthropy and the Hospitals of London, *The King's Fund, Clarendon Press, Oxford, Plate 2; originally published in the* Daily Mail, *27 November 1902)*

The voluntary hospitals' problems arose from a number of factors. First, the steadily improving capacities of medicine created a demand for better-equipped hospitals (Figure 5.4). Technical standards began to fall behind those in the USA. In the best American medical schools, *research* became an essential component of clinical medicine and hospital teaching after World War I; in Britain, such developments were slower to materialise.

Second, in British voluntary hospitals, the increased *salaries* of resident medical and nursing staff outstripped the growth in income from voluntary sources. The hospitals increasingly became dependent upon means-tested payments by patients, and upon payment from local authorities for treatment undertaken on their behalf. Hospital contributory systems were set up, but were expensive to operate. The Hospital Saturday and Sunday Funds (charities mentioned in Chapter 4) continued to supplement income. To meet increasing demand from would-be patients who earned above the £6 per week income limit, many hospitals expanded their wards for fee-paying patients. Even given these financial expedients, by the end of the 1930s, many of the voluntary hospitals were in financial difficulties, and the major teaching hospitals faced the worst of these problems.

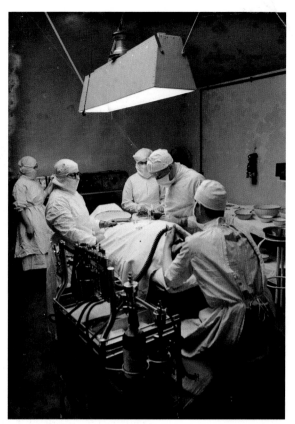

Figure 5.4 *Innovation in medical technology, for example in anaesthesia and blood transfusion, was stimulated by preparations for war. An operating theatre at Gravesend Hospital, Kent, photographed in 1939. (Source: Topham Picturepoint)*

- Look at Table 5.1. What changes strike you in the voluntary hospitals' sources of income between 1938 and 1947?

■ The proportion of income derived from donations declined and support from public authorities increased. The proportion derived from patient fees also declined, but remained a significant section of income.

The local-authority-based health service developed in a piecemeal way. The Local Government Act 1929 empowered local authorities to take over Poor Law infirmaries as *municipal hospitals*, but — outside London — the local authorities were slow to take up the opportunities offered by the 1929 Act.

Table 5.1 Sources of income of London voluntary hospitals, 1938 and 1947 (percentages).

Source of income	Percentage of income in 1938	1947
voluntary gifts	34	16
investments	16	8
public authority payments	8	46
other payments (patient fees, etc.)	42	30
total	100	100

Data from Eckstein, H. (1958) *The English Health Service*, Harvard University Press, Cambridge, Mass., p. 75.

5.2.3 Health-care finance in crisis

Finance was also a problem in the general operation of health services before World War II. The NHI scheme, based on the *approved societies* (which collected contributions and distributed cash benefits to claimants; see Chapter 4), faced increasing financial difficulties. The inter-war recession took a heavy toll on approved society finances, and by 1930, the huge profits revealed in 1925 at the second valuation had dwindled to virtually nothing. New support systems introduced in the early 1930s to help members who could not afford to keep up with contributions cost the societies huge sums. Even so, by 1934, over four million policies were in arrears.

The commercial approved societies were a powerful lobby and were not willing to 'pool' resources, as the 1926 Royal Commission had proposed. Even if this had been done, there would not have been sufficient funds to meet the needs of the working population. By the end of the inter-war period less than a dozen societies catered for nine-tenths of the insured population.

In addition, the number of Friendly Societies (to which workers might make 'sick club' contributions) fell sharply between 1918 and 1936 as almost one-third went out of existence. The health insurance system could do little other than survive; it failed to expand as its founders had hoped, mainly because of the political and economic climate within which it operated.

Although the operation of NHI has attracted much comment from historians (in part because of the debates about health insurance in the 1980s), the bulk of income for medical services in the inter-war period did not emanate from insurance funds, but from public authorities. Table 5.2 shows the major sources of revenue for health services in England and Wales in 1938–9.

● What strikes you about the patterns of funding revealed by the data in Table 5.2?

Table 5.2 Funding sources for health services in England and Wales, 1938–9.

Source of funding	£m	Percentage of total
Exchequer	3.0	4.6
rates (local property taxation)	40.3	61.1
NHI	11.2	17.0
voluntary sources	11.5	17.4

Data (rounded to the nearest decimal place) from C. Webster, previously unpublished, based on Treasury data.

■ The bulk of funding for health services was provided from the rates at the outbreak of war. Other contributions, including NHI, were roughly equal. (Note that the inter-war 'free market' system, often alluded to in policy debates around health-service funding in the 1980s, was in fact largely funded from public sources.)

5.2.4 Pressure for change

By the outbreak of war in 1939, a growing chorus of influential opinion demanded change to the chaotic and uncoordinated nature of British health services. The recently established *Socialist Medical Association* called for a free national health service administered by local authorities; and, as you will see shortly, the British Medical Association (BMA) also began to demand change.

Far more influential in terms of public opinion was a report published in 1937, by Political and Economic Planning, an independent and non-party group, on *The British Health Services* (PEP, 1937). The report attracted considerable attention, being welcomed on publication day by leading articles in eleven national and provincial daily newspapers. It also received a welcome from most of the specialist medical journals, and was subsequently republished in abridged form as a sixpenny Pelican paperback (PEP, 1939). The report concluded:

> The health services suffer greatly from confusion and overlapping, and in order to minimise this we propose their reorientation around the general practitioner, who should be enabled to bring the resources of the health services on the one hand into contact with the needs and peculiarities of the individual patient on the other … The general practitioner, however, cannot function satisfactorily unless he has behind him a range of better coordinated and less fragmentary health facilities of a specialised nature, to which cases can be readily referred where necessary … perhaps the most fundamental defect in the existing system is that it is overwhelmingly preoccupied with manifest and advanced diseases or disabilities and is more interested in enabling the sufferers to go on functioning in society somehow than in studying the nature of health and the means of producing and maintaining it. From this it naturally follows that millions of pounds are spent in looking after and trying to cure the victims of accidents and illnesses which need never have occurred if a fraction of this amount of intelligence and money had been devoted to tracing the social and economic causes of the trouble and making the necessary readjustments.
> (PEP, 1939, p. 205)

●   The PEP report identified the fragmentary and chaotic nature of the inter-war health system. What did it propose as solutions?

■   It placed emphasis on the role of the GP; on a coordinated specialist system backing up primary care; and on preventive as well as curative medicine.

The proposals in the report were in fact based on an extension of NHI; a completely free service was rejected on the grounds of cost.

5.2.5 The birth of the NHS

Change was in the air before 1939; but two crucial questions remain for us to consider: how much would have been achieved but for the impact of war? and what would have been achieved without the election of a Labour government in 1945?

The impact of war was certainly considerable. It led directly to the establishment of an *Emergency Medical Service*, planned before the war (and fully in operation by 1941) in order to cater for the large numbers of expected civilian bombing casualties (Figure 5.5 overleaf). Hospitals were run by existing authorities, but within a regional framework and with the Ministry of Health deciding what role each should play.

Figure 5.5 *Recovering military personnel take part in daily rehabilitative exercises on an Emergency Medical Service ward during World War II. (Source: Dunn, C. L., 1952,* Emergency Medical Services, *volume 1,* Plate XL, from the series, Medical History of the Second World War, HMSO, London)*

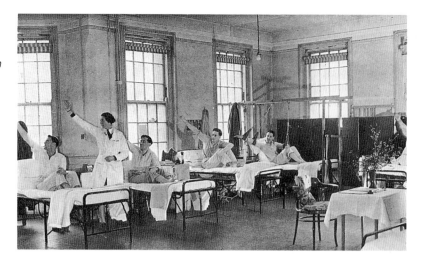

A further strong impetus to comprehensive proposals came with the publication of the Beveridge Report in 1942 on *Social Insurance and Allied Services* with its recommendations for a comprehensive health service. With the publication of the White Paper, *A National Health Service* (February 1944), the political temperature began to rise. The White Paper indicated the progress made since the outbreak of war. Whereas in 1941 the government had spoken only in terms of a *hospital* service, by 1944 a *comprehensive* service was planned, with free treatment financed from taxation.

> To ensure that everybody in the country — irrespective of means, age, sex and occupation — shall have equal opportunity to benefit from the best and most up-to-date medical and allied services available. To provide, therefore, for all who want it, a comprehensive service covering every branch of medical and allied activity. To divorce the case of health from questions of personal means or other factors irrelevant to it; to provide the service free of charge (apart from certain possible charges in respect of appliances) and to encourage a new attitude to health — the easier obtaining of advice early, the promotion of good health rather than only the treatment of bad. (Ministry of Health, 1944, p. 47)

However, it was becoming clear that one of the major planks of opposition to a national health service was the medical profession itself, and in particular the BMA. The latter resolutely opposed any move to a salaried medical service and local-authority control of health services for two reasons: first, the threat this offered to valued 'clinical freedom', and second, the echoes of nineteenth-century systems of lay control through the Friendly Societies and the Poor Law. The BMA also wanted an enhanced role for the voluntary hospitals and their consultants.

By 1945, the BMA had won substantial concessions on the 1944 White Paper. But the election of a Labour government and the arrival of Aneurin Bevan as Minister of Health changed the situation. Bevan espoused the *nationalisation* of the hospitals (bringing them into state ownership and control, under appointed local bodies) rather than local-authority control, which had been Labour Party policy until then. By doing so, he exploited already existing divisions within the medical profession between consultants and GPs, and, within the BMA, between the wealthier and the majority of poorly remunerated GPs. Although struggles between Bevan and sections of the medical profession continued even after the 'Appointed Day' for the inception of the **National Health Service (NHS)** on 5 July 1948, he had effectively won over both the influential consultants and the majority of GPs, neither of whom would have countenanced local-authority control.

The National Health Service Act 1946 established a nationally directed and financed *tripartite* system of (a) hospitals; (b) local authorities; (c) GPs, opticians and others. The plan for Scotland is shown in Figure 5.6; the equivalent for England appears in Chapter 6 (as Figure 6.5), where you will find further discussion of the tripartite system. Both the voluntary and local hospitals were nationalised and placed under the control of regional boards consisting of local-authority and voluntary hospital representatives. GP, dental, optician and pharmacy services were to be administered by Executive Councils, half professional and half lay. GPs remained **independent contractors** under the NHS in continuity with their status under the National Health Insurance scheme; each practitioner acted as an independent small business, contracting to supply defined NHI/NHS services to patients, in return for agreed *capitation* payments from the state, for each person opting to join the GP's list. Proposals for a salaried service were dropped. Counties and county boroughs retained responsibility for health centres, clinics and other services such as health visiting and ambulances.

The original intention was that health centres, provided by local authorities, would be the key coordinating agency between the three services. But, as you will see in Chapter 6, this proposal was abandoned; you will notice that health centres were not even featured in the pictorial plan of the new health services circulated in Scotland (Figure 5.6), while in England and Wales at this planning stage they were given a central place as the most important local authority function.

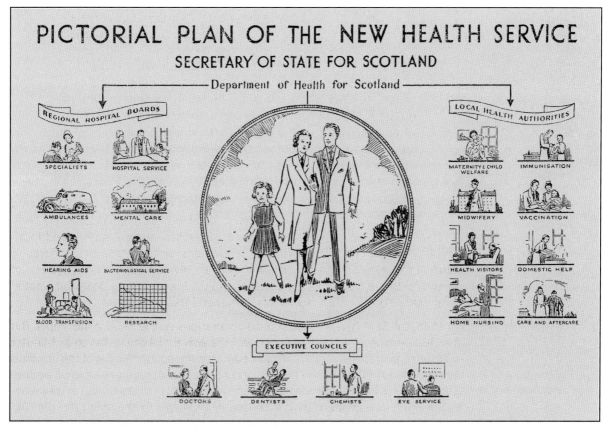

Figure 5.6   *Diagram produced in 1948 to explain the organisation of the new National Health Service in Scotland. Comparison with Figure 4.12 reveals how much of the Medical Officer of Health's former 'empire' in local government was transferred to the NHS. In Scotland, Teaching Hospitals were absorbed into the regional hospital organisations, whereas they were given separate status in England and Wales; and there were no arrangements for provision of health centres. (Source: Department of Health for Scotland, 1948,* Your Health Service: How it will work in Scotland, *HMSO, Edinburgh)*

Bevan's achievement was a considerable one. It is easy enough to think of the NHS as a 'natural' development from the pre-war discussions, but historical research has shown that the much trumpeted mood of 'war-time consensus' was largely illusory. Under the Labour Minister of Health, supported by key civil servants in the Ministry of Health, reform proceeded further and faster than it would have done under the 1944 White Paper.

The following memory of the arrival of the new service gives some indication of what it meant for poor families.

> I well remember our Brian being born. He was delivered by a doctor up at Oldham, a Scotsman, he got called up and killed in the war, so we never paid for Brian. The doctors were very good. You'd go to the doctor. He had your name and address. And after, you got a bill, and if you couldn't pay it, which very few people could, each doctor had his own collector. The collectors used to come round each week and you'd pay sixpence. My wife's father and mother used to say they'd never be straight in their lifetime. When the National Health came in all them doctors' bills were written off. The collectors always used to be the same type who were park keepers in them days — they'd be no use today, kids'd throw them in pond — but they were always little wizened fellers.
> (Gray, 1986, p. 88)

Some historians have argued that the establishment of the NHS was not unique, and that the principle of *regionalisation* (the regional planning and organisation of health services) was being established as a basic form of service organisation in many countries at this time. Certainly, in the period in which the NHS was being set up in Britain, parallel schemes were in operation or preparation elsewhere in Europe, Australia and the USA. But there were numerous differences of detail of funding and of access.

The European insurance-based systems were founded on non-governmental, non-profit-making public bodies, while in the USA insurance was provided by commercial companies. The British system was *unique* in its free and open access to all. All of the systems were dominated by hospital-based medicine. The unusual *nationalised* hospital system in Britain possessed certain advantages, but among its disadvantages were the fragmentation of the health system, an escalation of hospital costs, and a lack of democratic accountability. These drawbacks became increasingly apparent as time passed, as you will see in Chapter 6.

5.3   Lay care and boundaries with formal care: tipping the balance

You have seen how welfare systems were established in the inter-war period in a number of European countries. But the role of domestic, family and neighbourhood networks in providing health care remained central, in particular for poor families. The historian Elizabeth Roberts has collected memories of people living in Lancashire in the 1920s and 1930s. Here is one reminiscence. Mrs A. as a child, was part of a very large extended family in Preston. Her aunt, her mother's oldest sister, lived next door and was regarded as the family's expert:

> She was the one who, if we were ill, my mother always wanted guidance from. If anything was wrong with us it would be 'go and bring aunt Martha'.

The grandmother of the family had a stroke:

> She wasn't quite 71 and she was 77 when she died. She was in bed all the time. It paralysed her all down one side and she could get out of bed … but couldn't get back. So my auntie next door took her and she had her in the front room in the bed downstairs and my mother looked to her in the daytime and auntie looked to her at night. (Roberts, 1984, p. 51)

● Compare this description with the role of family members in health care today — what differences strike you?

■ Most obviously that there is no mention of any professional medical intervention in the home or any perceived role for institutional care. The old lady does not go to hospital or to a home; care is confined within the extended family.

● In Chapter 2 you read criticisms of the idea of a 'golden age' when every family looked after its own relations. How would you assess this quotation as historical evidence?

■ You should be aware of the limitation of oral evidence. This situation of informal care from the family was undoubtedly the case here, but may not have been universally the rule. It also ignores the contribution of lay care *outside* kinship networks, for example by friends and neighbours.

5.3.1 Establishing the boundaries

Traditions of lay care persisted, in part because of the limitations of existing formal services (see, for example, Figure 5.7a). The rudimentary statutory services were piecemeal, and the lack of service provision especially affected women and children. Only in a minority of cases would children's health problems be detected and treated under the school medical service (see Figure 5.7b).

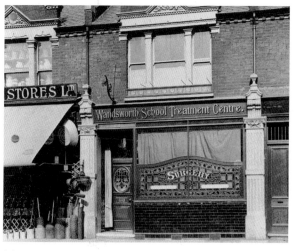

(a)

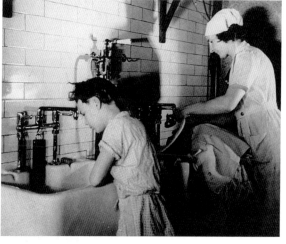

(b)

Figure 5.7   *(a) Wandsworth School Treatment Centre operating room, photographed in 1911. (b) A regular head inspection by the 'nit' nurse with her comb and bowl of disinfectant, was the way in which most children came into contact with the School Medical Service. (Source, both from: London Metropolitan Archives)*

- Can you recall why health care before the NHS was particularly inadequate for women and children?

■ The NHI scheme did not cover dependants, so women and children had no formal entitlement to 'panel' GP care.

It was customary in some working-class families to belong to the local hospital scheme, but this only covered emergencies and did not provide regular medical care. Maternity and child welfare clinics were established under local-authority control especially after the Maternal and Child Welfare Act of 1918, but provision of these was patchy and often encountered opposition from local GPs, who feared the competition emanating from the clinics.

There was also, at least in the period immediately after the war, a current of popular disbelief in the *efficacy* of formal health-care provision. Health visitors provide an instance where there are grounds for uncertainty over their effectiveness. During the interwar period, the professional status of health visitors increased and their training became formalised. They played a key part in the maternity and infant welfare services. The health visitor advised mothers and monitored the health of their infants. Sir Arthur Newsholme attributed to the work of health visitors, the greatly increasing 'knowledge of child hygiene and its wider application in the community' (Newsholme, 1925, p. 216). Health visitors certainly made some impact, but they were few in numbers, distributed inappropriately, and there was a limit to the effectiveness of their exhortatory methods. For instance, even in 1936 less than one third of expectant mothers received any advice from health visitors (PEP, 1937, p. 98). Where their services were available, health visitors seem to have become increasingly more humane and approachable. Therefore, they became less feared and more welcomed by poor women, but they were still liable to pay insufficient heed to the poverty which lay at the root of the difficulties faced by mothers and their infants.

Unqualified midwives also continued to be widely used: they were cheaper than qualified ones, they were generally thought friendlier and less 'starchy' and there was hardly any popular criticism of their competence. The Midwives Act of 1902 had made the training of new midwives and the registration of established ones compulsory, but untrained women continued to practise throughout the inter-war years. A coordinated midwifery service involving trained practitioners (see Figure 5.8) was not widely available until after World War II.

There was also a different working-class health 'culture'; and health beliefs were not the same as those in other sections of society. For example, there was a concern for death as well as for health. Almost all families would attempt to contribute to some form of death insurance. Elizabeth Roberts comments that:

> ... the strengths of working-class mores, and the demands of working class respectability, were such that the little surplus income there was, went, not towards health care for the living, but towards ensuring a decent funeral for the dead. (Roberts, 1980, p. 40)

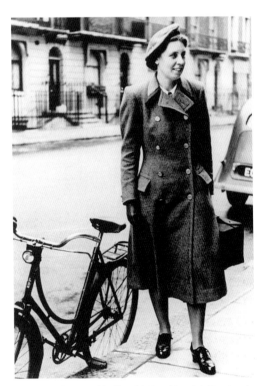

Figure 5.8 *A midwife with her bicycle, the classic image of the new trained and professionalised service. (Source: Royal College of Midwives)*

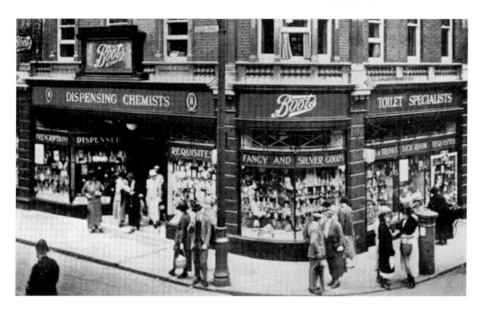

Figure 5.9 *This main branch of Boots in Pelham Street, Nottingham (photographed in 1935) was situated at a key city centre site, adjacent to the Council House (town hall). The imposing facade reflects the size of the market for self-medication and toiletries in the inter-war years. (Source: The Boots Company, plc, Nottingham)*

Self-medication was still the norm, as in the nineteenth century. Boots the Chemist continued its nineteenth-century expansion (see Figure 5.9) and Woolworths became the major supplier of spectacles in the United Kingdom.

There was also a widespread reliance on well-established popular remedies. Robert Roberts, who was brought up in a Salford slum, remembers what was used:

> At weekends people purged themselves with great doses of black draught, senna pods, cascara sagrada, and their young with Gregory powder, licorice powder and California syrup of figs … the working class had an awful fear of constipation … Pills sold at a penny a box, any doubts as to their potency being quieted by the venerable image of their maker smiling from the lid. He had cause for amusement. Nearly all the pills appeared to possess a dual purpose: they 'attacked' at one and the same the ills of two intestines 'Head and Stomach', 'Blood and Stomach', 'Back and Kidney', 'Back and Bladder' and indeed almost any pair of organs that could in decency be named. (Roberts, 1971, pp. 124–5)

● How could you investigate the extent of self-medication in the 1930s?

■ You could draw on your own or local experiences of self-medication now. You could talk to a sample of older people about the remedies that were most commonly used and how they were obtained. (You could also look at books listed in the References, such as Schweitzer, P. (ed.) (1985) *Can We Afford the Doctor?*, for reminiscences of self-medication.)

The role of local pharmacists in lay medical care was considerable. They frequently provided diagnosis and advice. One remembered in an interview:

> We were the first filter as it were … we had to do a bit of diagnosing in our own way and be responsible for it. Would they for example bring children in and say 'What is the matter?' Oh my goodness yes. What sort of things would be the matter with them? It might be just nettle rash, it might be measles — very often it was measles and teething trouble, a little feverish, constipation or something

like that, the usual childish ailments but we had to be very, very careful in case there was little yellow spots behind the throat and then write to the doctor.... You didn't charge for this advice? Oh dear no. Anything had to be inexpensive ... (Roberts, 1980, p. 45)

● What strikes you about the role of the pharmacist here by comparison with the occupation's present position?

■ In some respects, the current role of the pharmacist is not that different. (It is interesting that policy documents on pharmacy in the 1990s have emphasised the role of the pharmacist as a first-line practitioner.)

5.3.2 Rising aspirations

These patterns of lay care were in many respects little different from those we have described in the nineteenth century. But change was detectable in the inter-war period, in particular in *aspirations to health*. Higher standards of living and shorter hours of work, together with the extension of paid holidays to wider groups of workers, provided an impetus for an increase in almost every type of leisure activity. The widespread popularity of the cinema (a survey of Liverpool in 1937 found that 40 per cent of the population went at least once a week), radio and commercial magazines, served to raise social expectations and made information about health more widely available.

Active participation became the norm: sport, hiking, holiday camps (which had accommodation for more than half a million people by 1939), all found increasing popularity. Physical recreation and fitness was an aspiration for large numbers of working- and lower-middle-class people, although Britain was in general backward in providing state facilities for recreation, especially where they were needed most. Physical fitness was also an important part of preventive medicine in Germany and other central European states, for example Czechoslovakia. However, outside observers were suspicious of it as militaristic in intention.

5.3.3 Birth control and maternity services

In this period, family health and hygiene was promoted as a special part of a woman's 'role'. Under-population rather than over-population was seen as a threat, but reformers were also concerned about the *differential* birth rate. The fear was that the 'wrong' people (the poor and the unfit) would breed and might overwhelm the educated and upper classes of society. These 'eugenic' ideas have been a continuing theme in the birth-control movement, in addition to humanitarian concerns for women dragged down by endless pregnancies.

Organisations such as Women's Institutes and the Women's Co-operative Guild promoted birth control, hygiene and responsibility for family health among the working classes. The most important advocate of birth control and a more open attitude to sexual matters was Dr Marie Stopes. The popularity of her writings reflected a massive public demand for birth-control advice. In 1921, she opened her first clinic in Holloway Road, North London. In 1930, Stopes and others formed the National Birth Control Council, which in 1939 became the Family Planning Association.

Experiments in improving the diet of mothers were undertaken in the 1930s in South Wales and in the North East by the National Birthday Trust Fund and the

People's League of Health. These had an indeterminate effect on the maternal mortality rate, which continued to rise across the classes in the inter-war years, largely unaffected by improvements in maternity services. By 1939, however, sulphonamides were a more important means of reducing the death rate among women in childbirth.

● What does Figure 5.10 indicate about changes in the level of maternal mortality?

■ From 1900 to the mid-1930s there was little change in the rate. A steep and sustained decline followed. This, so it is argued, was associated both with effective drug therapies and with the increase in trained midwifery.

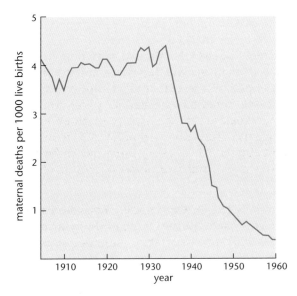

Figure 5.10 *The trend in maternal mortality in England and Wales, 1905–60. (Data from MacFarlane, A. and Mugford, M., 1984,* Birth Counts: Statistics of Pregnancy and Childbirth, *HMSO, London; graph from Loudon, I., 1991,* On maternal and infant mortality, *1900–1960, Social History of Medicine,* **4**, *p. 38)*

Changes in attitudes towards childbirth reflected wider changes in lay attitudes towards formal health services. The trend was towards medicalised childbirth; in 1927 only 15 per cent of births took place in hospital, but by 1946, this had risen to 54 per cent. This trend gave obstetrics a new status; it was also supported by women who recognised the need for more aseptic procedures. It thus reflected both medical and consumer demand and also developments taking place in the USA and across Europe (although not in the Netherlands, where home births remained the norm).[2]

In itself, hospitalised childbirth was not an essential component of maternal and infant health. In the inter-war period in the United Kingdom, most births still took place at home, but here, too, there was a less fatalistic attitude to childbirth and a lessening of women's role in assisting at the event. The help and advice of outside trained experts — the doctor, health visitor and clinic — were increasingly referred to instead of relatives and neighbours. The final tipping of the balance towards professional help came only after the establishment of the NHS in the late 1940s.

[2] The trend towards hospital births in the UK, and the continuation of home births in the Netherlands, persists to the present day, and is discussed further in *Birth to Old Age: Health in Transition* (Open University Press, 2nd edn 1995; colour-enhanced 2nd edn 2001), Chapter 3.

5.4 Public-health services: in search of an identity

The reluctance of the laity to seek professional help may have been prolonged by a significant mismatch between the issues that working people saw as affecting their own and their family's health — low pay, unemployment, poor housing and nutritional standards — and the concerns of public-health doctors and the services they controlled.

In the nineteenth century, environmental issues were central to public health, and were the responsibility of the emergent **public-health profession** advising governments or local authorities. In the twentieth century such environmental issues did not disappear, as you will see from the following discussion of housing, incomes and nutrition. But they became less central to the *work* of the MOH and other public-health doctors employed in local government, and to the *ideology* of public health to which these doctors adhered. The inter-war years were, in one sense, a 'golden age' of public health, when public-health doctors had more responsibility at the local level than before or since. In another sense, they were a period of crisis when the profession and the ideas of public health failed to adapt themselves to the realities of poverty and unemployment in the Depression.

Despite a dramatic growth in the statutory powers of public-health departments in local authorities, the nineteenth-century concern to deal with all aspects of the environment and housing as a means of promoting health and cleanliness gradually disappeared. Increasingly, public-health departments focused on what the *individual* should do to ensure personal hygiene; for example, the instruction of women in family hygiene at the infant welfare clinics mentioned earlier. Public health justified its emphasis on clinic work with mothers and children as 'applied physiology', a kind of preventive clinical medicine. Both before and after the transition to the NHS, this brought MOHs into competition with GPs, who also claimed control over this work.

Public health established itself substantially at the local level in the inter-war years. As indicated in the previous chapter, especially by Figure 4.12, public-health departments assumed an ever-widening range of responsibilities. Between 1918 and 1939, some twenty pieces of legislation extending the remit of *local-authority health services* were passed. By 1939, local authorities were providing maternal and child welfare services; the school medical service; TB clinics and treatment; infectious disease, ear, nose and throat and VD services; even embryonic social worker services; and *health centres* — the most elaborate being that built by Finsbury Borough Council in 1938 (Figure 5.11; see also Figure 5.1).

In addition, the Local Government Act of 1929 allowed local authorities to take over the Poor Law hospitals. Finally the Cancer Act of 1939 placed responsibility on local authorities for the development of regional cancer schemes. This was a substantial increase in power and influence, but, as the historian Jane Lewis has argued, it also meant that public-health practice had no clear guiding philosophy during the inter-war years. The *aims* of public health were formulated according to the functions *actually being carried out*. Public-health departments added to their responsibilities without questioning what was distinctive about public health.

Looking back in 1939, R. M. F. Picken, Professor of Preventive Medicine at the Welsh School of Medicine, felt that the profession of MOH had gone down the wrong path:

> Public health might have developed on very different lines. It might well have remained purely preventive, grown out of sanitation to

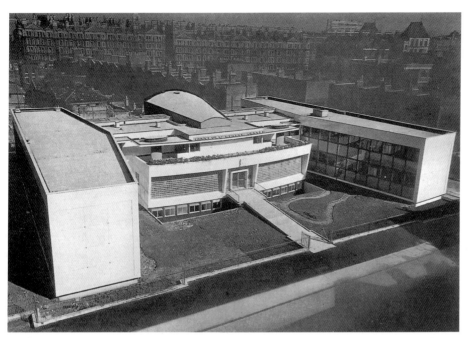

Figure 5.11 *Finsbury Health Centre, designed by the avant garde Russian architect Berthold Lubetkin (also famous for the modernist penguin pool at London Zoo), was completed by Finsbury Borough Council in 1938. It became a symbol of the possibilities for developing positive health (as Figure 5.1 demonstrates), and was operated by the local authority, which made it symbolic in a different way since, in the event, the NHS programme for local-authority health centres in England and Wales was abandoned until the 1960s. (Source: Allan, J., 1992, Berthold Lubetkin: Architecture and the Condition of Progress, RIBA, London. By kind permission of John Allan)*

> be concerned mainly with the problems of the nutrition of the people, their physical fitness, and public education generally, and kept away from any sort of medical advice and treatment of the individual … (Quoted in Lewis, 1986, p. 29)

● Picken thought that public health should have kept away from individual medical advice and treatment. What was his suggestion for public health?

■ His view, although broader than questions of medical treatment, is still focused on prevention of disease at the *personal* level and *individual responsibility* for health rather than the environmentalism of nineteenth-century public health.

5.4.1 The neglect of social causes of ill-health

One result of public health's 'administrative focus' during this period was its relative neglect of sources of danger to the people's health. Public-health doctors were on the whole little involved in the debates on the effects of *unemployment* on health. They did not bring to public notice the large number of cases of *malnutrition* in the depressed areas, or the widespread sickness among *childbearing* women.

British people during the 1920s and 1930s did experience some overall improvement in living standards. Average life expectancy was up and mortality down; and inter-war surveys found poverty levels lower than in the late Victorian investigations. But social class and regional disparities persisted and in some cases worsened. This was demonstrated through surveys of *diet and nutrition*. Sir John Boyd Orr's study,

Food, Health and Income, published in 1936, showed that a tenth of the population, including a fifth of all children, were chronically ill-nourished. Dr George M'Gonigle, the MOH for Stockton-on-Tees, found that in 1936 the death rate among the poorer section of the local population (families with an income of 25–35 shillings per week) — who spent only 3 shillings a head per week on food — was twice that of the more affluent (families with an income of 70–80 shillings per week), whose food expenditure was 6 shillings a head.

● Figure 5.12 is taken from M'Gonigle's report. What general point does it illustrate? And what cautionary note should we bear in mind when interpreting these data?

■ M'Gonigle's data make a strong connection between poor diet and poor physical condition. He relates 'unsatisfactory' diet to the incidence of a large range of physical defects (he discounted diarrhoea, which was the result of infection, but is in fact exacerbated by under-nutrition). However, he has used his own definition of satisfactory and unsatisfactory diets, and has neglected the effects of repeated illness on general health.[3]

DIAGRAM 2   TABLE 10   EFFECT OF DIET ON PHYSICAL CONDITIONS

KEY. GROUP WITH SATISFACTORY DIET
GROUP WITH UNSATISFACTORY DIET
DIFFERENCE BETWEEN GROUPS

BONE DEFECTS
31%
55%   DIFFERENCE   24

PHARYNGEAL CONDITIONS
10%
24%   14

DENTAL DECAY
18%
37%   19

SQUINT
1%
6%   5

ANAEMIA
22%
41%   19

DIARRHOEA
40%
39%   −1

BRONCHITIS
33%
40%   7

OTORRHOEA
9%
14%   5

The association between *unemployment*, poverty, under-nutrition and health during this period is also controversial, as it remains today[4] (see Figure 5.13). In the 1930s, a general overall improvement in health disguised a tremendous regional diversity. As always, ill-health and malnutrition had the greatest effect on women and children.

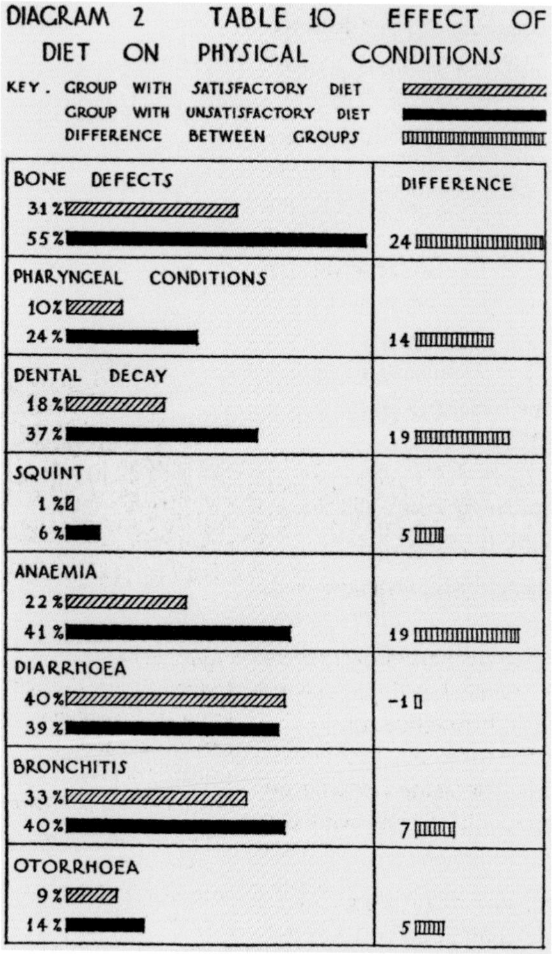

Figure 5.12 *Dr M'Gonigle's tabulation of the relationship between diet and poor physical condition. (Reproduced from M'Gonigle, G. and Kirby, J., 1936,* Poverty and Public Health, *Victor Gollancz, London, p. 98)*

[3] Problems associated with defining an 'adequate' diet and distinguishing the health-damaging effects of under-nutrition from those of repeated infections, particularly in childhood, are discussed in World Health and Disease (Open University Press, 3rd edn 2001), Chapter 11.

[4] See World Health and Disease (Open University Press, 3rd edn 2001), Chapter 10 for a full discussion.

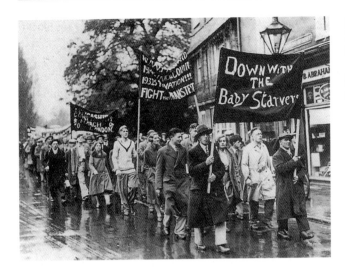

Figure 5.13 *Supported by students, the Lancashire contingent of the hunger marchers leave Oxford for High Wycombe, 22 October 1932. (Source: From Laybourne, K., 1990, Britain on the Breadline, Alan Sutton Publishing, Gloucester)*

5.4.2 Housing and health

Regional diversity was also evident in the attempts to improve *housing conditions* — part of the public-health mandate in the nineteenth century. Slum clearance got under way to a significant extent after World War I, although progress was patchy. Rents were controlled and subsidies offered for private house-building.

Between 1931 and 1939, local authorities built over 700 000 houses, supposedly rehousing four-fifths of existing slum dwellers (the numbers in the slums were actually underestimated). In Leeds, the Quarry Hill Scheme saw 2 000 slum houses demolished and 938 new flats built at a cost of £1.5 million. New standards for space and design were laid down. But the most dramatic developments took place in private house building, and poor housing remained one of the most pressing social issues.

New council estates (see Figure 5.14) tended to be occupied by skilled and white collar workers, leaving behind the poor in rapidly deteriorating housing stock. London had one of the worst problems: a survey in 1933 revealed that almost half a million people in the capital were suffering from overcrowding.

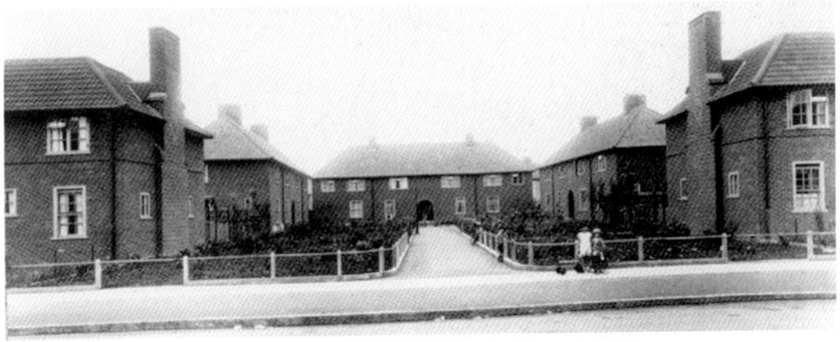

The lead in raising the questions about the complex relationship between housing, unemployment, low pay and nutrition in the 1930s came from political lobby groups such as the Children's Minimum Council, not from within the public-health profession. In the 1940s, moves were made to reorientate public-health practice round the new academic discipline of **social medicine**. This aimed to link the *planning* of health and social services to the *needs* of the population. Social medicine became an academic specialty, its flagship the Oxford Institute of Social Medicine, with the philosopher clinician, John Ryle, as Professor.

Figure 5.14 *This London County Council estate at Dagenham provided a good standard of new housing in the inter-war period, typical of the house-building programme of the time. (Source: London Metropolitan Archives)*

However, this initiative failed to influence the medical schools and medical education, and was alienated from the practice of public health. Ryle's chair at Oxford was not filled when he died in 1950, by which date social medicine was seen as a failed experiment, a telling indication of the declining importance of environmental issues and public health. As you will see in the next section, the tension between academic clinicians and the MOHs was just one of many boundary disputes among health-care occupations.

5.5   Formal health-care occupations: disputed boundaries

5.5.1   Regulating the 'para-medical' professions

Health-care occupations in general underwent considerable development in the inter-war years and there was increasing professionalisation among what (by the 1960s) had become known as the **professions supplementary to medicine**[5]: opticians, dentists, radiographers, chiropodists and physiotherapists. Whatever their many differences, health-care occupations were, and remain, similar in their quests for occupational monopolies. Some of the supplementary professions attracted medical patronage, but their ambitions soon began to clash with those of groups of physicians and surgeons also intent on shaping their own specialist fields.[6]

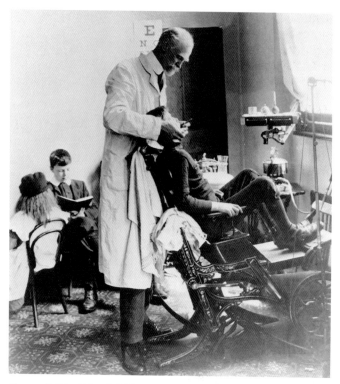

Figure 5.15   *School children undergoing dental inspections in 1911; dentists were not state registered until 1921. (Source: London Metropolitan Archives)*

These clashes mounted, particularly after the 1914–18 war. The new Ministry of Health and the medical professional bodies were forced through several stages of response. The sociologist, Gerald Larkin, has characterised these as follows:

> … the initial stage was an often contemptuous dismissal of 'auxiliary' ambitions by the Ministry and medical profession; this was followed by the offer of a compromise by the Ministry and the doctors, usually involving lower status alternatives to an occupational monopoly; and finally came the eventual collapse of this alliance of medical and Ministry interests and the concession of the case for further forms of state registration. (Larkin, 1987, pp. 51–2)

The evolutionary process defined by Larkin began in the 1920s. The final establishment of registration and monopolies took place in the 1950s and will be discussed in Chapter 6.

Nurses and dentists (Figure 5.15) were successful in securing state registration respectively in 1919 and 1921. This encouraged smaller groups such as the opticians to emulate these achievements. But the Ministry and medical officials worked together to frustrate claims which, in their view, meant licensing inferior alternatives to medical practice. Ophthalmic opticians, for example, expressed their aspirations for professional status through the 1920s, but their claims to share the sight-testing

[5] See *World Health and Disease* (Open University Press, 3rd edn 2001), Chapter 10 for a full discussion.

[6] Moves by the medical profession to exclude or to incorporate (in a subordinate role) other health-care professions are also discussed in *Medical Knowledge: Doubt and Certainty* (Open University Press, 2nd edn 1994; colour-enhanced 2nd edn 2001), Chapter 2.

market were side-tracked into a Ministry of Health Committee of Enquiry, dominated by medical interests.

Similarly, a 1928 chiropody bill was opposed. Limited recognition was achieved in the 1920s by radiographers who were allowed 'to describe the appearances of X-ray plates' to doctors, but not to attempt diagnosis. Physiotherapists were also advanced via a royal charter, granted in 1920 through the aristocratic connections of early masseuses; but this also expressly forbade treatment without medical referral.

By 1928, the BMA council had decided on a policy of shaping, rather than automatically rejecting, auxiliary ambitions in order to establish the doctors' authority over the other groups. In the 1930s, the BMA worked for a Board of Registration of Medical Auxiliaries, which was set up in 1936 under BMA control. Its constitution had two features: a permanent medical voting majority; and a duty for all affiliated to it to work *exclusively* under medical direction and supervision. But the Board failed and was unable to reconcile a number of dilemmas. Expansion of its remit was opposed by existing affiliates because this diluted the scarcity value of medical expertise. There were, in fact, few requests for affiliation because the entry terms required a thorough subordination to BMA interests in order to satisfy demands for medical control.

After World War II, as the inception of the NHS came closer, the BMA pressed for the Board's inclusion as an instrument of management under its own control. But there was considerable government opposition to this course of action. In the ten years after the NHS was established (as you will see in Chapter 6), the BMA failed to secure its policy, while the state was pushed into a more immediate managerial responsibility for qualified health-care workers within the NHS.

The BMA, as you can see from this brief history of its relationship with the 'para-medical' professions, was growing in power as the trades union representing doctors. The BMA also aspired to influence national health policy and developed its views on the evolution of the health services. It aimed to put the National Health Insurance panel at the centre of health-care organisation. The BMA joined the debate on the health service when it issued its proposals for *A General Medical Service for the Nation* in 1930. This suggested a system of health insurance for virtually all adults and their dependants. By 1938, when a revised version was issued, it had almost been overtaken by events. But its basic principle was a faithful reflection of the more idealistic approach to health care which was gaining acceptance at this time:

> That the system of medical science should be directed to the achievement of positive health and the prevention of disease no less than to the relief of sickness. (BMA, 1938, p. 8)

5.5.2 The role of the general practitioner

The BMA's version of a national health service put the GP centre stage. The NHI panel scheme suited GPs well. By 1938, 90 per cent of all GPs were participating. At this date the scheme covered low wage earners, but in 1942 it was extended to a substantial group of non-manual workers.

A striking feature of the BMA's 'trades-union' activities in the run-up to the NHS was its defence of GP panel practice. Doctors had come to appreciate the NHI scheme because it provided a firm basic income for those practitioners who could expect to earn least from private practice, for instance the small fees that they could recover from the dependants of insured persons on their list

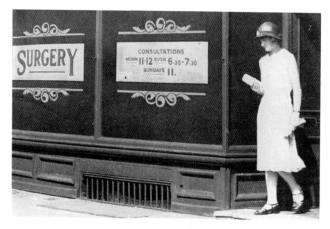

Figure 5.16 *A patient leaving a GP panel practice surgery in the 1930s. Panel practices were generally in less well-to-do districts. When a panel doctor sold his practice to another GP, the patients usually remained on the panel of the purchaser. (Source: Dorien Leigh/The Pilot Press)*

(see Figure 5.16). Those GPs in more affluent areas treated their NHI fees as a sideline to lucrative prizes available from their private practice. Thus there existed big income differentials in general practice, which explains the strong resistance by better-off practitioners to salaried service, which they asserted would destroy the incentives to excellence in the existing competitive situation. The advocates of salaried service retorted that the competitive system penalised those doctors attempting to provide a decent level of service to the poor. Table 5.3 shows the pattern of GP earnings in the inter-war period.

● What strikes you about the trends shown in Table 5.3?

■ GPs were showing a substantial increase in earnings, which was proportionately higher than that for most other groups, particularly in the period of the Depression in the 1930s.

Table 5.3   GP earnings in the inter-war period, compared with average earnings in selected professions and occupations.

	1913–14 £	1922–4 £	1936–8 £	Change 1913–14 to 1922–4 %	Change 1922–4 to 1936–8 %
higher professionals					
GPs	395	756	1 030	91	36
barristers	478	1 124	(1 090)[1]	135	−3
solicitors	568	1 096	(1 238)	93	13
dentists	368	601	676	63	12
clergy	206	332	370	61	11
army officers	170	390	205	129	−47
engineers	292	468	n/a	60	n/a
chemists	314	556	512	77	−8
higher professionals[2]	328	582	634	77	9
lower professionals[2]	155	320	308	106	−4
all men (including manual workers)	94	180	186	91	4

[1] Figures in brackets are more uncertain. [2] Average weighted by the constituent numbers employed in corresponding years. n/a = data not available (Data from Digby, A. and Bosanquet, N., 1988, Doctors and patients in an era of National Health Insurance and private practice, 1913–39, *Economic History Review*, **41**, p. 77, Table 3)

The pay structure of GPs at this time is well illustrated by Dr G. L. Pierce, who practised in a mining valley in South Wales and gave evidence to the Spens committee on GP pay in 1946. He varied his private fee according to the patient: a more prosperous person might be charged half or even 1 guinea for a service while a poorer person would pay 3s 6d or 5s for the same service. This system was sometimes referred to as 'climbing over the backs of the poor into the pockets of the rich'. It was an argument used later to justify the existence of pay beds in NHS hospitals; these were said to subsidise access by non-paying patients.

The GP panel system, although it suited doctors well in some respects, also led to a sense of poverty and insecurity among many GPs and demanded long working hours (in England one half day off during the week and an early finish on Sunday was common practice).

The relationship between general practice and the hospital system had its difficulties. The growth of hospital contributory schemes (already discussed earlier in this chapter) worried GPs. By admitting patients directly to hospital, it threatened to short-circuit the referral system they had established at the turn of the century. Many GPs resorted to establishing *cottage hospitals*, the numbers of which expanded from fewer than 200 at the turn of the century to over 600 by 1935. This ensured that GPs continued to be involved in surgery; in fact, we still call their premises the 'surgery'. In 1938–9 it was estimated that 2.5 million surgical operations were performed by GPs — an average of three per doctor per week. (Since the health service changes of the 1990s, the amount of 'day surgery' carried out by GPs has again been on the increase.)

In Europe, the relationship between general practice and hospitals developed differently. Sickness insurance schemes meant that patients had direct access to specialists rather than being referred by their GP as in Britain. Specialists often developed their own elaborate private clinic facilities rather than being hospital-based. Specialism thus developed further in the rest of Europe during this period. For example, families would consult a paediatric specialist about their children's ailments — the 'family doctor' in the British sense, caring for all family members, was less common in Europe except in rural areas. In the USA also, specialisation of doctors persisted (as Open University students should recall from the Reader article by Rosemary Stevens,[7] which you read when studying Chapter 4).

5.5.3 The crisis in nursing

The NHI system had greatly enhanced the prestige of the medical profession, but the status of other health-care professions was more indeterminate. This is emphasised by the deepening crisis which beset *nursing* in this period.

Registration of nurses — achieved in 1919 — was not the hoped-for solution in terms of occupational monopoly and status. Many practising nurses failed to meet the requirements for registration and yet still regarded themselves as nurses. The state had become a substantial employer of nurses and so had an interest in the matter. It did not want to grant **registered nurses** a monopoly when it was possible to keep the ranks of nursing more open and costs down. The issue of who should and should not be on the register continued to be an area of contention in this period and one in which the Ministry of Health played an important role. It is clear that the advance of the public sector led to improvement in the status of nurses because of the imposition of standardisation of conditions and terms of employment. Nurses came to enjoy the benefits of other local government employees. Certification was helpful for grading nurses on the local government wage scales.

---

[7] 'The evolution of the health-care systems in the United States and the United Kingdom: similarities and differences', in *Health and Disease: A Reader* (Open University Press, 2nd edn 1995; 3rd edn 2001).

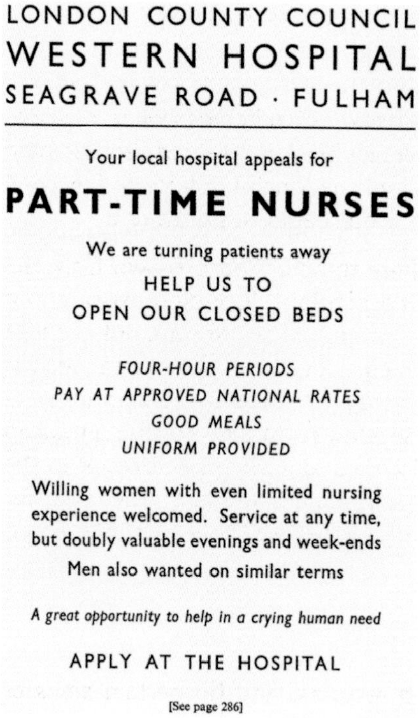

Figure 5.17 *A typical 'window card' used by London County Council hospitals in 1947. (Source: Ross, J. S., 1952,* The National Health Service in Great Britain, *Oxford University Press, London, p. 287)*

LONDON COUNTY COUNCIL
WESTERN HOSPITAL
SEAGRAVE ROAD · FULHAM

Your local hospital appeals for

PART-TIME NURSES

We are turning patients away

HELP US TO
OPEN OUR CLOSED BEDS

FOUR-HOUR PERIODS
PAY AT APPROVED NATIONAL RATES
GOOD MEALS
UNIFORM PROVIDED

Willing women with even limited nursing experience welcomed. Service at any time, but doubly valuable evenings and week-ends

Men also wanted on similar terms

A great opportunity to help in a crying human need

APPLY AT THE HOSPITAL

[See page 286]

During the 1920s and 1930s, as hospitals expanded, the *nursing shortage* dominated the period. Unregistered nurses were hired in increasing numbers (Figure 5.17) and trade union militancy spread among them for better conditions and pay. On the eve of World War II, the Athlone Committee recommended that a second level of nurse, the **enrolled nurse**, be trained and recognised. This marked a step towards the emergence of a formal hierarchy of nursing grades (see Figure 5.18). The struggle between the Ministry of Health and the College of Nursing over the status and grading of nursing continued in the post-war years and indeed the debate continues to the present day.[8]

We conclude this analysis of the period between the World Wars by looking beyond the parochial concerns of health care in Britain, to health care in the colonial territories governed by Britain and other European powers.

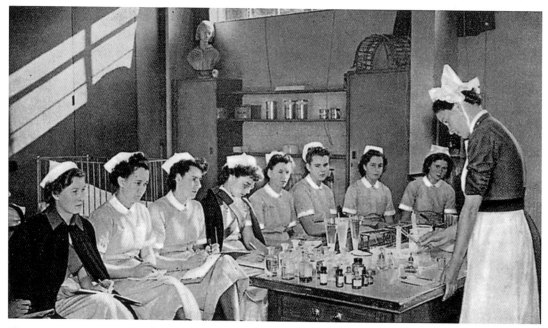

Figure 5.18   *A class for student nurses at the Nightingale Training School at St Thomas's Hospital, London. Links with historical tradition are emphasised by the bust of Florence Nightingale and the archaic starched bonnet of the teaching Sister. Photographs of this kind were used in the national drive to recruit more nurses; the white, middle-class image of nursing was preserved in publicity photographs until well into the 1970s. (Source: from Graves, C., 1947,* The Story of St. Thomas's 1106–1947, *Faber and Faber Ltd, London, p. 70)*

[8] See *Dilemmas in UK Health Care* (Open University Press, 3rd edn 2001), Chapter 5.

5.6   Empires and exchanges: the limits of paternalism

The years 1918–48 witnessed crucial changes in Europe's relations with its overseas colonies. Prior to World War I, former settler colonies like Australia had been granted the status of self-governing *Dominions*, and in India nationalist politics had reached a new pitch, with an intensification of violent protest against British rule.

The 1914–18 war did much to accelerate these trends. Troops drawn from the colonies to fight in Europe returned with new aspirations, including expectations of democratic reform and better social provisions such as health care. But in only a few cases did indigenous peoples benefit from collective health provisions such as those described earlier in this chapter. Even where more extensive provisions were made in the colonies, they were, as in Europe, severely constrained by the prevailing mood of financial conservatism in the late 1920s and 1930s. Health care in the colonies also remained paternalistic, although in India and some other colonies indigenous peoples began to play a greater role in the health services established by the colonial state.

5.6.1   India: devolution and diversity

In India, political reforms in 1919 devolved responsibility for certain areas of administration — including health care — upon provincial governments which had by then become responsible to a majority of elected representatives. For the first time, Indians began to play a major role in decision-making in medical policy and matters of public health.

At first sight, the 1919 reforms appear to have provided a stimulus to the provision of health care in India, with provincial government expenditure on health rising substantially betwe en 1919 and 1939, and more rapidly than other areas of revenue expenditure. However, provincial governments continued to operate within strict financial limits, particularly during the economic depression of the early 1930s.

The Indian economic historian V. R. Muraleedharan has argued that the Government of Madras was 'far more concerned about reducing its financial commitments' than providing adequate health care, and that it showed a 'lack of concern for the efficiency and effectiveness of the measures taken' (Muraleedharan, 1987, pp. 333–4). Figure 5.19 shows the causes of death in British India, 1928–1937, many of which were preventable. Although respiratory diseases and fevers were responsible

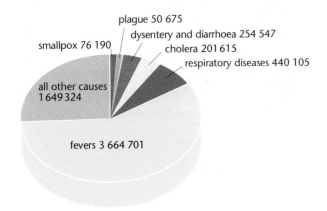

plague 50 675
dysentery and diarrhoea 254 547
smallpox 76 190
cholera 201 615
respiratory diseases 440 105
all other causes 1 649 324
fevers 3 664 701

1928–37 total deaths 6 337 157

Figure 5.19   *Causes of death in British India, 1928–1937. Many of the large number of deaths from 'fevers' were due to malaria, which probably rose in this period due to new irrigation programmes for agricultural developments in previously arid areas, such as the Punjab. Respiratory diseases such as TB were a particular problem amongst migrant labourers employed in textile mills. (Source: data from Sorsby, A., 1944,* Medicine and Mankind, *Watts and Co., London, Figure 21, p. 89)*

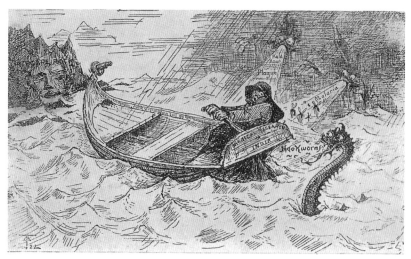

Figure 5.20 *A cartoon from the* Indian Medical Gazette *of June 1923, showing the risk that 'Medical Research in India' ran of being wrecked by the policy of the Inchcape Commission. The Commission recommended drastic reductions in research personnel and in the amount of money allocated to medical research. The sea monsters are labelled 'plague', 'malaria' and 'hookworm'. (From Balfour, A. and Scott, H. H., 1924,* Health Problems of the Empire, *Collins, Glasgow, p. 134)*

for the vast majority of deaths among Indians, they received comparatively little attention from the colonial government. It concentrated nearly all its resources on preventing epidemic diseases such as cholera, which could have serious political and economic ramifications. Retrenchment also adversely affected medical research in India, its budget being cut drastically in the 1920s and 1930s (see Figure 5.20).

One other feature of health care in India between the wars, which it had in common with other colonial countries, was the durability of *indigenous medical systems*. It is difficult to assess the precise impact of colonial rule on indigenous medicine, although it is certain that traditional systems like *ayurveda* and *unani* (which you encountered in Chapter 2) enjoyed something of a renaissance around the turn of the century, as a result of attempts by some nationalists to revive Indian culture, and with the expansion of the middle-class market for medical services. Many new colleges were established to train practitioners in both Islamic and Hindu medicine, gradually replacing the old system of training by apprenticeship.

However, much of the funding for these institutions came from private sources, with the provincial governments, including many Indian representatives, ambivalent or even hostile to traditional Indian medicine. Many 'modernising' nationalists, who drew their inspiration from the West, denounced Indian medicine as 'unscientific', creating a debate on the relative merits of the two systems which persisted beyond political independence in 1947.

The fate of *folk medicine* under British rule is harder to gauge and appears to have fluctuated greatly according to local economic conditions. In general, it seems that specialist remedies such as bone-setting were in many areas displaced by Western medicine, but that non-specialist traditions, such as the use of local plants for medicinal purposes, continued to thrive. Health care in the colonies, as in Britain, remained essentially pluralistic.

● Why might indigenous medical systems continue to thrive at a time when Western medical intervention was also increasing?

■ Western medical provisions were still limited and often unacceptable because of their links with an alien regime. Indigenous systems were more widespread, were not hindered by cultural obstacles, and, in many cases, were equally effective.

5.6.2 Africa: the 'great campaigns'

The Indian experience of health care between the wars was, however, untypical. Western forms of health care in Africa and other colonies usually remained in the hands of the European authorities, in conjunction with non-governmental organisations (such as the Rockefeller Foundation) sponsoring medical research and the prevention of disease. Such programmes were geared not so much to the health needs of Africans — they usually ignored diseases associated with poverty — but to the economic and medical requirements of the colonial state. According to the historian of Africa, Megan Vaughan:

> In the first half of the twentieth century, any contact which the majority of Africans had with colonial medicine was likely to have been in the form of a 'great campaign'. [In these campaigns] Africans were conceived of as an undifferentiated mass, part of a dangerous environment which needed to be controlled and contained. (Vaughan, 1991, pp. 39–40)

Attempts to eradicate diseases such as sleeping sickness could, however, be promoted as acts of imperial beneficence, and used to justify or rationalise European domination. This was particularly true of those regimes, like that of the Belgian Congo, which had been heavily criticised in the British press earlier in the 1900s for its treatment of indigenous peoples.

Similar motivating forces propelled the work of non-governmental organisations such as the Rockefeller Foundation. Having begun its work in the United States, the Foundation became increasingly involved, between the wars, in funding overseas medical programmes against so-called *tropical diseases* like hookworm and bilharzia. Figure 5.21 illustrates the vast geographical range of the Rockefeller Foundation's 'medical empire'. The trustees of the Rockefeller Foundation saw Western medicine

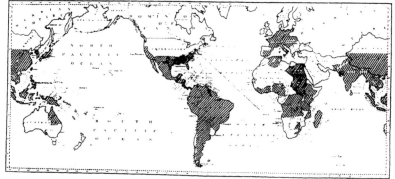

Figure 5.21   *Field of operations of the Rockefeller Foundation's International Health Commission in 1916. (Courtesy of the Rockefeller Archive Center)*

as a vehicle for American commercial expansion as much as for humanitarian endeavour. It was hoped that medical campaigns in the colonies would present Western culture and capitalism in a good light.

Yet it cannot be denied that these military-style campaigns had some beneficial effect. In her study of sleeping sickness in the Belgian Congo, Maryinez Lyons records that by 1930 the state medical service had examined 3 million people and had treated 104 000 for sleeping sickness. By 1940, 5 million had been examined, and by 1955 the number had risen to 6.6 million. Since the population of the colony in 1951 was only 11.7 million, Lyons concludes that, from the point of view of organisation at least, the sleeping-sickness campaigns were impressive.

However, like the majority of recent writers on disease in colonial Africa, Lyons maintains that these campaigns were little more than 'justification after the fact' (Lyons, 1988, p. 253), since the problem of epidemic sleeping sickness had itself been created by upheavals caused by colonisation.

5.6.3 Colonial medicine in transition

The great campaigns typified the paternalistic approach which had, until this time, dominated the provision of health care in the majority of European colonies. But, by the 1930s, and in some cases even earlier, there was increasing recognition that health programmes could be made more effective by encouraging the active participation of indigenous peoples.

In the Cook Islands, for instance, the New Zealand government began nurse training programmes for the islanders in 1917, and after World War I, a more ambitious scheme for the training of rural health workers was inaugurated by an American, S. M. Lambert, who was director of the Rockefeller Foundation's health programme in the Pacific. At the same time, in Africa, the colonial state began to employ village headmen as vaccinators and 'sanitary police'. By the 1930s, Africans were far more likely to encounter Western medicine via indigenous personnel than through the 'white doctors' of the Colonial Medical Service. This trend gradually gained pace and underpinned the primary health-care revolution in developing countries in the 1970s, which will be considered in Chapter 8.

Although the chief objective of medical education in the colonies was to supply subordinate medical staff for missions or government service, there were also limited opportunities to study for a medical degree. In India, indigenous peoples had had access to Western medical education since the 1830s, and a medical career was an attraction second only to law among the new Western-educated elite. After World War I, medical education in India expanded rapidly, and the number of medical graduates per annum rose from 800 in 1905 to over 2 000 by 1934.

However, in British eyes, education in the Indian medical schools was inferior, particularly in midwifery, and in 1924 the General Medical Council refused to recognise medical degrees from Indian universities, agreeing to do so only in 1930, after certain reforms had taken place. At the same time, medical education in Britain became an increasingly attractive option for those Indians who could afford it.

Another major development of the inter-war years was the establishment of health programmes focusing specifically on women and children, who had so far benefited little from the health policies of colonial governments. In the years after World War I, in the light of concern over child welfare in Britain, the spotlight came to rest on high levels of maternal and infant mortality in the colonies: a source of growing embarrassment to colonial apologists and a barrier to colonial development.

Initiatives to reach women and children began in India in the mid-1880s, with the establishment of the Dufferin Fund, which sought to provide female medical personnel for the treatment of women. As late as the 1930s, according to the Indian Medical Service officer Henry Holland, the seclusion of women was still so widely practised that:

> ... rather than allow a man doctor to attend the women of the household, the family would often let a patient die. (Holland, 1958, p. 178)

Treatment usually centred on the dispensary, where women and children were treated as out-patients for eye-diseases, dysentery and diarrhoea, and other ailments that were endemic in many parts of India. But dispensaries were educational as much as therapeutic institutions, and were the main conduit for Western notions of hygiene, diet and child-care. Where they succeeded in reaching indigenous peoples, such measures undoubtedly had beneficial consequences for the health of women and children, but the underlying causes of ill-health — poverty and malnutrition — were, in this period, seldom addressed.

5.6.4 Malnutrition in the colonies

Research into the physiological effects of malnutrition began in India before World War I by an Indian Medical Service officer, Robert MacCarrison, who first published his research on goitre and *deficiency diseases* in 1921. By the mid-1920s, more general nutritional surveys were being conducted in Africa, first among livestock and then among indigenous peoples.

These investigations, which were primarily concerned with the effects of malnourishment on labour efficiency, eventually led to international recognition of the problem. In 1933, the full Assembly of the League of Nations considered a *Report on Nutrition and Public Health* drafted by its Health Organisation, which argued that nutrition ought to be made an integral part of public-health policy. As the historian Michael Worboys has noted, these claims signalled the impending emergence of nutrition as a discipline in its own right (Figure 5.22 overleaf).

Many of those associated with this emerging discipline held radical political views, critical of imperialism, and attributed malnutrition to economic inequalities created by colonialism itself. But, as Worboys points out:

> ... the technical dimensions of this problem allowed for this radicalism to be lost as the definition changed from one of inappropriate structures to one of inadequate knowledge ... Colonial malnutrition was rapidly reconstructed from ... an epidemic problem to an endemic one, for which colonialism had little responsibility and over which it could exercise little control. (Worboys, 1988a, p. 222–3)

The political dimensions of colonial and post-colonial malnutrition remained submerged until after World War II, when they were again exposed through the efforts of organisations such as OXFAM.

The 1918–48 period, then, brought significant changes in the nature and extent of health-care provision in the colonies, with the increasing participation of indigenous peoples in Western systems of health care, and the growing involvement of philanthropic organisations such as the Rockefeller Foundation. But the intervention of these bodies, and of the colonial state, continued to be motivated largely by self-interest, which meant that many important areas of health remained untouched.

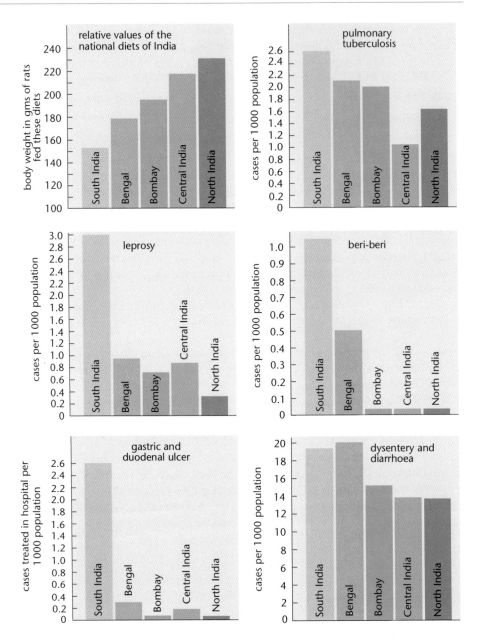

Figure 5.22 *These data were collected in India between the World Wars and reflect both the growing interest in malnutrition in the British colonies in this period and the increasing influence of 'nutrition' as a scientific discipline (note the use of rats to estimate the nutritional value of human diets). The link between regional diets in India and the diseases shown is unclear, except for beri-beri (a vitamin-deficiency disorder which damages the cardiovascular system, nerves and muscles, causing intense pain) in Southern India and Bengal, where the use of highly-polished rice removed vitamin B$_1$. (Data derived from Sorsby, A., 1944,* Medicine and Mankind, *Watts and Co., London, Figure 10, p. 35)*

This was particularly the case in relation to malnutrition, where European governments and medical practitioners chose to ignore the economic causes of ill-health. You will recall from earlier in this chapter that in Britain too, the effects of the Depression were underplayed in favour of an emphasis on individual responsibility for health. All this was to change after World War II, as Britain mobilised for total welfare.

OBJECTIVES FOR CHAPTER 5

When you have studied this chapter, you should be able to:

5.1 Define and use, or recognise definitions and applications of, each of the terms printed in **bold** in the text.

5.2 Use examples to illustrate the chaotic nature of health services in Britain and their funding in the inter-war years.

5.3 Assess the variety of forms in which lay medical care manifested itself; and the shifts which took place between lay and formal care in this period.

5.4 Describe the changing emphasis of public health in the inter-war years.

5.5 Analyse the tensions and conflicts in the moves towards greater professionalisation among health-care occupations prior to and during World War II.

5.6 Describe the new developments in colonial health care in this period and explain why many fundamental medical problems had still not been addressed.

QUESTIONS FOR CHAPTER 5

1   (*Objective 5.2*)

In 1920, the Consultative Council on Medical and Allied Services, chaired by Sir Bertrand Dawson (Lord Dawson of Penn), recommended the 'close coordination' of preventive and curative services and spoke of:

> ...the increasing conviction that the best means of maintaining health and curing disease should be made available to all citizens. (Consultative Council on Medical and Allied Services, 1920, p. 3)

What in fact happened to health services and their funding in the inter-war years?

2   (*Objective 5.3*)

Read the following extract from an interview conducted in 1979 with an elderly Englishwoman, Mrs Cooper:

> My father you know, he worked for a licensed vet ... he learned a lot ... all about these medicines ... He used to send me ... to the chemist in Golborne Road, N. Kensington and buy three penn'orth of laudanum, three penn'orth of red lavender and three penn'orth essence of peppermint. Well that was for dysentery, diarrhoea and all that. The neighbours used to come to him for that. (Mrs Cooper, quoted in Berridge, 1979, p. 51)

What does this quotation tell you about lay care and self-medication in the inter-war years? What was happening in general to lay care?

3   (*Objective 5.4*)

How did public health differ in practice and in theory in this period from nineteenth-century public health and what criticisms have been made of the inter-war approach?

4   (*Objective 5.5*)

What problems affected the moves towards greater professionalisation of nursing during this period?

5   (*Objective 5.6*)

In India, wrote R. Palme Dutt, a Marxist critic of British rule:

> ... provision for the most elementary needs of public hygiene, sanitation or health is so low, in respect of the working masses in the towns or in the villages, as to be practically non-existent. (Dutt, 1940, p. 79)

From what you have read in this chapter, how justified do you think Dutt was in making this claim, and to what extent might his remarks apply to other colonies between 1918 and 1948?

CHAPTER 6

Mobilisation for total welfare, 1948 to 1974

6.1 **Welfare capitalism**   168

6.2 **Health services for all**   169
   6.2.1 The post-war NHS   169
   6.2.2 Containing the cost of services   171
   6.2.3 Establishing medical specialities   172
   6.2.4 The rise of hospital medicine   173
   6.2.5 Barriers to coordinated services   174
   6.2.6 Pressure for reorganisation   176

6.3 **Lay care and the welfare state**   178
   6.3.1 Community care   178
   6.3.2 Lay care and family life   181

6.4 **The changing division of work in health care**   183
   6.4.1 Working in hospitals   183
   6.4.2 Proliferation of occupations   184
   6.4.3 The general practitioner: decline and revival   185
   6.4.4 Public-health doctors: loss of an empire   187

6.5 **Campaigning for public health**   189
   6.5.1 'Single-issue' campaigns and the growth of health activism   189
   6.5.2 Public-health failings of the welfare state   191

6.6 **'Scientific' medicine and the 'Third World'**   192
   6.6.1 International initiatives   193
   6.6.2 Importing European health care   194

Objectives for Chapter 6   196

Questions for Chapter 6   196

Study notes for OU students

This is the first of the chapters discussing health care in the period since World War II. Sections 6.2–6.4 are concerned with the British National Health Service (NHS) — a vast and complex organisation, eventually employing about 1 million persons. You will need to pay particular attention to the terminology introduced to describe the modern health service; this chapter provides the historical background to subjects treated in *Dilemmas in UK Health Care* (Open University Press, third edition 2001). For reasons of simplicity the description of the health service in the present chapter largely refers to England and Wales; the position in Scotland was discussed in Chapter 5. It will also be helpful for you to read again the article by Rosemary Stevens, which was discussed in Chapter 4; it appears in *Health and Disease: A Reader* (Open University Press, second edition 1995; third edition 2001).

6.1   Welfare capitalism

The return of peace to Western Europe when World War II ended, the inception of political stability, and prolonged and exceptional economic growth, created a contrast with the dismal events that followed World War I. This new expansionist climate was conducive to demands from the underprivileged for a more egalitarian social order, and for concessions from the elite. Whether arising from altruism or necessity, wide consensus was achieved for decisive measures to secure economic stability and social harmony. There was broad agreement on basic means to prevent a renewed slide into economic depression and the rebirth of Fascism.

In Britain, the new spirit was epitomised by adoption of the economic principles of John Maynard Keynes and the social programme of William Beveridge, which implied:

- commitment to full employment;
- economic planning; and
- active state investment in industry and welfare.

The world order after World War II was of course strikingly different from the pre-war system. The Soviet bloc adopted its own path to social progress. Western Europe entered into the closest economic, political and military integration with the USA. Paradoxically, owing to more favourable indigenous traditions and appropriateness of existing institutions, welfare regimes developed on a more ambitious scale in Europe than proved practicable in the USA, despite the latter's incomparably greater intrinsic wealth.

As indicated in Chapter 5, the groundwork for more systematic state provision for welfare was laid before World War II, but the final construction was a product of the post-war settlement. Social insurance provided an expanding proportion of funds for health and other welfare services, such as pensions and unemployment protection, in Britain and other countries before World War II (Figure 6.1). Western states varied enormously in the mechanisms employed, but all participated in what Abram de Swaan called 'mobilisation for total welfare'. The period between 1948 and 1974 seemed to witness exponential growth on all fronts. He concludes that 'after 1945, democratic society everywhere seemed to imply a welfare state' (de Swaan, 1988, pp. 223–4). (In Chapter 1, we discussed his analysis of 'modernisation'.)

The era of the **welfare state** involved action across a wide front, including income protection, housing, economic and urban planning, education and social services. Formal health-care provision constituted one of the prime areas of commitment. Although the services developed took on a vast diversity of forms, they shared certain common features. De Swaan describes the welfare state as a:

> … vast conglomerate of nationwide, compulsory and collective arrangements to remedy and control the external effects of adversity and deficiency. (de Swaan, 1988, p. 218)

Although it would be a mistake to see this development as an expression of unmitigated altruism, the arrival of the welfare state conveyed undoubted benefits to the 'working classes', as a result of which they became protected from the vagaries of the capitalist system better than ever before. In the rest of this chapter you will see that the positive gains and the dysfunctions of the welfare mechanisms are well illustrated by the health services. Although modest in their scale at the outset, the Western health services gradually emerged as one of the most dominant, expensive and indispensable elements in the modern welfare regime.

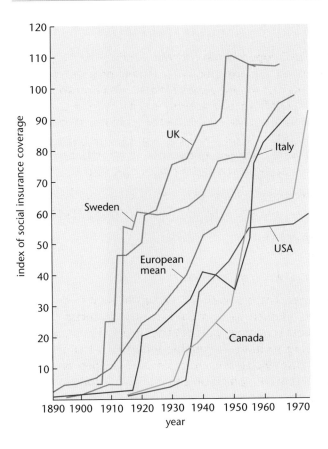

Figure 6.1 *The growth of social insurance coverage in Western Europe, 1890–1975. The proportion of insurance provision in both Britain and Sweden was well above the norm for Europe, whereas that in North America lagged behind. However, the insurance contribution to health care spending in the UK, especially after 1948 when the tax-funded NHS began, has never been more than a minor factor. (Subsequent trends in insurance-based health schemes are discussed in Chapter 9.) (Source: Flora, P. and Heidenheimer, A. J. (eds), 1981,* The Development of Welfare States in Europe, *Transaction Publishers, Piscataway, New Jersey, USA, p. 85)*

6.2 Health services for all

Between 1945 and 1964, all sixteen countries in Western Europe greatly extended collective responsibility for health care. Most of the services were components of compulsory insurance-based schemes for social security (Figure 6.1), developed in linear descent from the Prussian social security reforms instigated under Bismarck. Consequently they generally involved connection between payments and benefits, and organisation on a decentralised and highly bureaucratic basis. Of the European schemes, that in Sweden approximated most closely to the United Kingdom model, but its universal scheme was not established until 1955. Even then the range of services was less comprehensive and it involved a higher level of direct payments from patients.

6.2.1 The post-war NHS

It is notoriously difficult to draw definitive conclusions about the performance of the rival systems of health care in Europe. However, it is safe to say that the British system was one of the most generous in its basic design. On the other hand, the NHS possessed intrinsic weaknesses that have never been effectively corrected, and which, when combined with relative resource starvation, have prevented the British health service from fulfilling the high ambitions of its architects (Figure 6.2).

The NHS introduced in Britain by the post-war Labour government was an ambitious conception. However, the initiators of the NHS were only dimly aware of the nature of the commitments into which they were entering. Speculations concerning the likely *cost* of the health service expressed at the outset represented a spectrum of

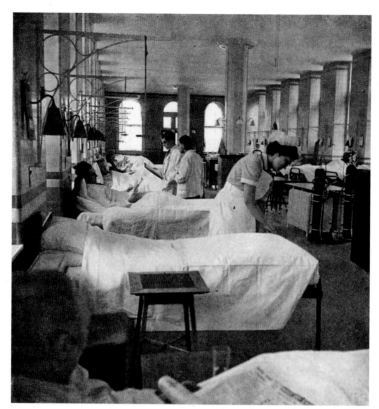

Figure 6.2   *St Thomas's Hospital, within sight of the Houses of Parliament, was a forceful reminder of the scale of the post-war problems. Buildings were dilapidated because of intrinsic building faults, and had been severely damaged during World War II. Here, Nuffield Ward is shown when it re-opened in 1947, after restoration from bomb damage. Facilities were neglected because of lack of capital investment. (Compare this with Figure 6.8.) (Photo: by Mr and Mrs Holliman, from Graves, C., 1947,* The Story of St Thomas's 1106–1947, *Faber and Faber, London, plate facing p. 61)*

opinions which find their modern counterparts. The Labour Cabinet and the civil servants thought that the new service would involve *cosmetic* adjustments of the inherited system. Beveridge subscribed to the somewhat naive, but widespread fallacy, that the health service might constitute a *diminishing* drain on public funds as the service progressively cleared up avoidable problems of ill-health within the workforce.

However, Aneurin Bevan, as the Minister responsible for the new health service in England and Wales, was in no doubt that the nation was embarking on an expensive venture, on account of previous under-funding, a great backlog of untreated conditions, and massive prospective liabilities associated with rising expectations, an ageing population, and the high cost of medical innovation. Taking Bevan's argument to an absurd extreme, critics of the NHS argued that the government had unleashed uncontrollable demands for health care, which would result in escalation in costs, economic ruin and political dislocation. Such polemicists as Dr Ffrangcon Roberts argued that the 'Welfare State will surely end in the Totalitarian State' (Roberts, 1952, p. 193).

With respect to its formal commitments, the new health service decisively turned its back on the multitude of limitations and discriminations inherent in the previous system. From the outset it was determined that the service should be universal and comprehensive:

> The proposed service must be 'comprehensive' in two senses — first that it is available to all people and second, that it covers all necessary forms of health care. (Ministry of Health, 1944, p. 9)

● In what ways was the NHS improving on the National Health Insurance scheme (NHI) in its coverage and range of services?

■ The NHS was universal, whereas NHI was effectively confined to manual wage earners and provided no coverage for dependants. NHI provided for GP care but not for specialist or hospital services.

The NHS made available for the first time, and to the whole population, treatment for defects of teeth, eyes and hearing. Indeed the most publicised aspect of the early NHS was the massive supply of dentures, spectacles and hearing aids. The NHS thus contributed significantly to transforming the quality of life of elderly people.

Aneurin Bevan was committed to making a decisive break with the ethos of services associated with charity, means-testing and the Poor Law. The new service was therefore completely free of *direct charges* to patients, and designed to provide the highest quality of care — what he called 'universalising the best'. He was conscious that the nation was embarking on 'the biggest single experiment in social service that the world has ever seen undertaken' (quoted in Webster, 1991, p. 140). The enlightened ethos of the new health service is indicated by the text of the introductory leaflet shown in Figure 6.3.

6.2.2 Containing the cost of services

In the event, even in the expansionist atmosphere of the post-war decades, it proved impossible to summon the political will to commit resources on anything like the scale required to fulfil Bevan's remit for the NHS. After a hesitant start, the Labour government pegged down NHS expenditure, imposed direct charges for spectacles and dentures, and prepared the ground for the prescription charge. Thereafter, both Conservative and Labour governments gradually expanded these charges. (The proportion of total cost of the NHS raised by charges to patients between 1974 and 2000, under successive governments, is discussed in Chapter 9 of this book.)

Until 1960, NHS expenditure was rigidly contained, to the extent that its share of national wealth, measured as Gross Domestic Product (GDP) actually *fell* — so contradicting the apocalyptic forecasts of critics like Ffrangcon Roberts. The low cost of the NHS was

THE NEW
NATIONAL
HEALTH
SERVICE

*

Your new National Health Service begins on 5th July. What is it? How do you get it?

It will provide you with all medical, dental, and nursing care. Everyone—rich or poor, man, woman or child—can use it or any part of it. There are no charges, except for a few special items. There are no insurance qualifications. But it is not a "charity". You are all paying for it, mainly as taxpayers, and it will relieve your money worries in time of illness.

Figure 6.3 *Front page of the NHS introductory leaflet, prepared by the Central Office of Information for the Ministry of Health in 1948 (the version shown here is a replica produced to mark the 50th anniversary of the NHS). This leaflet was distributed to every home and provided details of the services available. (Source: Public Record Office, CAB 21/2035, by permission of HMSO, Norwich)*

independently confirmed by an interdepartmental committee established by the Conservative government (the 'Guillebaud Report').

Eventually the imposition of a severe regime of economy on the NHS proved untenable. By 1960, political embarrassment was being caused by such factors as long waiting lists, the slow pace of improvement of services, and the antiquated state of hospital buildings. The backwardness of the health service was also evident in the light of obvious comparisons with the rapidly expanding educational sector, or against health services in other Western states. The dreary, overcrowded atmosphere of the typical out-patient department demonstrated that in reality the NHS was slow to adjust to the best modern practices and rising expectations.

The evident shortcomings of the NHS led to unavoidable pressures for increased expenditure, as a result of which the NHS share of GDP rose from 3.9 to 5.5 per cent between 1960 and 1975. This boost reflected sporadic responses to crises by both Conservative and Labour governments. Modest increments in expenditure allowed the launching of urgently-needed initiatives, the most expensive being the Hospital Plan, the large hospital rebuilding programme launched in 1962 (Ministry of Health, 1962).

6.2.3   Establishing medical specialities

From the outset, the main priority was establishing a comprehensive specialist service, and the resources of the NHS were heavily concentrated on this task. The scale of this undertaking is described by Sir George Godber, one of the chief planners of the system:

> The result … was an immediate and large increase in the amount of specialist time available, especially in hospital centres outside the large cities. By the end of 1949 there had been a substantial increase and the equivalent of the whole-time three and a half thousand consultants was provided by the five and a half thousand individuals available in England and Wales. This process was to continue and by the end of 1970 there was two and a half times as much consultant time and double the number of medical staff in all grades. In the same period the number of nursing staff including the number of trained nurses doubled; the hospital professional and technical staff, other than doctors and nurses, increased more than two and a half times and included many new technologies and skills.

> General medicine and general surgery were the largest medical specialties in 1948 but increased little after the first few years while other specialties were established and grew rapidly. Neurosurgery, thoracic surgery, and plastic surgery which had been established in a few centres were quickly provided by the Health Service in every region. Regional radio-therapy services separate from diagnostic radiology were established. The deficiencies in pathology and diagnostic radiology had been exposed by wartime needs and partly remedied, but needed expansion and re-equipment. Anaesthesiology developed rapidly into the largest specialty followed by pathology and psychiatry. The increase in consultants was thus not only in numbers, but much more importantly in range of expertise. Geriatrics and child psychiatry

developed from almost nothing; urological and cardiological units were established at least in main centres, pathology became subdivided; orthopaedic surgery became predominantly concerned with repair of trauma and defects at birth or of ageing. But rheumatology and rehabilitation were often neglected. (Godber, 1975, pp. 27–8)

6.2.4 The rise of hospital medicine

It was a massive and genuine achievement to make available the most advanced diagnostic and treatment facilities for the entire population. However, because of the shortage of resources, the **acute hospital sector** (i.e. the secondary level of health care, catering for short-stay patients suitable for immediate treatment, including maternity care) was developed at the expense of everything else.

Given the revolution in the capacities of high-technology medicine from the mid-century onwards, it is understandable that the new health service should place the first emphasis on acute hospital services. There was an urgent need to bring Britain's old-fashioned and under-resourced hospitals up to the standards existing elsewhere in the advanced economies, modernise the conditions of employment of hospital doctors, and remove obstacles of access to patients.

The aim was to provide such basic functions as safer and effective accident and emergency services, properly equipped operating theatres (Figure 6.4), X-ray and pathological laboratory diagnostic facilities, and a comprehensive blood transfusion service. There was also increasing demand for hospital childbirth. The acute services were politically the easier priority because hospitals were under direct state control. This also met the expectations of the public, who were inundated with media publicity about advances in hospital medicine.

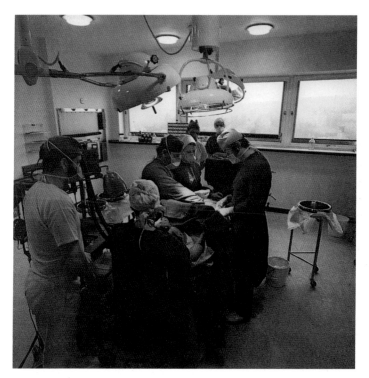

Figure 6.4 *The modernisation of hospitals and acute services took precedence over other sectors of health care in the 1960s. This photograph of an operating theatre in Torbay Hospital — one of the first of the new District General Hospitals built under the 1962 Hospital Plan — was used by the Department of Health and Social Security to promote the image of the 'modern' health service. (Compare this with Figure 5.4.) (Source: courtesy of the King's Fund)*

The acute services absorbed the increasing resources made available to the NHS in the 1960s. Also they took up an increasing slice of the total expenditure, as Table 6.1 shows.

● Examine Table 6.1 for evidence of gains and losses in the competition for NHS resources between 1949–50 and 1964–5.

■ The hospitals enjoyed an increase of just over 13 percentage points, at the expense of general medical, dental, ophthalmic and other services. The great majority of the increased spending was on current expenditure, i.e. the cost of running the hospitals.

Table 6.1 Comparison of the percentage expenditure on parts of the NHS financed by central government in England and Wales, 1949–50 and 1964–5.

	1949–50	1964–5
Hospitals		
current	49.6	58.5
capital	2.3	6.7
(*subtotal*)	(51.9)	(65.2)
Executive Council Services		
general medical	10.6	8.5
pharmaceutical	7.8	12.0
general dental	10.9	6.2
general ophthalmic	5.6	1.8
(*subtotal*)	(34.9)	(28.5)
other	13.2	6.3
total	100.0	100.0

Data from C. Webster, previously unpublished, based on Treasury data.

You will notice from Table 6.1 that spending on new buildings and refurbishment of hospitals (capital expenditure) was always at a low level in the first fifteen years of the NHS, but this Table indicates a small increase in 1964–5, which marks the beginning of the implementation of the Hospital Plan. Between 1965 and 1975, the gathering pace of hospital development was responsible for further reducing the share of NHS resources devoted to the family practitioner services administered by Executive Councils, which today we would refer to collectively as *primary health care*. (You will find in Chapter 7 that the above trend was reversed in the 1980s.)

The pattern of expenditure recorded in Table 6.1 contributes to the view that primary health care, community, preventive and health promotion services, were cut off from the mainstream of advance concentrated in the acute hospital sector of the NHS. From the outset, the NHS failed to capitalise on the potentialities of preventive and primary care, a defect which has never subsequently been completely corrected.

6.2.5 Barriers to coordinated services

In principle, under the NHS, GPs treated all members of the family on an equal basis and gave access to modern drugs. However, the majority of patients were seen by over-stretched and doubtfully competent GPs, working from poorly equipped and inadequate accommodation, a situation little different from the pre-NHS practice described in Chapter 5.

During the first two decades of the NHS there was no specific training for general practice in medical schools and no systematic post-graduate education. Older GPs were therefore increasingly out of touch with developments in chemotherapy and diagnosis, and they were not likely to be informed about new approaches to such problems as psychosomatic illness, alcohol and drug abuse or tobacco addiction.

An expert on health administration, Gordon Forsyth, noted the static character of general practice:

> In terms of organisation, there has been undoubtedly no change as a result of the NHS. Admittedly, partnerships have been

encouraged by financial incentives; but many partnerships are financial fictions, not operational realities.... We still talk about coordinating the family doctor with the district nurse, the health visitor and the social worker, but we have failed to provide the institutional framework within which these services might be coordinated. The Health Centres never materialised. The family doctor is still the independent self-employed entrepreneur that he was in the 19th century. (Forsyth, 1963, p. 10)

● Examine Figure 6.5 and consider ways in which the *actual* organisation of the NHS provided the barriers to coordination mentioned by Gordon Forsyth.

■ You will notice especially that *health centres* were supposed to provide the coordinating link between services administered by Executive Councils and those provided by the local authorities. Abandonment of the health-centre plan severed the vital connection between the GP and community services.

Later in this chapter, you will find out more about changes within general practice. First we consider the hospitals inherited by the NHS. Not all the hospitals shared in the advances experienced in the acute sector. The worst defects of the NHS were hidden from sight in the vast conglomeration of asylums, mental deficiency

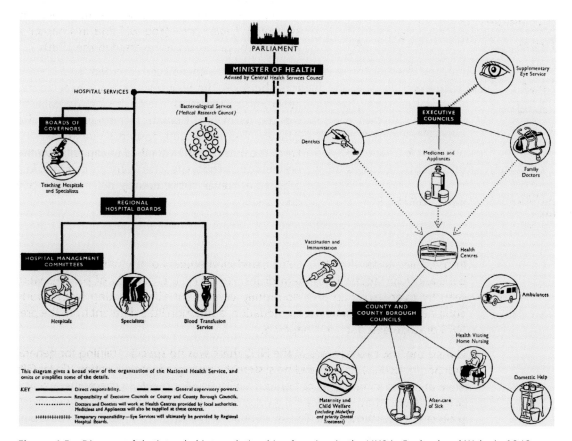

Figure 6.5   *Diagram of the intended inter-relationship of services in the NHS in England and Wales in 1948, taken from a pamphlet,* The National Health Service, *published by the Central Office of Information at the time. The services provided by Executive Councils and by County and County Borough Councils were supposed to be linked through health centres. Abandonment of the plan for health centres removed the opportunity for integration. (Source: Ministry of Health and Central Office of Information, by permission of HMSO, Norwich)*

institutions, and workhouse infirmaries taken over by the NHS and converted into mental hospitals, mental handicap[1] hospitals, and geriatric hospitals (all parts of the *chronic* sector). In 1948, these institutions housed about 300 000 patients and constituted more than half of the bed capacity of the NHS; with good reason they became known as the 'Cinderella services' of the health system. This massive sector lapsed into a neglected backwater until a series of public scandals erupted in the 1960s. An extract from one of the more restrained reviews of the problem gives an insight into the true horror of the situation.

> A very great number of elderly people sit waiting for death in mental hospitals where they have no business to be. They are there because the mental hospitals are being used as a dumping ground for the elderly, whose mental problems are caused by untreated physical illness. The mental hospital staff cannot possibly give them proper care, let alone rehabilitate them. There are not enough staff, not enough money, no facilities. The buildings in which they are expected to work are shameful. We cannot dodge the accusation that we, as an advanced and civilized country are treating a very great number of our old people in a manner that is far worse than merely barbarous. (Editorial in the *Nursing Times*, 10 June 1966)

6.2.6 Pressure for reorganisation

It was increasingly realised that the problems of the NHS could not be entirely solved by higher expenditure. The structure of its administration came under increasingly critical scrutiny. No sooner was the ink dry on the 1946 NHS legislation than the question of *reorganisation* of the health services emerged, and it soon joined expenditure as the major policy obsession. Reorganisation was expected to bring about greater harmony, unity and cooperation, thereby unlocking gains in efficiency. Although presented as the result of deliberate planning, the original administrative structure adopted for the NHS was an untidy compromise (for reasons indicated in Chapter 5), designed to reconcile a wide variety of conflicting groups. These demands forced the government to abandon its scheme for a *unified* service. Instead a divided service was adopted, involving three entirely different forms of administration:

- hospital services, administered by Regional Hospital Boards and Boards of Governors;
- local government services, administered by County and County Borough Councils;
- family practitioner services, administered by Executive Councils.

As noted in Chapter 5, this came to be called the **tripartite system** of health care, based on the accidental parallel with the post-war tripartite system of secondary education. The health system was further complicated by lack of uniformity between the parts of the United Kingdom. The organisation of the NHS at its inception in Scotland was shown in Figure 5.6 in the previous chapter; you have already examined the contemporary representation of the complex 1948 structure in England and Wales in Figure 6.5. Apart from changes in terminology, local government and family practitioner services represented continuations of pre-NHS administration, except that local government was stripped of its hospital responsibilities.

[1] The term 'mental handicap' was commonly used during the period covered by this chapter. It has since been replaced in literature from more enlightened sources by less-pejorative terms such as 'learning difficulties' or 'learning disabilities'.

The real innovation in the Labour government's scheme was the *nationalisation* of all hospitals, and the creation of a new form of *regional* hospital administration with Hospital Management Committees at the periphery. However, although *teaching* hospitals in England and Wales were nationalised along with the rest, they each retained independent management, outside the regional structure. This represented a concession to the voluntary hospital tradition and it anticipated the formation of self-governing NHS Trusts in the 1990s.

The new health system was therefore a failure as an exercise in unification, simplification and rationalisation. In England and Wales alone there were more than 400 hospital authorities and a total of about 700 (and in Scotland 170) administrative authorities involved in the health service. Arrangements for cooperation worked badly, even within the hospital sector. In certain respects the NHS constituted a step back from the degree of coordination obtaining in the larger local authorities before 1948. Coordination and efficiency were impaired and there was no mechanism for decisively improving the situation.

- Again examine Figure 6.5. Indicate the separate authorities responsible for providing care in an imaginary provincial town in England and Wales possessing a medical school.

- The Hospital Management Committee of the Regional Hospital Board would provide general hospital services; the Board of Governors would supply more specialist teaching-hospital services; the Executive Council would superintend the family practitioners (the GPs, pharmacists, dentists and opticians); and finally the County Borough Council would provide a miscellaneous range of preventive and community services.

Although the existing system was universally accepted as detrimental to the best interest of patients, there was a reticence to displace the delicate balance achieved by the 1948 compromise arrangements. However, the many illogicalities and inefficiencies of the system suggested that reorganisation was unavoidable.

Planners were faced with two alternatives for improving the organisation of services. One idea was unification of the health services under local government, a possibility enhanced by the imminence of local government reform. However, this arrangement was unacceptable to the medical profession, and was against the trend of events. The alternative was unification under expanded hospital authorities, continuing the trend begun in 1948.

During the 1960s, pressures from all sides mounted for reform and the prospect emerged of a radical simplification of the existing service — perhaps unifying all health and personal social services under as few as 40 new area health authorities in England and Wales. A Green Paper making this suggestion was issued by the Labour government in July 1968, shortly before the Ministry of Health was amalgamated with the Ministry of Social Security to form the Department of Health and Social Security (DHSS). There was then a delay before the second Green Paper of February 1970. Further delay was occasioned by a change in government. The Conservative consultative process then began in May 1971 and was concluded with the reorganisation which took effect in 1973 in Northern Ireland and in April 1974 in the rest of the United Kingdom.

As you will see in Chapter 7, any expectation that this reorganisation would contribute decisively to solving the problems confronting the health service was rapidly dispelled.

6.3 Lay care and the welfare state

The coming of the NHS in 1948 and increased access to formal medical services for women could have dispensed with the role of lay care. But the situation in the post-war years, which is discussed in this chapter and in Chapter 7, turned out to be rather different.

6.3.1 Community care

Lay care, defined as care by *informal family networks*, became entwined with the concept of **community care**. This concept became a prominent policy goal of governments of both the main political parties after World War II. But despite widespread agreement about the necessity for 'community' rather than institutional care, no consistent meaning has been applied to the term. The social policy analyst, Alan Walker, has commented that the attractiveness of the term 'community care' owes much to its manipulation to encompass the widest possible range of constructions — it is all things to all politicians and policy makers.[2]

Community care, so far as it can be defined, developed a number of broad and interrelated strands, some of which have implications for lay care. Care in the community could be provided formally or informally. It is thus possible to distinguish between formally-organised care given primarily by health and personal social services; formal and quasi-formal care by voluntary organisations; and informal care by neighbours, friends and kinship networks. The concept has also been taken to mean different things at different times and in relation to different groups in need. Many of the terms used in this chapter (and Chapter 7) for people who provide community care, are euphemisms for 'women'. As you will see, the development of community-care provision has taken for granted women's role as 'natural carers'.

Behind the development of community-care policies lay a post-war change in the age-structure of the population. On the one hand, the birth rate was lower and the children that were born were healthier. But there was also a huge growth in the proportion of elderly people in the population.[3] The numbers of elderly people had been growing rapidly between the wars as well, but the potential scale of their demand on the contemporary welfare system had been disguised by the crisis over unemployment during the Depression.

When Seebohm Rowntree conducted his first survey of York, published in 1901, the proportion of the British population aged 65 and over stood at 4.7 per cent. In his 80s, he returned to the town in 1951 to make a last survey. The proportion of the population over 65 was then 11 per cent and rising. Rowntree found that the elderly population dominated his tables: old age accounted for 68 per cent of the causes of poverty, with sickness the next largest category at 21 per cent; unemployment failed to register at all (Vincent, 1991, p. 135).

The initial concern of government was with questions of labour shortage, in particular the shortage of skilled labour. From the mid-1950s, in an attempt to maximise the available workforce, the Ministry of Labour launched a vigorous and

---

[2] Community care in the 1990s, particularly for elderly or disabled people, is discussed further in *Dilemmas in UK Health Care* (Open University Press, 3rd edn 2001), Chapter 4.

[3] Demographic trends in the age of the population of the United Kingdom are described in *World Health and Disease* (Open University Press, 3rd edn 2001), Chapter 2, and the effects of an ageing population on disease patterns are discussed in Chapters 9 and 10.

unprecedented campaign to create a positive image of the older person (those in their later 60s). But the campaign was an entire failure. Since the late nineteenth century, the proportion of the workforce who retired in their mid-60s had been gradually increasing, and in the post-war period this trend accelerated.

The age-structure of the elderly population had implications for patterns of care. The rising numbers of elderly people — and in particular those in their 70s and 80s — added to the build-up of pressure in the **chronic hospital sector** (the long-stay wards and institutions). Proposals for community care of the elderly population were developed; in 1958, the Minister of Health stated that:

> ... the underlying principle of our services for the old should be this: that the best place for old people is in their own homes, with help from the home services if need be. (Quoted in Townsend, 1962, p. 196)

The same policy was also developed in the field of mental health and the Royal Commission on Mental Illness in 1957 recommended a shift in emphasis from hospital to community care for people diagnosed as mentally ill and mentally handicapped. This was also one of the first uses of the term 'community care' in the official literature.

The principles of community care in policy statements in the immediate post-war period can be summarised as:

- ensuring individuals remained integrated with their families and neighbours;
- a pattern of non-institutional care;
- the provision of support in the home from a wide range of services.

In theory, the structure of health services at the local level and in particular the local-authority-based **domiciliary services,** was sufficient to achieve this aim. But, as you saw earlier, coordination within the fragmented tripartite structure of the NHS was poor. The idea of *domiciliary teams* comprising a range of health-related occupations was widely discussed in the 1950s. The work of home nurses, home helps, health visitors (who were beginning to work to an increasing extent with elderly people) and social workers, as well as the 'meals-on-wheels' service undertaken largely by voluntary agencies (Figure 6.6), were seen as important in maintaining older people in their homes. But these domiciliary services were generally inadequate and their extension insufficient to meet the needs of the ageing population. The home-help service, for example, which was recommended but not obligatory under the 1946 NHS Act, remained small in relation to the size of its client groups. Inevitably, lay carers (usually women) filled the gap.

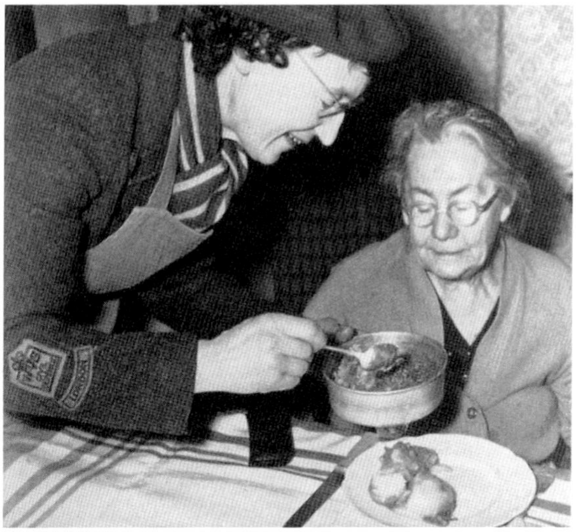

Figure 6.6 *Since the 1950s, the delivery of 'meals-on-wheels' by volunteers has been assisting elderly or disabled people to remain in their own homes rather than enter residential care institutions. (Source: Fox Photos Ltd., from Ministry of Health, 1963,* Health and Welfare: The Development of Community Care, *Cmnd.1973, HMSO, London)*

In the 1950s and 1960s, 'community care' was also redefined to encompass **residential care** in the community. Local authorities developed the more traditional alternative of building residential homes for elderly people. By 1960, such residential accommodation housed a total of 84 000 persons, including 39 000 in homes opened since 1948 (Figure 6.7 overleaf). Residential homes were provided mostly for elderly people, but a small number of homes were given over to

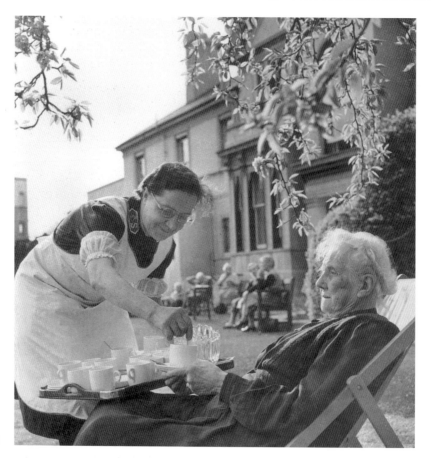

(a)

(b)

Figure 6.7   *The policy ideal of caring for frail older people in 'homes' in the community, contrasted with the reality that many experienced. (a) Tea is served to residents in the garden of the Alder Bank Eventide Home, Clapham, London, April 1958. (Source: Erich Auerbach, Hulton Getty Picture Library); (b) Residents of a local authority home in the 1950s. (Source: Peter Townsend, from Townsend, P., 1962,* The Last Refuge, *Routledge and Kegan Paul, London, plate 3)*

handicapped people and other groups. Residential homes of the model type with places for about 60 residents received much publicity. Community care became what the sociologist Philip Abrams called *community treatment* (Abrams, 1980).

Peter Townsend, a sociologist, questioned the whole philosophy of this development in his book *The Last Refuge: A Survey of Residential Institutions and Homes for the Aged*, which was published in 1962. In his view, the expansion of residential homes was an illustration of the absence of clear policy and detailed planning around the concept of community care.

Coordination between separate services quickly became a dominant policy theme and this, rather than the expansion of domiciliary services and the closure of out-dated institutions, became the primary goal of community-care policy. Policy was, however, ambiguous. In the DHSS White Paper, *Better Services for the Mentally Handicapped*, published in 1971, it was argued that the services in need of greatest expansion included residential homes for children and adults, and a target increase of 15 per cent was set for the number of mentally-handicapped persons in residential care. But planning forecasts for domiciliary services were completely omitted.

It was only in relation to elderly people that the need to support families caring for dependants, and for shared responsibility between the family and domiciliary services, was recognised. Initially, in this period, lay care was not given the dominant role in community care which it came to occupy later.

6.3.2 Lay care and family life

The tendency in other areas of health care, most obviously childbirth, was for the formal health service to exclude the lay carer. The pre-war trend towards the increased *hospitalisation of childbirth* continued and accelerated in the 1950s and 1960s (Figure 6.8). In 1927, 85 per cent of births were at home; in 1961, this had

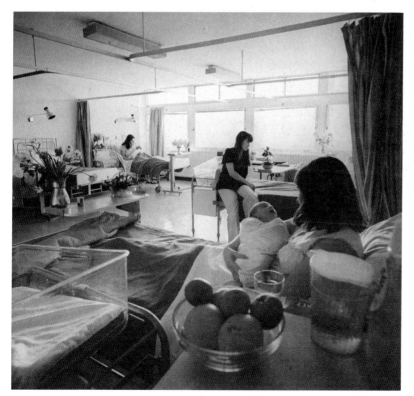

Figure 6.8 *Maternity ward, St Peter's Hospital, Chertsey. Childbirth was increasingly taking place in hospital rather than at home in the 1960s. Initially many women welcomed the opportunity to have access to pain relief and medical care, but by the 1970s, strong objections to the medicalisation of childbirth began to be heard. (Source: courtesy of the King's Fund)*

fallen to 32 per cent; and in 1980, only 1.3 per cent of confinements took place there. And within the hospital, the extent to which women gave birth without intervention from a doctor or midwife also changed, as Table 6.2 shows.[4]

Table 6.2   Trends in obstetric intervention: estimated percentage of all deliveries in England and Wales[1], 1953–78.

Year	Induction of labour or artificial rupture of membranes	Caesarean section	Instrumental delivery[2]	Episiotomy[3]
1953	–	2.2	3.7	–
1958	–	2.3	4.4	–
1963	8.9	3.1	5.3	–
1968	18.0	4.0	7.9	–
1973	34.9	5.0	11.0	44.0
1978	36.3	7.3	13.3	53.4

[1] Includes women resident outside England and Wales. [2] Forceps or vacuum extraction. [3] A small cut made to enlarge the vaginal opening. (Data from MacFarlane, A. and Mugford, M., 1984, *Birth Counts: Statistics of Pregnancy and Childbirth*, HMSO, London, p. 575, Table A7.32a)

● Looking at Table 6.2, what developments do you notice in childbirth in the immediate post-war period, and in the 1960s and 1970s?

■ In the 1950s, the number of medical interventions in childbirth increased only slightly, but in the 1960s and 1970s they rose much more quickly: overall, the rate of Caesarean sections and instrumental deliveries more than trebled, and two interventions (induction and episiotomy) became commonplace.

However, family support and advice on health matters continued to play a major role in working-class lives. In the mid-1950s, two sociologists, Michael Young and Peter Willmott of the Institute of Community Studies, spent three years observing working-class family life in Bethnal Green and a new housing estate, Greenleigh, where many of the families were rehoused during this period. In what has become a classic study, they demonstrated the continuing role of family involvement in childbirth and child health. Mrs Banton, for example:

> I take more notice of my mum than I do of the welfare. She's had eight and we're alright. Experience speaks for itself, more or less, doesn't it? If you're living near your mother, you don't really need that advice. You've got more confidence in your mother than you would have in the advice they'd give you … (Young and Willmott, 1962, pp. 53–4)

Lay diagnosis and treatment outside the professional medical sector remained important throughout this period. A 1950s study of a working-class housing estate found two-thirds of the people interviewed were taking some self-prescribed medication, often in addition to a prescribed drug. Laxatives and aspirins were most commonly self-prescribed (quoted in Helman, 1990, pp. 72–3). At the end of the 1960s, the same pattern was evident. A major study was undertaken in 1969

[4] Trends in the place of birth in England and the 'medicalisation of childbirth' are discussed in *Birth to Old Age: Health in Transition* (Open University Press, 2nd edn 1995; colour-enhanced 2nd edn 2001), Chapter 3.

by two sociologists, Karen Dunnell and Ann Cartwright, who found that 80 per cent of a large sample of the population drawn from across the country said that they had taken some medicine in the two weeks prior to the interview. Self-prescribed medicines — aspirin again and tonics, skin preparations and antacids — outnumbered those prescribed by doctors by two to one.

At the end of the 1960s, lay care both in terms of informal care and assistance and non-professional advice and self-medication, was thriving. This was despite the advent of a formal welfare state which, at least in theory, could have superseded it. In the 1970s and 1980s, however (see Chapter 7), lay care assumed a new and growing importance as the foundation of government community-care policies.

6.4   The changing division of work in health care

Bevan's nationalisation of the hospitals in 1948 had been facilitated by the support of the influential hospital consultants. The voluntary-hospital consultants and the leaders of the medical profession were well pleased with the 1948 settlement, which gave them security, prestige and high remuneration, while also permitting the continuation of private practice. In the post-war period, the process of incorporation of the profession as a whole in the structure of decision-making by the state continued and expanded. But there were also changes within the medical profession.

The division of labour, relative role and status of hospital doctors and GPs changed; there were boundary shifts between doctors and nurses, and between nursing and ancillary workers within hospitals. The 1980s have been associated with the rise of 'managerialism' in health administration but, as you will see, this is a tendency that had its origins in the 1960s. Management, so it has been argued, has replaced the power of doctors in the health service and health policy-making. Whether that is the case still remains to be seen.

6.4.1 Working in hospitals

The status and areas of competence of the hospital-based occupations underwent significant change. As Chapter 7 describes, the successive reorganisations of the NHS and management changes between 1974 and the present have altered relations between categories of workers, and nowhere more so than in the hospital service.

Initially, as the sociologist Margaret Stacey has commented, the NHS was composed of three occupational hierarchies; medical, nursing and administrative. Nursing 'served' medicine, and administration facilitated the services of both doctors and nurses. Hospital doctors were at the top of the power structure, but both nurses and administrators had some areas of control. The alternative power base of the matron in a hospital, in charge of all nursing services, was considerable (Figure 6.9).

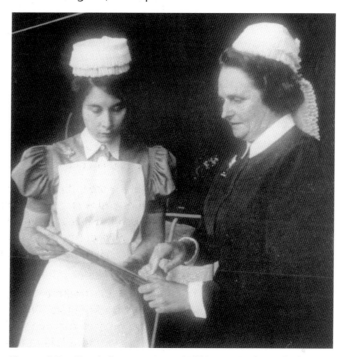

Figure 6.9   *Hospital matrons were held in awe in the early decades of the NHS, but their role was gradually replaced by managerial grades in the 1970s; crises in the NHS in the 1990s led to calls to 'bring back matron'. Here, the matron of the Royal London Hospital, inspects a chart, 1969. (Source: Royal London Hospital Archives)*

The general tendency since the 1960s has been to seek *organisational* solutions to problems of health service costs and control. The application of the managerial ethos led to changes in the distribution of power between the three hierarchies. Nursing was the first to be affected.[5] The 1966 Salmon Report led to a new managerial structure for nursing, by which managerial grades were instituted above the ward sister and superseded the hospital matron. The work of nurses employed by local authorities was reorganised on similar lines. The Salmon Report greatly increased the hierarchy of management in nursing.

Moreover, the Salmon reorganisation effectively blocked career opportunities in *clinical* nursing; the only route to upward mobility for a nurse was to leave the bedside and take a management post. The new structure had the effect of further dividing nurse leaders from the great bulk of the nursing rank and file. At that level there was increasing militancy and unionisation from the 1960s onwards, as government efforts at cost containment focused on nursing salaries, the largest sector of the health-care budget.

At the same time, within hospitals, what was termed *functional management* was introduced, i.e. an appraisal of the functions that different occupational groups carried out, which led in some cases to reallocation of tasks and responsibilities. Nurses became more conscious of the distinction between direct *nursing* care of patients and other commonly undertaken duties which came to be seen as *outside* nursing; for example, domestic services were separated out from nursing, and laundry was organised on an area basis.

The progressive dilution of nursing by the development of lower-level staff to carry out less technical aspects of care continued with the unplanned growth of the *nursing auxiliary* in the 1950s and 1960s. By 1958, these unqualified nurses in general hospitals exceeded registered nurses by 50 per cent. The registered nurses' hostility to their use was consistent in this period. Nurses have been criticised for the elitism that this hostility invoked. For example, Robert Dingwall, a medical sociologist who has studied the nursing profession, complained that:

> The obstruction of more systematic training and a properly defined role for auxiliaries under the supervision of registered nurses merely denied patients such benefits as more skilful practical carers could have brought them. (Dingwall *et al.*, 1988, p. 116)

6.4.2 Proliferation of occupations

The use of auxiliaries underlined a more general development in this period — the increased number of divisions in health-care labour. In general, the range of non-medical workers, scientists, technicians and workers in the para-medical professions expanded in the post-war period. By 1960, all the para-medical professions had achieved state registration (the opticians through a 1958 Act and the remainder through the Professions Supplementary to Medicine Act of 1960). Some commentators thought this marked an 'end to medical hegemony'. But there were also powerful arguments against this point of view. Not all changes went against doctors.

Changes in obstetric practice and the moves from home to hospital-based childbirth reduced the status of midwifery. Gender divisions between female midwives and (largely male) doctors complicated questions of division of labour. The sociologist

[5] Strategies for increasing the status of nursing in the 1990s are discussed in *Dilemmas in UK Health Care* (Open University Press, 3rd edn 2001), Chapter 5, which also refers to other health workers in occupations generally designated as 'allied to medicine', e.g. radiographers and physiotherapists.

Gerald Larkin, in his analysis of the relationship between medicine and para-medical occupations, argues that recognition of para-medical skills did not imply a dilution of medical hegemony; it was a matter of redrawing the boundaries without equalising all the parties. At the end of the 1960s little had yet effectively challenged overall medical dominance.

6.4.3   The general practitioner: decline and revival

Consultants may have been satisfied with the 1948 settlement, but for GPs the situation was much less clear cut. GPs had fought off the threat of a whole-time, salaried service and retained their status as 'independent contractors', i.e. each practitioner acted as an independent small contracting business. But this gain was offset by the blow to their morale and professional status through the gathering pace of their exclusion from specialist work in hospitals.

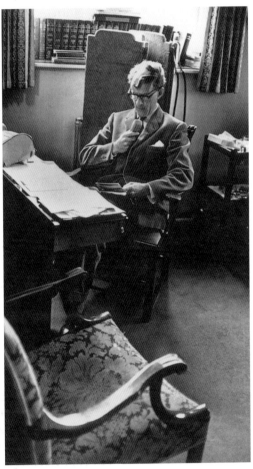

GPs had been partially excluded from major hospitals in the inter-war years. The NHS made this process more absolute by forcing a choice between a general practice or a hospital career, and by placing what one commentator called an 'antiseptic barrier' between the two branches of the profession. Obstetrics remained a battleground where GPs retained some rights to hospital access and care of their patients; but, in general, few GPs found a role in hospitals in the post-war decades.

This was in sharp contrast to the American system of health care, where many GPs passed completely into the specialist category and the boundaries between hospital and general practice were much less clear-cut. (OU students should think back to the Reader article by Rosemary Stevens that you read during your study of Chapter 4.)

●   What reasons does Stevens give for the different patterns of development of the professions in health-care systems in Britain and the USA?

■   Stevens places emphasis on the systems of checks and balances which emerged from the pre-specialisation era in Britain. The old social division between branches of practice have continued in the separate functions of primary and secondary care. In the USA, in contrast, there were no medical guilds; no national focus for an elite; and, until the 1870s, relatively few hospitals.

In Britain, the status of the post-war GP was in decline and their image was fusty and old-fashioned (see Figure 6.10). Access to the new laboratory-based diagnostic techniques remained under the control of hospital specialists; GPs were not allowed to use them until the 1960s. Loss of hospital work had severely reduced the status of GPs, who had seen their exercise of surgical skills as conferring prestige. Above all, they were overwhelmed, so it seemed to them, by trivia.

Figure 6.10   *The post-war GP typically worked alone from a private house, usually his (rarely her) own home, as in this practice in the Forest of Dean. Secretarial help in record-keeping and booking house-calls was often provided by the GP's wife. (Contrast this with Figure 7.19, the GP in 2001.) (Source: Jean Mohr)*

One GP interviewed by the sociologist Ann Cartwright in 1964, complained:

> We're swamped with trivialities. This isn't the sort of work one spent years at university preparing oneself for. There's the utter futility and humiliation of a professional man who feels his training is wasted. The GP has no status because he doesn't do medicine. (Quoted in Tudor Hart, 1988, p. 85)

Few medical students in the 1960s actively wanted to be GPs. In 1968, the Royal Commission on Medical Education found that only 23 per cent of final year medical students favoured a career in general practice, but 50 per cent ended up there, having failed as hospital trainees.

After a hesitant beginning, the GP has in fact gained new status and power under the NHS. How did this come about? Two factors need to be stressed. A new vision of general practice emerged from doctors themselves; and general practice became an important 'front-line' health service to governments who were increasingly conscious of the costs of a hospital-dominated service.

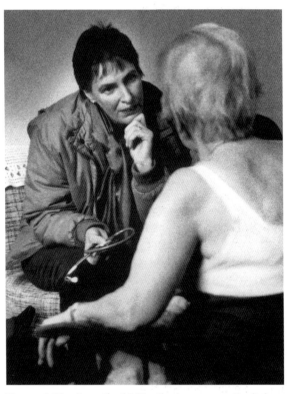

Figure 6.11 *From the 1950s, the 'new conception' of the family doctor began to celebrate the GPs' detailed personal knowledge of their patients from the cradle to the grave. Home visits were part of the service. (Source: Paul Schatzberger)*

The internal rejuvenation of general practice was inspired by what Margot Jefferys and Hessie Sachs, in *Rethinking General Practice* (1983), have called the 'rehabilitation of trivia'. The GP's importance as a friend, guide and counsellor began to be stressed (Figure 6.11). In 1950, the newly formed section of general practice of the Royal Society of Medicine held a discussion on 'what is general practice?' It concluded:

> The essence of general practice is to live amongst your patients as a definite cog in the whole machine, knowing them so well both in health and in sickness, and from birth until death. (Quoted in Armstrong, 1983, p. 80)

● This quotation describes the 'new conception' of the family doctor. Think back over the development of general practice described in Chapters 4–6; how have the GPs' functions changed over time?

■ In the nineteenth century, the GP could also have undertaken some salaried work, such as Medical Officer to a friendly society or Poor Law Medical Officer. In the inter-war period, some ran their own cottage hospitals. In the post-war period, they lost hospital access, but gained a wider role in the community.

The history of general practice was reconstructed to promote a vision of a distant era in which deep insight into the family life and character of patients was the very essence of good practice; the idea of the 'family doctor' was revived. The work of Michael Balint and his book *The Doctor, His Patient and the Illness* (1956), provided GPs with a holistic model of medical practice which refuted the mind/body dichotomy of much of hospital medicine. The influence of Balint, in particular among GPs active in the newly established *College of General Practitioners* (founded in 1952), was substantial.[6] John Horder, later its President, describing the work of Balint, claimed he had taught GPs that:

> ... since every patient is unique, diagnosis must be like biography and is inseparable from treatment. (Quoted in Armstrong, 1983, p. 81)

To this internal rethinking of the role of the GP was added a concern for general practice in the government health departments in the 1960s. A more prominent role for general practice was seen as vital for containing the mounting costs of acute hospital care, for facilitating the run down of mental hospitals, and therefore, in general, for shifting the focus of care away from hospitals. The *Family Doctor's Charter*, devised by a group of GPs in 1965 and ratified by the profession and the government in the following year, became the blueprint for the further development of general practice for the next twenty-five years.

Doctors were to work in common premises, and to employ support staff. They were encouraged to use hospital diagnostic services and to have opportunities to refresh their professional expertise with funding from their postgraduate education allowance. The attachment of other health workers to general practices was encouraged; GPs were to be 'king pins in a hierarchy of dependent occupations' (Jefferys and Sachs, 1983, p. 326). The idea of *health centres*, which had lain dormant since they had failed to become the intended fulcrum of the new NHS after 1948, was revived in the 1960s. New terms and conditions for GPs removed their objections to working with local authorities, which provided the funds for health centres, and GPs became enthusiastic 'leaders' of multidisciplinary teams delivering primary care from multipurpose facilities.

Regular training posts for doctors entering general practice and a qualifying examination were instituted. The non-specialist role of the GP was then accordingly reconstituted as a form of specialism. The boundaries between hospital and general practice changed as a result; GPs clawed back some of the medical work from hospitals, in particular through the moves to community care discussed earlier and to which we return later in the chapter. The GP became an established and important part of the panoply of community health and welfare services.

6.4.4 Public-health doctors: loss of an empire

With the establishment of the NHS in 1948, the primary role of public-health doctors in hospital administration was abandoned. Although local-authority control of all health services had originally been Labour Party policy, Bevan secured the nationalisation of the hospitals as a condition for the acquiescence of consultants in the fledgling service. The voluntary hospital system became the dominant model for the rest of the hospital service. At a stroke, public-health doctors lost the hospital empires that they had built up in the inter-war decades.

Local authorities were left with substantially reduced responsibilities for a range of services — maternal and child welfare, midwifery, health visiting, home nursing, home helps and so on. Public-health doctors were gloomy and despondent about their role in the new service. But, as historian Jane Lewis has commented, they

---

[6] Balint's work is discussed more fully in *Medical Knowledge: Doubt and Certainty* (Open University Press, 2nd edn 1994; colour enhanced 2nd edn 2001), Chapter 9.

bore some responsibility for the outcome in 1948. Their vision of public health in the inter-war years had been too limited:

> ... public health doctors were happy to extend their activities in whatever direction the Ministry permitted and anticipated that eventually this gap-filling exercise would be transformed into a fully-fledged state medical service in which they would play a dominant role. It was a dream doomed to disappointment, for neither the Ministry nor the medical profession shared it ... (Lewis, 1986, p. 49).

The public-health profession could have been a unifying force in the tripartite fragmentation of the health service. But it was buffeted in this period between the rest of the medical profession and local government structures. The public-health empire in local government began to disintegrate and relationships with GPs remained difficult.

The Medical Officer of Health (MOH) could have acted as the coordinator of community health services under the developing policies of community care. The role of health visitors as providing the link between general practice and public health was also an important one. But from the 1960s onward, cooperation was achieved by attaching health visitors to GPs. Health centres, which expanded from the late 1960s, operated not as the original intention had been, as a means of providing *integration* of the health services and community care, but as a focus for the establishment of *group general practices*. The volume of clinic work for local-authority doctors declined, as much of this work gradually passed to the GPs. There were tensions between the two groups of doctors as a result.

The position of public health as a specialty within the local authorities also caused problems. By the late 1960s, the idea of the MOH based in the local authority as the coordinator even of community services was no longer a practical possibility. Parts of the public-health empire were beginning to break away. Sanitary inspectors had begun to claim autonomy in the 1950s and had their own specialist training; they were renamed *public-health inspectors* in 1956. A major defection a decade later was that of the *social workers*. In 1968, the Seebohm Committee recommended the removal of social work from local-authority public-health departments and the setting up of separate social work departments.

A new definition of public health was beginning to emerge in the late 1960s. This was the concept of **community medicine** and of the *community physician*, replacing the role of the old MOH. These ideas were also developed in the late 1960s in a number of policy documents, in particular the Todd Report on medical education of 1968. The local-authority role of public-health doctors had gone, but a range of policy documents published in 1972 predicted an important new role for them as community physicians within the NHS. However, that role was poorly specified.

The twin components of community medicine were seen as *epidemiology* (the study of patterns of disease in populations)[7] and *medical administration*. But how these functions would operate in tandem, and how the community physician would operate *within* the NHS, remained unclear. Notice that, despite their title, community physicians were not at all involved in community *care*. As you will see in Chapter 7, the fate of public health was closely bound up with the larger issue of NHS reform.

[7] The methods and philosophy of epidemiology are taught in another book in this series, *Studying Health and Disease* (Open University Press, 2nd edn 1994; colour enhanced 2nd edn 2001), Chapters 7, 8 and 10, and further exemplified throughout *World Health and Disease* (Open University Press, 3rd edn 2001).

6.5   Campaigning for public health

● How did the ethos of public health change in the early part of the twentieth century (as described in Chapters 4 and 5)?

■ Public health concerned itself much more with questions of individual behaviour and lifestyle, rather than looking at the structural and economic issues involved in the health of the people. In the inter-war years public-health doctors took on the administration of hospital services, a role which gave them considerable powers, but they failed to take the lead in raising questions about the relationship between health and social issues such as housing, unemployment, low pay and poor nutrition.

As you saw earlier, public health as a profession suffered by comparison with the rise of the GP in the post-war period and by the loss of MOH direction of both social workers and sanitary inspectors. In 1971, social workers gained autonomy in entirely new Social Services Departments of local government. Then, in 1974, in the context of NHS reorganisation, sanitary inspectors became upgraded to environmental health officers, in newly-created local government Environmental Health Departments. This opened the way, at least in theory, for public-health doctors to take the lead in campaigns to improve public health on a broad range of issues. But this opportunity was not grasped. In the 1970s, the transition to community medicine saw public health redefined with a narrower, rather than a broader, focus.

6.5.1 'Single-issue' campaigns and the growth of health activism

In the 1950s and 1960s, environmental and public-health issues tended to be dealt with as **single-issue campaigns** for action against a particular cause of ill-health or for the introduction of a certain treatment or policy. Such campaigns were advanced by pressure groups, not by public-health doctors.

You will recall from Chapter 2 that air pollution was already an issue in London in the early seventeenth century; the severe toll on health from industrial smoke and fumes was illustrated in Chapter 3, in relation to the 'Potteries' (Figures 3.1 and 3.2) in the nineteenth century; and the cartoon by Barlach (Figure 1.4) reminds us that smoke pollution was regarded as a particularly potent hazard at the beginning of the twentieth century. But in the UK it was not until the 1950s that air pollution was confronted with any seriousness. The 'great London smog' of 1952 brought matters to a head (see Figure 6.12). From 5 to 9 December, London was subjected to a dense smoke-polluted fog of catastrophic proportions, responsible for at least 4 000 deaths. Deaths on this scale had not been seen since the 'flu epidemic of 1918–19. The Clean Air Act of 1956, passed in part because of this and other 'smogs', established smokeless zones and controlled domestic smoke emissions for the first time.

But the passing of the Act was the result of pressure from the National Society for Smoke Abatement, a cross-party group of MPs — and a few committed MOHs. The Act played a

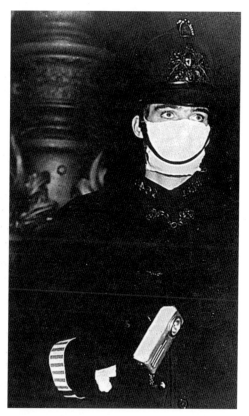

Figure 6.12   *A London smog in the 1950s. Police on duty were forced to wear smog masks. (Source: Hulton Getty Picture Collection)*

substantial part in the reduction of air pollution. Two million tons of smoke were discharged into the atmosphere in 1954; by 1971 this had fallen to 700 000 tons, a reduction of 65 per cent. This was a successful environmental campaign, although of course, this specific measure of control left the growing problem of air pollution from vehicle exhaust and other sources completely unresolved. In the period covered by this chapter, it became recognised that air pollution was being exacerbated by exhaust fumes from motor vehicles, but it was not until the 1980s that action was taken to impose statutory controls over constituents like lead in exhaust emissions.

In the 1940s, exhaust fumes were suspected of being responsible for the rise of lung cancer, which in 1951 overtook tuberculosis as a cause of death in the UK. Then, in the 1950s, tobacco was established as the culprit. Chapter 7 briefly considers the lethargic response of governments to this major threat to public health.

Another area of public health with which the public-health profession had little to do was the struggle to establish *birth control*. The post-war 'baby boom' and the reassertion of the importance of women's prime role as wife and mother in the home (via the writing of John Bowlby and others), led to services promoting contraception being given low priority. A breakthrough came in 1955 when the Family Planning Association celebrated its silver jubilee and received its first official recognition with a visit from Ian Macleod, then Minister of Health.

Between 1955 and 1960, despite opposition from some quarters, the battle for respectable contraception was largely won. At the Lambeth Conference in 1958, the Anglicans came out firmly in favour of birth control, which was accepted as a 'right and important factor in Christian family life'.

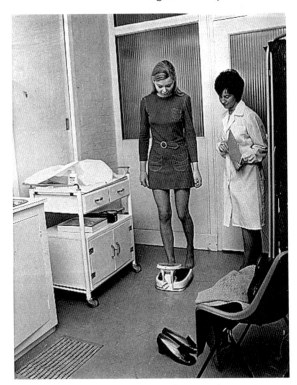

Figure 6.13 *This photograph of a client at a Family Planning Association consultation in the 1960s was used to promote the 'modern' image of contraception among young women. (Source: Brook Advisory Centre)*

Another key development was the advent of the contraceptive pill, approved by the Medical Advisory Panel of the Family Planning Association in 1961 (Figure 6.13). By 1964, there were about 480 000 women on the pill in Britain. The pill was 'scientific' and available only on prescription, and this put contraception for the first time firmly in the hands of the medical profession. As the historian, Barbara Brookes, has commented:

> ... the pill and medical control ensured matters of fertility control became an integral part of medical practice rather than a separate moral issue. (Brookes, 1988, p. 128)

The prospect of universal access to contraception drew attention to the limited role of the NHS in family planning. At first the pill was available on private prescription, although without charge in the case of clinics run by voluntary organisations. Beginning in the mid-sixties there was a campaign to make contraception available free on NHS prescription. This was finally conceded by the Labour government in 1974. Mass publicity methods were used in the 1970s, for example the poster shown in Figure 6.14.

Even greater controversy attended the campaign for *abortion reform*, stimulated by public outrage at the thalidomide disaster (in which prescription of an anti-morning-sickness drug caused malformations in the fetus and large numbers of children were born with deformities), and at the lengths women had to go to obtain an abortion. The key pressure group in this campaign was the Abortion Law Reform Association, which saw the Abortion Act of 1967 as a victory. The Abortion Act opened the way to the development of NHS abortion facilities. However, within the NHS this was left entirely to local discretion, with the result that either on grounds of policy or principle, in many areas abortion remained effectively unavailable under the NHS. Accordingly, those requiring this service were often dependent on charities and private agencies. Some historians have pointed out that both abortion reform and the development of the contraceptive pill gave the medical profession greater authority over women's lives.[8]

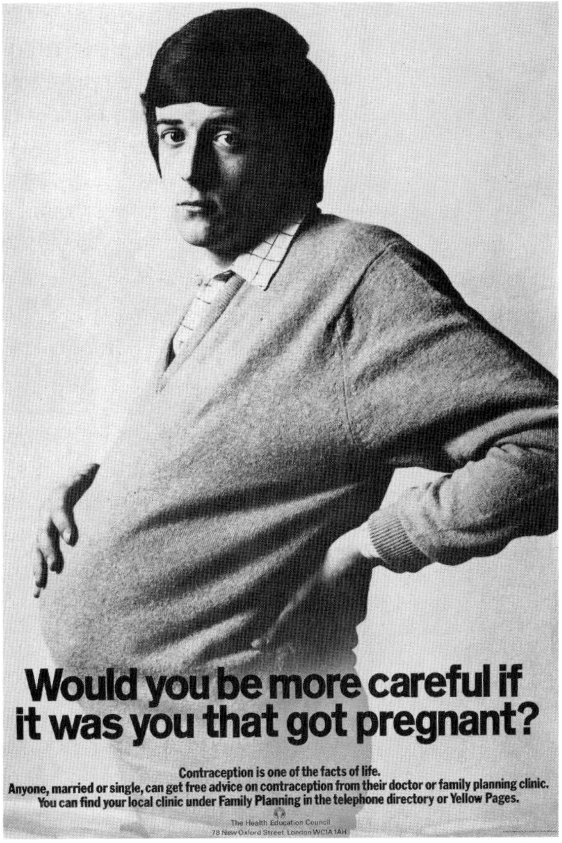

Would you be more careful if it was you that got pregnant?

Contraception is one of the facts of life.
Anyone, married or single, can get free advice on contraception from their doctor or family planning clinic. You can find your local clinic under Family Planning in the telephone directory or Yellow Pages.

The Health Education Council
78 New Oxford Street, London WC1A 1AH

Figure 6.14 *The Family Planning Association's 'pregnant man' poster attracted widespread publicity in 1974–5. (Source: Science and Society Picture Library, London)*

The single-issue campaigns relating to smoke pollution, family planning and abortion were representative of the wide range of such movements that sprang up to press the case for reform in areas relating to public health. As in the case of thalidomide, some of these pressure groups were newly established; in other cases, long-established charities were reorganised to meet the challenges of the future. For instance in 1959, with the decline in tuberculosis, one of the big charities — the National Association for the Prevention of Tuberculosis — became the Chest and Heart Association. The process of evolution continued until this organisation became the British Heart Foundation, which is active in the public health sphere in combating tobacco smoking, and encouraging a healthy diet and physical fitness.

Long-established and influential organisations increasingly adopted short titles (e.g. MIND in 1970; MENCAP in 1981), in order to increase their public profile. The newer campaigning organisations such as Action on Smoking and Health (ASH), reflected a new lifestyle orientation in public health. Also indicative of growing sensitivity to consumerism was the increasing involvement in public health issues of the Consumers Association.

6.5.2 Public-health failings of the welfare state

The prominence assumed by campaigning groups underlined the limitations of the health service, and the welfare state more generally, in meeting the needs of vulnerable groups and in responding to new threats to health. Indeed, as illustrated by housing policy, some of the biggest investments of the welfare state generated as many problems as they solved. In the post-war period, the Labour Party consistently tried to increase the stock of council housing, while the Conservatives

[8] The increasing intervention of medicine into matters of fertility, infertility and contraception is discussed in *Birth to Old Age: Health in Transition* (Open University Press, 2nd edn 1995; colour-enhanced 2nd edn 2001), Chapter 7.

gave priority to expanding owner-occupation. Under the Conservatives, from 1954 to 1964 a greater proportion of private houses were built. This balance of construction also continued under Labour as a result of the impact of the 1967 devaluation of the pound on public expenditure programmes.

By the mid-1970s, the overall standard of housing had considerably improved. But 'new slums' had been created in the high-rise council estates of the 1960s. In the medium term, these became the foci of deprivation and social degeneration, exacerbating instead of diminishing health inequalities.

Even before the economic crisis of 1973, serious doubts were emerging about the sustainability of the welfare state. The Conservative government of 1970–4 began to mount a reaction against the apparently inevitable extension of the interventionist state. Many of its measures had public-health implications. Increases in prescription charges and the price of school meals, and the abolition of cheap welfare milk were among the first assaults on the welfare state. In the 1980s, as you will see in Chapter 7, the erosion of welfare gathered momentum and had further implications for public health.

But before considering our own more recent past, we turn to health issues in the colonial, and former colonial, territories held by Europe at the end of World War II. As you will see, a more nineteenth-century construction of public health was still in practice there.

6.6 'Scientific' medicine and the 'Third World'

Up to the 1940s, international public health had been strongly influenced by the association made in colonial times between tropical medicine and the study and treatment of parasitic diseases. Expatriate civil servants, military personnel and managers were threatened by tropical diseases that were non-existent in Europe, or of limited importance. As a result, several important parasitic diseases including malaria and schistosomiasis (bilharzia) received considerable attention, and huge strides were made in understanding their causes and their natural history.

As you will recall from earlier chapters, schools of tropical medicine, established in Europe at the beginning of the twentieth century, took over from the predominantly military schools of medicine. As a more stable basis for research was needed, laboratories were established in colonial territories in what was then referred to collectively as the *Third World*: the Dutch specialised in Indonesia, the Belgians in Zaire, Rwanda and Burundi, the Germans in what was then Tanganyika. Britain and France's interests were more widespread because of their colonisation patterns. The American Rockefeller Foundation also played a dominant role in supporting research institutions in a number of developing countries.

The early 1940s were characterised by great confidence in medical science and its ability to challenge disease. The advent of sulphonamides, penicillin and the wide-spectrum antibiotics between 1930 and 1950 gave Western medicine what were described as *magic bullets*, i.e. synthetic and naturally occurring drugs which could destroy infectious organisms without harming the living host.[9] In Africa, the use of penicillin injections to cure the infectious disease yaws and sexually transmitted diseases made an indelible impression that injections were the best medicine for any ill.

[9] The mechanisms by which infectious organisms produce disease symptoms in people, and the effect of antibiotics on bacteria are discussed in another book in this series, *Human Biology and Health: An Evolutionary Approach* (Open University Press, 3rd edn 2001), Chapters 5 and 6.

The synthesis of the pesticide DDT and its application to control malaria-carrying mosquitoes seemed equally magical. By the 1950s, vaccines that gave protection against many important infectious diseases gave added impetus to the triumph of medical science and its wonder drugs. Such pharmaceutical advances strengthened expatriate beliefs that indigenous systems of health care were unscientific and potentially harmful, further undermining alternative traditional methods.

6.6.2 International initiatives

Medical confidence was paralleled by a social climate of reform in the wake of the 1930s recession and World War II. In the late 1940s, in a wave of idealism and wish for global peace, a number of new organisations were established to form the United Nations system. The agency with a major responsibility for health was the *World Health Organisation* (WHO), with headquarters in Geneva, and six regional offices around the world. Its main aim was to promote international cooperation in the field of health. It evolved from an earlier agency of the League of Nations, established in 1923. Another UN agency closely involved with health was *UNICEF* (United Nations Children's Fund), its target group including both mothers and children.

Countries became members of WHO in order to gain from its expertise and influence policy on health. This exchange at the international level was important in terms of influencing thinking about health policy. For instance, one of the earliest programmes supported and initiated by WHO and a number of big donor agencies was against *malaria*. World War II had drawn attention to the powerful influence of this disease, which in Asia and the Pacific area caused far more illness and deaths among military forces, than occurred as casualties of war. Largely as a consequence of this world-wide sensitivity to an old problem, WHO launched a malaria eradication programme in 1955 (see Figure 6.15).

This programme was a great success in parts of Europe and North America where malaria was endemic and in some parts of South America and the Western Pacific.

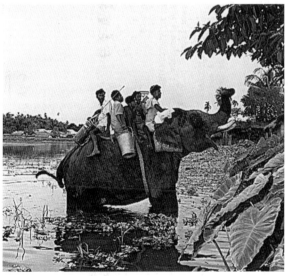 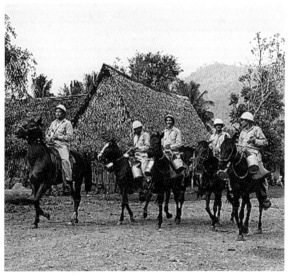

(a)   (b)

Figure 6.15   *Illustration of the WHO malaria eradication campaign, launched in 1955. (a) In India, a malaria team makes its way into the depths of the forest through marshes and across lakes. (b) In Mexico, the campaign was launched with the thoroughness of a military organisation and spray teams were deployed as though they were combat troops. In this picture the 'malarial cavalry' set out from Jacaltepec to climb the bridle-paths into the High Sierras. (Sources: (a) WHO/photo by P. N. Sharma; (b) WHO/photo by Eric Schwab)*

By 1968, about 1.1 billion[11] people were protected from malaria as a result of environmental measures. But by then the momentum of the eradication programme was slowing down: DDT, which had successfully killed off strains of mosquitoes in some areas, was increasingly seen to have environmentally negative effects, and resistant strains of mosquitoes evolved which were immune to spraying.

In the poorer tropical countries, the eradication campaign illustrates how difficult it is to sustain public-health measures when there is no basic rural infrastructure of health facilities to carry out essential activities (for example, spraying houses regularly; cutting down bush near homes; preventing stagnant pools of water in order to discourage mosquitoes breeding, and treating people with anti-malarial drugs when they were ill). The name of the programme changed from 'eradication' to 'control'; successful eradication of disease implies a significant measure of social reform.

6.6.3 Importing European health care

Social reform was also manifest in thinking about improving state provision of health services. Many of the ideas embodied in the Beveridge report in the United Kingdom were shared by others. The ex-colonies of South Africa and India set up Commissions in the British tradition, to explore how to organise health systems that would more effectively meet people's needs. The Bhore Commission in India explicitly looked towards a socialised system of health services in which public health predominated, and eventually replaced private medical practice. The Bhore report was radical in its recognition that nutrition and general living standards were major determinants of health, and that 'it is the tiller of the soil on whom the economic structure of the country eventually depends' (quoted in Jeffrey, 1988, p. 113). The report therefore recommended, among other things, the establishment of a health system in India that emphasised preventive measures and was based on salaried workers in a public-health service that linked villages to district health centres. The Gluckman Commission in South Africa was asked to advise on an:

> ... organized national health service in conformity with the modern conception of 'health' which will ensure adequate mental, dental, nursing and hospital services for all sections of the people of South Africa. (Gluckman, quoted in Marks, 1988, p. 8)

However, only a few of the recommendations of the Bhore and Gluckman reports were implemented. This was partly due to the political and administrative structures of those countries, which gave considerable responsibility for health care to the states or provinces, with the central government retaining only minimal control over policy. But it was also due to political tensions, the resistance of the medical profession to radical change, and the beginning of the 'Cold War' during which any ideas that seemed socialist or communist in origin were viewed with suspicion in the West.

In developing countries around the world, the medical establishment encouraged the founding of medical schools and training curricula modelled on those in the industrialised world. Universities and research institutions were set up, often in partnership with universities from the 'mother country'. There was a strong emphasis on comparability of standards and building up 'centres of excellence' which would equal the best of the medical schools and teaching hospitals of Britain, France, Italy and Germany. Curricula were imported from European schools, and medical students were taught about the chronic diseases of Europe rather than the infectious and other more relevant conditions (at the time) of their own countries.

---

[11] Throughout this book, 1 billion is taken to equal 1 000 000 000 (one thousand million).

Moreover, because of the emphasis on professional comparability, many doctors and nurses left developing countries for further training in the industrialised world (Figure 6.16), and many never returned (a topic to which we return in Chapter 9). The international ramifications of the 'brain drain' were analysed in the 1960s. The key findings were that it represented a huge donation from poor to rich countries. By 1982, the Philippines alone had lost a total of 14 000 doctors and 89 000 nurses, mostly to the USA. In the industrialised countries, these health workers filled important gaps in the less prestigious hospitals and specialties.

In order to emulate the medical systems of the industrialised world, disproportionate amounts of health budgets went on teaching hospitals, importing diagnostic and therapeutic technology and medicines that were extremely costly (see Figure 6.17). By the 1960s, it was clear that what the expert in tropical diseases among children, David Morley, has called the 'three-quarters rule' was true all over the developing world: three-quarters of spending on health care was for high-technology care in *urban*-based hospitals and staff (he called them

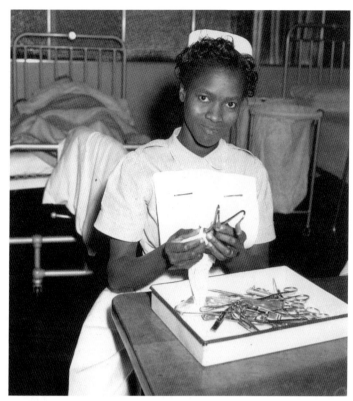

Figure 6.16   *A Nigerian nurse cleans surgical instruments at Brook General Hospital, Blackheath, London, in 1958; thousands of nurses (and doctors) from many developing countries came to work in Western hospitals from the 1950s onwards. (Source: George W Hales/Hulton Getty Picture Library)*

'disease palaces'), although three-quarters of the population lived in the *rural* areas, and three-quarters of all *deaths* were due to conditions that could be prevented by relatively *simple and inexpensive measures* (Morley *et al.*, 1983).

By the 1970s, health policies that had encouraged the importation of Western or industrialised models of health care were increasingly criticised, and developing countries themselves were experimenting with alternative systems of care. In Chapter 8, we look at how these changing ideas and experiences laid the basis for a revolutionary change in policy — the introduction of the *primary health-care* approach in the 1970s — and at its gradual demise in more recent decades.

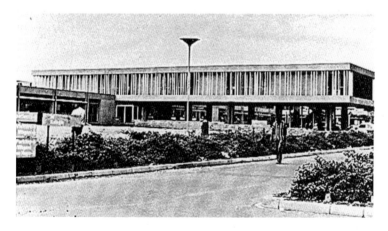

Figure 6.17   *The Kenyatta National Hospital in Nairobi (photographed in 1974) compared well with hospitals in the industrialised world, but absorbed a huge proportion of Kenya's total health budget. (Source: Diesfeld, H. J. and Hecklau, H. K., 1978, Kenya: A Geomedical Monograph, Springer-Verlag, Berlin)*

OBJECTIVES FOR CHAPTER 6

When you have studied this chapter, you should be able to:

6.1 Define and use, or recognise definitions and applications of, each of the terms printed in **bold** in the text.

6.2 Describe the principal innovative features of the NHS and identify its intrinsic organisational weaknesses as it was originally established.

6.3 Analyse the development of the concept of 'community care' in Britain in the period 1948–74, and its interaction with continuing patterns of lay care.

6.4 Describe the changes in the relative status and areas of competence of the medical profession in Britain in this period and the changes in the health-care division of labour.

6.5 Use examples to illustrate the changing nature of 'public-health issues' in Britain in this period and their relationship to the formal public-health profession.

6.6 Describe some of the ways in which health systems in developing countries mirrored those of the industrialised world in this period, and how far such emulation undermined their own needs.

QUESTIONS FOR CHAPTER 6

1 (*Objective 6.2*)

What factors led planners to concentrate their energies on building up the acute hospital services of the NHS? What effect did this policy have on the range of services available under the NHS?

2 (*Objective 6.3*)

Aneurin Bevan argued that: '… the undertaking to provide all people with all kinds of health care … creates an entirely new situation and calls for something bolder than a mere extension and adoption of existing services' (quoted in Webster, 1991, p. 41). To what extent was the NHS in practice unable to break free from the pattern of health care inherited from the past?

3 (*Objective 6.3*)

What did community care mean in the period 1948–74? How did it relate to patterns of lay care in Britain at this time?

4 (*Objective 6.4*)

List the factors involved in the change in status of GPs in Britain in 1948–74.

5 (*Objective 6.5*)

How did the function of public health change in Britain in the post-war decades? Cite examples of some public-health campaigns in this period and comment on the involvement of the organised public-health profession.

6 (*Objective 6.6*)

Describe the main post-war influences on emerging health systems in developing countries that stemmed directly from the industrialised world.

CHAPTER 7

Caring for health in the UK, 1974 to 2001

7.1   **Introduction**   198

7.2   **Containment and crisis of welfare**   198

     7.2.1   Political landscape in the UK   199

     7.2.2   Feeling worse   200

     7.2.3   Institutional inertia   201

7.3   **The NHS: management of crisis**   204

     7.3.1   Size of the system   204

     7.3.2   Management change   208

     7.3.3   Reorganisation   212

     7.3.4   The internal market   214

     7.3.5   Integrated care   216

7.4   **Care by the community**   220

     7.4.1   Policy development   220

     7.4.2   Who cares?   224

     7.4.3   Informal networks of care   226

     7.4.4   Complementary and alternative medicine   228

7.5   **Upheavals in the health-worker hierarchy**   231

     7.5.1   Hospital clinicians   231

     7.5.2   GPs and the primary health care team   233

     7.5.3   Nurses   236

7.6   **Promoting the public health**   240

     7.6.1   Fragmentation of public health   240

     7.6.2   Prevention and inequality   242

     7.6.3   Health promotion and the 'new public health'   245

     7.6.4   Communicable diseases   247

     7.6.5   Health of the Nation   247

     7.6.6   Our Healthier Nation   248

Objectives for Chapter 7   250

Questions for Chapter 7   250

Study notes for OU students

This chapter is the longest in the book. It has a dual function in the course: within the framework of the themes for this book as described in Chapter 1, it takes forward the history of health care in the UK from 1974 to 2001. And it also provides the foundation for the whole of the next book in the course, *Dilemmas in UK Health Care* (Open University Press, third edition 2001), which explores issues of major contemporary importance in UK health care. Section 7.3 is the longest part of this chapter and the most complex; consequently, we suggest that you allocate about a third of the study time for this chapter to it. During Section 7.4.2, you will be asked to read an article entitled 'The carer at home', by Michael Young and Lesley Cullen, which appears in *Health and Disease: A Reader* (Open University Press, third edition 2001); this article was optional reading for an earlier book in the course, *Birth to Old Age: Health in Transition* (Open University Press, second edition 1995; colour-enhanced second edition 2001).

7.1 Introduction

This chapter analyses the complicated developments in health care in the UK that have taken place between 1974 and the start of the new millennium. It is organised as a sequence of five separate and partly chronological surveys, each on a specific topic and each ranging over the period covered here.

Section 7.2, *Containment and crisis of welfare*, gives a short overview of the political, economic and institutional problems that have affected health care in the UK in this period. Section 7.3, *The NHS: management of crisis*, is the longest part of the chapter and comprises a detailed discussion of the complex changes to the management and organisation of the NHS since 1974. Section 7.4, *Care by the community*, is concerned with developments in community and informal networks of care, and also the rise in use of complementary and alternative medicine. Section 7.5, *Upheavals in the health-worker hierarchy*, discusses the main shifts in the roles, status and responsibilities of three groups of health workers: hospital clinicians, GPs and nurses. Lastly, Section 7.6, *Promoting the public health*, deals with the emergence of evidence concerning inequalities in health since the 1970s, and policies to prevent disease and promote the public health.

7.2 Containment and crisis of welfare

1974 is the date of the first major reorganisation of the UK National Health Service (NHS). It also marks a more general watershed, indeed one of the most important points of global economic and social transition in the twentieth century. The impact of this moment of change was all the more significant because it took the developed world almost completely by surprise.

Since World War II the Western economies had enjoyed an unparalleled period of prosperity. As already described in the previous chapter, this enabled Western powers to confound the sceptics and embark on ambitious programmes of welfare, apparently without exercising adverse effects on their economies. In retrospect, social analysts regard the period ending in 1974 as the 'Golden Age of the Welfare State'. Among the member states of the Organisation for Economic Cooperation and Development (OECD: that is, the Western industrialised nations), between 1960 and 1974, welfare expenditures as a whole expanded at an average rate of about 6.5 per cent a year. This represented a rate of expansion that has never been surpassed before or since. Spending on medical services represented one of the most buoyant of these welfare commitments.

The courtship of welfare by Western states was more reckless than was realised at the time. Especially in Northern Europe and the USA, expansion was carried out heedless of the economic consequences. The point was inevitably reached when the mounting burden of welfare became insupportable. The fragility of Western economies was suddenly exposed in 1973 when the Organisation of Petroleum Exporting Countries (OPEC), mainly representing developing nations, and at that date dominated by the Middle East, embarked on a policy of aggressively increasing the price of oil. This was merely the catalyst to a crisis that had profound and permanent effects. The Western economies as a whole experienced a big decline in growth, a rise in unemployment, a balance of trade deficit and a sharp rise in inflation. It was abundantly clear that expansion of welfare expenditures could not continue at the previous rate, and indeed that it was necessary to go into reverse.

The American social analyst Hugh Heclo noted that:

> ... complacency about the momentum of the welfare state gave
> way to doom-mongering by many in the intellectual elite. (Heclo,
> 1981, in Flora and Heidenheimer, p. 399)

Suddenly the welfare state was turned from virtuous prize into a kind of Frankenstein's monster. From this point onwards, confronting the perceived 'crisis' of the welfare state became a major preoccupation of Western governments. The former consensus on welfare strategies fragmented, with different solutions being tried in different countries.

7.2.1 Political landscape in the UK

As one of the weakest economies in post-war Northern Europe, the UK experienced only moderate expansion of its welfare and health expenditures before 1974. Thereafter, in common with its Western neighbours, the UK has experienced the greatest difficulty in sustaining its welfare and health programmes. The UK felt the full impact of the oil crisis, and the Labour government elected in 1974 was forced to turn to the International Monetary Fund (IMF) for support. In return the IMF required immediate cuts in welfare and health spending. Reflecting the failure of the government to adapt successfully to this new situation, Labour suffered a general election defeat in 1979 and a long political decline. This contributed to the Conservatives retaining power for an unprecedented period, indeed until 1997.

The Conservative administration of the 1980s, headed by Margaret Thatcher, was armed with a radical prospectus. It seemed likely that the government would take the axe to all welfare programmes in a crusade to rein back public expenditure and reduce the role of the state. Big changes of policy were introduced, and the state drastically cut back its role in areas such as housing. However, when the Conservatives left office in 1997, spending on health and social security constituted one of the biggest elements of the economy. Indeed, the combined expenditure on health and social security in the UK increased from about 20 per cent of Gross Domestic Product (GDP)[1] in 1975 to about 25 per cent by 1997. The Conservatives were therefore unsuccessful in their mission to reduce the share of GDP absorbed by the welfare programme as a whole. Nevertheless, their policies profoundly altered the characteristics of the welfare state. As you will see in the course of this chapter, no sector of the health service was left in the form inherited from the Labour administrations of the 1970s.

During their long spell in opposition (1979–1997), Labour politicians attacked every Conservative policy intervention in the health and social services and promised to return to the spirit of the welfare state introduced by the 1945 Labour government. Labour's promises of restitution were particularly vehement with respect to the health service. In practice, by 2001, the 'New' Labour government returned in 1997 had modified Conservative policies only to a limited extent. The Conservatives had by trial and error found various means of containing most aspects of spending on the welfare state. A viable welfare system no longer seemed incompatible with a stable economy. New Labour invested its energies in consolidating this course of action.

With respect to some of the biggest social welfare programmes at least, the prophets of doom of the 1970s seem to have been confounded. Although the UK has spent much less of its national resources on health care than its Western counterparts,

---

[1] Gross Domestic Product (GDP) is a measure of the wealth of a country; its relationship to spending on health care is discussed in Chapter 9.

there has been a steady rise in investment in health care. This additional funding, together with a rolling programme of reforms extending over the entire period since 1974, seems to have contained costs and created a framework for successful modernisation of the entire health service. From the 1990s onwards the public relations machinery of government worked in overdrive to promote this positive conclusion. In the rest of this chapter, we will examine the process of modernisation, taking special care to avoid the 'triumphalist fallacy' highlighted in Chapter 1.

7.2.2 Feeling worse

As you can see from the above summary (which is amplified in Chapter 9), since 1974 all of the Western economies have experienced the greatest difficulty in sustaining growth in spending on health care to meet the unavoidable pressure of demand for resources, which has been created by such factors as demographic change and medical innovation. Increased demand associated with the rising numbers of elderly or disabled people within the population, modern achievements of high technology medicine such as scanning devices, or the ever increasing availability of powerful new drugs for treatment of major diseases such as cancer, have almost invariably entailed escalation of costs. Only rarely do they give rise to cost savings.

This dramatically changing situation has inevitably called for a more rapid pace of policy review, sometimes implying a total redesign, affecting every sphere of health care. It is therefore evident that health services throughout the West have been plunged into the massive task of adaptation, requiring much more than increased resources. As indicated below, in most key problem areas, the twin issues of *policy* and *resources* were often inextricably mixed together.

Although throughout the OECD region, health care has been pursued as a high priority of governments, the air of crisis that overtook health care in 1974 has never been entirely dispelled. This perception of crisis has been particularly prevalent in the UK because of such factors as relatively low levels of funding and inherent weaknesses in organisation and management. The ominous alarmist headlines that repeatedly appear in the press are a reminder of the acute anxiety surrounding the state of Western health-care systems. As you will see in Chapter 8, the situation in low- and middle-income countries of the developing world has consistently given even greater cause for concern.

Although the NHS has enjoyed certain special advantages — for example until the mid-1980s it had particularly low administrative costs — these were insufficient to compensate for the adverse position of the UK in the international league table of health-service expenditure. (This handicap is considered in some detail in Chapter 9.)

As already noted in Chapter 6, resource constraint plagued the NHS from the outset, with the result that the UK health service was slow to embark on urgent tasks of modernisation. The UK dragged behind other Western nations in evolving up-to-date care programmes for major patient groups. The *Hospital Plan* was not launched until 1962. As a consequence, hospital modernisation had made little headway by the time it became slowed down by the cuts imposed in the wake of the oil crisis. This meant that the district general hospital services, upon which the whole system turned, were housed in dilapidated accommodation, thereby impeding the introduction of more efficient new services and causing wastefulness in the use of scarce resources. The inadequacy of the buildings used for modern hospital purposes is illustrated by Figure 7.1 (see also Figure 1.3g).

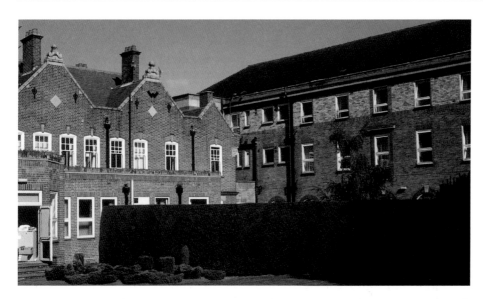

Figure 7.1 *The West Norwich Hospital is an example of the patchwork of unsatisfactory buildings added at different dates, which has been typical of the piecemeal approach to NHS hospital provision. (Source: Robert Moore)*

Lack of capital investment in acute hospitals was paralleled by delays in the development of acute hospital specialisms such as day surgery and advanced forms of care. From the beginning of the NHS to the present, experts in the health-care field and client-group lobbies have been vociferous in complaining about the backwardness of facilities across the board, for instance inadequately staffed accident and emergency or outpatient departments, the lack of high-technology facilities to deal with kidney failure or heart disease, and poorly coordinated services for treating cancers. Common to all complaints is the assertion that services in the UK are inferior to those existing elsewhere in the European Union, and that outcomes for patients are substantially worse.

7.2.3 Institutional inertia

In the last quarter of the twentieth century it became increasingly apparent that the NHS was less effective than most of its Western counterparts in keeping up with the demands of modernisation. Lack of resources was conventionally cited to explain the shortcomings. However, it was increasingly clear that certain inherent features of the NHS undermined efforts to bring about improvement and, in consequence, restricted resources were not being used to best advantage. Successive governments have expressed determination to overcome this institutional inertia, only to be frustrated by the indifferent results of their efforts at reform.

Among its shortcomings the NHS has failed to achieve equity in the distribution of resources or uniformity in the delivery of services. This is perhaps particularly surprising given the egalitarian objectives of the NHS. Consequently there have always been, and still persist, substantial and irrational differences in the level of service provided between one district and another. In the 1990s this endemic tendency to geographic inequity became known as the **postcode lottery**. With the emergence of powerful but expensive new treatments for intractable health problems, denial of access has inevitably attracted media attention. For instance, in the course of the last few weeks of 1999, the headlines were caught by stories of postcode lotteries with respect to the treatment of various types of cancer, coronary heart disease, motor neurone disease, Alzheimer's disease, depression, obesity and infertility.

Embarrassment and frustration over the failure to establish services on a par with others among Western neighbours has provoked expressions of resentment, not only from patient groups, but also from experts in the field. For instance Professor

Gordon McVie, the Director General of the Cancer Research Campaign attracted media headlines in 1999 following his lecture pointing out the inadequacy of resources to meet present and likely future needs for cancer care (Figure 7.2). Professor McVie itemised characteristic failings of cancer services.

> We are not delivering state-of-the-art treatment to everybody with cancer in the UK. We have been shouting and screaming and protesting for five years, ever since our data showed the difference in outcomes according to where you live … This has resulted in disgraceful cancer mortality figures in the UK, probably the worst in Western Europe and certainly worse than in the United States … New drugs such as Taxol, which can extend the lives of young women with ovarian cancer, were not being funded. Radiotherapy machines were 20 years out of date. And the Calman–Hine review of cancer care, which recommended that patients should see cancer specialists in centres of excellence instead of general consultants at district hospitals, was not being fully implemented. Health Authorities and Trusts are sitting there doing nothing. (McVie, 1999, quoted in *The Guardian*, 21 October)

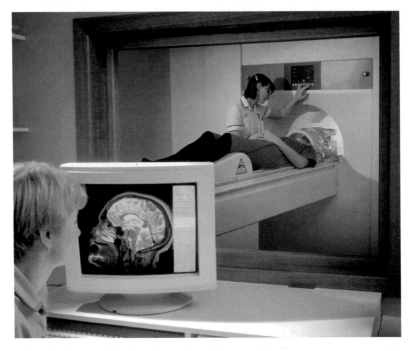

Figure 7.2 *Magnetic Resonance Imaging (MRI) scanners are extensively used in the diagnosis of cancer. The shortage of modern equipment of this kind, together with the shortage of specially-trained staff and properly organised regional cancer centres, lies behind the relatively poor record of the UK in cancer treatment. (Source: Geoff Tompkinson/Science Photo Library)*

● Where does Professor McVie place the blame for shortcomings in cancer services?

■ Many of the difficulties he cites can be directly related to resource limitations, but he also strongly complains about inertia within the health service; both central government and NHS management are censured for their failure to respond appropriately to the crisis.

Professor McVie was specifically concerned about failure to implement the Calman–Hine review of cancer services, which dates from 1994. However, the strength of his words reflects a deeper frustration. The Calman–Hine review was itself necessary because of the failure of a succession of earlier reforms of cancer services. Indeed, the idea of concentrating services in regional oncology centres dates back to a report of 1970, which was accepted as policy by the 1970–74 Conservative government under Edward Heath. An expert in this field comments that this initiative collapsed owing to 'procrastination ... lack of planning, lack of finance, and no indication of the scale of the operation' (Austoker, 1988, p. 311). The performance of the UK cancer services is not uniformly inferior, but the endemic weaknesses have been sufficiently pronounced to explain the frustration of Professor McVie and his colleagues.

Cancer services are not an isolated instance. Similar endemic shortcomings have been cited in areas such as cardiovascular surgery, stroke treatment and renal care. The government's own Performance Indicators confirmed in 2000 the seriousness of the shortcomings, including the extent of the postcode lottery. Confidence in hospital services was further damaged by evidence concerning the incompetence or negligence of health-care professionals, ranging from medical personnel to those interpreting the results of routine tests such as cervical smears.

Echoing past scandals about the state of long-stay hospitals, and more recent publicity over the deficiencies of community care, the same problems of resource shortage and incompetent planning are endemic in services affecting elderly, mentally ill or mentally disabled people. A review of mental health policy since the 1970s (Rogers and Pilgrim, 1998), complained about inertia of policy in central government and neglect by health-service administration. Contrary to stated policy, hospital care continues to absorb 90 per cent of spending, while community mental health services remain in a primitive state and are patchy in their development (ibid., p. 197).

Since its election in 1997, the Labour government has conceded the justice of complaints about the shortcoming of services. For instance, addressing the Royal College of Surgeons in May 2000, Alan Milburn, Secretary of State for Health, frankly accepted that the NHS was 'too slow, too inconvenient and too unresponsive' and he complained that as a result of systems failures the service habitually 'conspired to place the wrong patient in the wrong place at the wrong time' (quoted in *The Independent*, 2000, 19 May). As an earnest of a new level of determination to address these problems, in 1999 the government appointed 'Czars' to head expert teams charged with spearheading action to reform the cancer and heart services.

The 'feeling worse' perception due to shortcomings of medical treatment was reinforced by mounting fears about public health issues.

●   What lapses in public health have caused alarm in the UK since the 1980s?

■   You may have suggested the arrival of HIV/AIDS; the BSE crisis and the identification of variant Creutzfeldt–Jakob disease (vCJD) in humans; fatal outbreaks of *E. coli* and *Salmonella* food poisoning; the emergence of antibiotic-resistant strains of TB; untreatable infections acquired in hospital, partly attributable to lapses in hospital hygiene; hazards to health from environmental pollution — including from the burning or burial of animal carcasses during the foot-and-mouth disease outbreak in 2001; and damage to the ozone layer. Many of these problems are global in their occurrence, but some, such as BSE, were rooted in the UK.

None of these examples of shortcomings detract from the benefits derived from the substantial resources invested in the NHS. Indeed, in some respects the NHS has performed better than its counterparts elsewhere. Nevertheless, evidence of defects within the system gives few grounds for complacency. Public anxieties, often echoed in the media, are supported by expert opinion on the inadequacy of resources and failings of policy, which have tended to undermine public confidence in the health service. These same experiences have also contributed to a more questioning attitude to Western scientific medicine in general (a point we return to in Section 7.4.4).

7.3   The NHS: management of crisis

For reasons cited in the previous section, the UK has experienced some particular difficulties in managing the crisis that has affected Western health care. Although the UK health services might have benefited from such potential advantages as funding from central taxation, low administrative costs, and from the economies of scale possible in large, integrated organisations, in practice health care has not derived the full benefit from these characteristics.

● Summarise the factors (outlined in Section 7.2) that have contributed to the particular difficulties faced by the NHS in recent decades, compared with its Western counterparts.

■ Lower spending on health care compared with other OECD nations; failures in central command over policy or practice in the field, resulting in slow response to innovations or improvements in care; failure to iron out inequities in the allocation of resources between areas and programmes; and difficulty in meeting expectations resulting from the obligation to offer comprehensive services to the entire population, free at the point of delivery.

7.3.1 Size of the system

Although state provision of medical care has predominated in the UK since 1948, it has never extinguished other forms of medical provision. The many agencies supplying medical services outside the NHS will frequently be mentioned in this chapter. For example, since 1974 there has been such a sharp rise in private dentistry that in many areas it is difficult to locate dentists accepting new patients under the NHS. Also, by 1995, about 12 per cent of the population had taken out private health insurance, compared with 4 per cent in 1975 (we consider this trend further in Chapter 9). Private purchases of pharmaceutical products, many of them relating to complementary and alternative therapies, are also increasing rapidly.

These examples are all significant social phenomena, but their quantitative impact is relatively small compared with the scale of spending on the NHS. In 1995 private health care (mainly private medical insurance), and individual spending on pharmaceutical products, amounted to about 15 per cent of the level of spending on the NHS, compared with about 10 per cent in 1975. As Chapter 9 explains, the UK is exceptional in the dominance of its tax-funded health-care arrangements.

In practice reliance on central taxation proved a doubtful asset, since spending on health care was exposed to the vagaries of political interference and made dependent on the performance of the economy. Under its tax-based system, the UK drifted inexorably down the OECD league-table of health spending. As noted earlier, in the course of the 1990s it became evident that levels of spending were insufficient to support a modern health service.

Responding to the perceived state of crisis, in February 2000, the Prime Minister pledged the government to raise spending on the NHS to the European average. In the March 2000 budget this was translated into a pledge to increase spending on the NHS to twice the historic average. For the first time since 1948 it seemed that funding would be sustained at a level proportionate to the needs of the vast organisation that comprised the NHS. Time will tell how this commitment is fulfilled.

From the outset, the hospital sector has absorbed the largest slice of funds available to the NHS, its share being dictated by the labour-intensive nature of the hospital service. If anything, the increasing pace of medical advance has added to this labour intensiveness. The changing character of the Hospital Services sector is reflected in the numbers employed in various staff groups (Table 7.1).

Table 7.1 Number of staff (thousands) employed in NHS Hospitals by category, UK, 1973–1997.

Year	Medical and dental	Nursing and midwifery	Scientific and technical	Admin. and clerical	Domestic and ancillary	Total
1973	32.9	392.4	47.8	69.2	231.1	772.1
1978	41.5	445.6	69.0	120.4	258.6	927.4
1983	46.6	506.6	82.5	132.3	252.4	1007.3
1988	49.7	516.4	98.5	144.5	180.3	989.4
1993	56.8	470.2	112.9	189.6	128.3	957.8
1997	66.8	373.1	111.2	187.6	98.8	837.4

Nursing and midwifery includes full-time and part-time staff numbers, and unqualified staff grades (mainly nursing assistants and auxiliaries) who comprise about one-quarter of the total. (Data from Office of Health Economics, 1999, *Compendium of Health Statistics*, 11th edition, Chapter 12, Table 3.3. Note that data are given in 5-year intervals until 1993, concluding with 1997, the most recent year for which data were available.)

● Describe the main trends in hospital staff numbers shown in Table 7.1, starting with the total employed. Which groups have seen the largest increases or decreases over time in relative terms?

■ The total number of hospital staff peaked in 1983 at over one million and has since fallen back below the 1978 level. The largest sector, the nurses and midwives, mirrored this trend, growing to over half a million in 1983 and 1988, but declining sharply thereafter, until by 1997 they had fallen below their numbers of 24 years earlier. In relative terms, the largest cuts have occurred among domestic and ancillary staff (Figure 7.3a, overleaf), whose numbers have more than halved since their high-point in 1978. The largest gains have been in administrative and clerical staff, whose numbers multiplied to 2.7 times their 1973 level, and in scientific and technical staff (up 2.3 times over the period, Figure 7.3b, overleaf), but both staff categories appear to have passed their peak level and have declined in recent years. Medical and dental staff numbers have doubled since 1973 and the increase is continuing.

The footnote to Table 7.1 refers to the fact that the numbers quoted for nurses and midwives include unqualified staff, mainly nursing assistants and auxiliaries working on the wards. Their employment increased substantially during the 1990s; consequently the fall in the numbers of qualified nurses working in hospitals has been much greater than it appears from the table. The decrease in hospital nurses and midwives has stemmed from recruitment difficulties and falling retention rates,

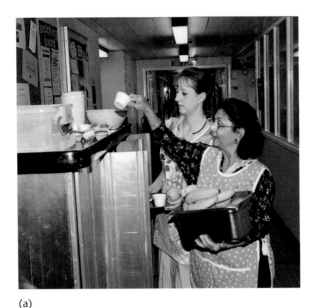

(a)

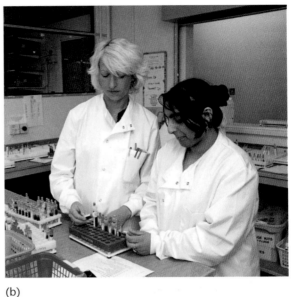

(b)

Figure 7.3 *(a) Hospital domestic and ancillary services were extensively 'privatised' in the 1980s, more than halving the number of staff in this category directly employed by the NHS; (b) By contrast, scientific and technical staff more than doubled over the same period, although this remained insufficient to meet service requirements. (Source (a) and (b): Mike Levers)*

which have led to staff shortages in some critical skill groups. The fall in domestic and ancillary staff is due to policy changes that have privatised functions such as maintenance, catering, cleaning and laundry services, previously undertaken by personnel directly employed by the NHS.

Alterations in the NHS labour force will be further discussed at various points in the rest of this chapter. For the moment it is sufficient to note that staff shortages impose severe limitations on the volume and safety of work within the NHS. That is why hospital nursing staff numbers are often taken as a barometer of the 'health' of the NHS. It was a matter of acute concern that nursing staff numbers remained in decline as the new millennium approached. For example, in England, the crucial number of whole-time equivalent Qualified Nurses had remained at about 246 000 since 1995. The growing adverse impact on services forced the government to take special action to improve recruitment. In May 2000, with some relief, the Department of Health reported that nurse numbers in September 1999 had risen to 250 000.

● Why are static or falling numbers of hospital nurses, midwives and scientific and technical staff likely to impact adversely on the performance of the NHS?

■ Because increasing numbers of these highly trained groups are needed to deal with the rise in emergency admissions, the need for intensive care, and the greater range of high-technology activities within acute hospitals.

The changing character of the NHS is also indicated by data concerning the provision of hospital beds within different medical specialties (Figure 7.4).

● You can see from Figure 7.4 that the rate of decrease varies between specialties. Can you account for any of the differences by drawing on your general knowledge of trends in health care in the UK?

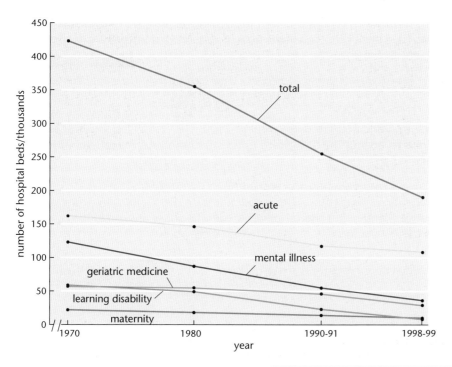

Figure 7.4 *Number of beds (thousands) in NHS Hospitals by category 1970–1999, England. (Data derived from Department of Health, 2000,* Shaping the Future NHS: Long Term Planning for Hospitals and Related Services, *Table 3.1)*

■ The fall in the number of NHS beds for patients with mental illness, learning disability or needing geriatric medical care is associated with their transfer to community care, including nursing and residential homes outside the NHS. The fall in acute care beds reflects the increased use of day surgery and the introduction of treatments allowing more rapid turnover of patients. The fall in maternity beds results from the rise in short-stay admissions and 'same day' discharges.

From 1970 to the end of the millennium there was a decline in acute care and maternity beds from 5.2 to 3 beds per 1000 population, which is considerably less than most other European nations. Of the OECD countries, only Sweden has substantially fewer hospital beds than the UK. The question naturally arises whether the decrease in beds has gone too far. The shortage of intensive care beds, often caused by shortages in the specialist nurses required to support them (Figure 7.5), attracts most attention during the winter crises that regularly affect the NHS.

A further effect of the bed and staff shortages is cancellation of planned operations. The

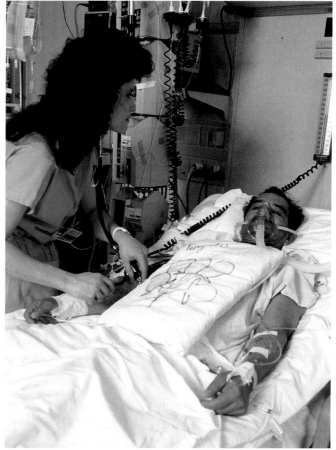

Figure 7.5 *The shortage of intensive care beds is frequently made worse by the shortage of specialist nurses to staff them. (Source: Custom Medical Stock Photo/Science Photo Library)*

National Audit Office reported that in the year to September 1999, some 57 000 operations had been cancelled at the time of admission of the patient (Comptroller and Auditor General, 2000).

Plans for new hospitals under the Private Finance Initiative (to which we return in the next section), have resulted in further pressures for bed reductions. In September 1998 increased tensions over this issue resulted in establishment of the National Beds Inquiry, which reported in February 2000 (Department of Health, 2000). It called for a reversal of the downward trend, an immediate increase of 4 000 NHS hospital beds and a further increase of 25 000 beds by 2020.

The data concerning staffing and bed numbers demonstrate that the NHS is by no means a static organisation. The period since 1974 has not only witnessed big quantitative changes, but also major organisational upheavals and indeed a general cultural transformation.

7.3.2 Management change

In the course of the 1970s it was appreciated that administrative changes in themselves were insufficient to improve the performance of the NHS. This led to an increasingly voiced conclusion that the NHS was 'over-administered and under-managed'. Attention therefore gradually shifted to management and indeed the 1974 reorganisation was designed as both an administrative and management solution. Management consultants played a leading role in designing the reorganisation, which involved an especially radical change — the introduction of **consensus management** throughout the system. This gave medical, nursing and management personnel a joint role in framing decisions.

Although embodying some attractive elements — for instance giving nurses greater authority in decision-making — in practice consensus management merely added to the extreme complexity and confusion of the system. Reaching a decision at the district operational level relied on achieving agreement in the whole management team; it also needed compliance with teams operating at the local and regional levels in the hierarchy, not to mention advisory Medical Committees operating at every level. The 1974 changes therefore demonstrated that the management problem was not going to be solved by a one-shot reorganisation.

Cash limits and direct charges

Some important management changes of lasting influence were rooted in the 1970s. For instance, a big impact was made by the introduction of the system of **cash limits** in 1976. This meant that each NHS authority was granted a specified amount of cash to spend on Hospital and Community Health Services (HCHS) in a given financial year, which comprised a limit that local managers were not allowed to exceed.

● What do you think were the consequences of cash limits?

■ Since the basis upon which the cash limit was calculated was likely to be less than that required to meet such liabilities as staff pay rises, NHS authorities were forced in the course of each financial year to make economies that in effect reduced the volume of resources available for patient care. On the positive side, the cash limit forced authorities to try to improve their efficiency.

The biggest anomaly in the cash-limits system was exclusion of family practitioners on the grounds that their services were **demand-led**, i.e. their level was determined by quantitative and qualitative patient demand upon which it was not possible to place a ceiling. This exclusion from cash limits has helped to protect the Family Health Services (FHS) from the annual expenditure crisis that tended to afflict the HCHS. The cash-limit distinction helps to explain why the HCHS : FHS spending ratio has drifted from 3.1 in 1975 to about 2.3 in 1999. This represents a major shift of resources from hospitals to primary care, which has largely been due to increased spending on expensive new drugs and a rise in the number of GPs and their support staff.

Following the imposition of cash limits in the HCHS sector, the government was alarmed by the potential for an uncontrolled rise in FHS spending. Particularly after 1979, they turned to methods of limiting demand by such devices as regular increases in the prescription charge, expanding charges for dental services to a large proportion of the cost of the service, and restricting free eye services to people on benefits, the young and certain restricted medical groups. Elderly people were absolved from prescription charges, but they were required to pay for eye tests and dental checks. All of these policy changes were unpopular and politically controversial.

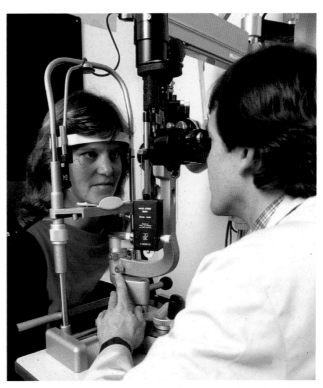

Figure 7.6 *Presentation for a routine eye test. Even though charges for spectacles were introduced in 1950, and were then periodically increased, eye tests remained free until 1989. (Source: Ed Young/Science Photo Library)*

Perhaps the most unpopular measure of all dated from 1989, with imposition of charges for eye tests (Figure 7.6) and dental checks. As illustrated further in Chapter 9, charges for eye tests drove down the numbers of people presenting for tests. Labour capitalised on the unpopularity of these charges by promising their abolition, and accordingly scrapped charges for eye tests for those above the age of 60 in 1999. But the Labour government's undertaking to review charges for dental checks was deferred indefinitely.

● Why were charges for eye tests and dental checks regarded as particularly offensive?

■ There were three main reasons: they constituted a disincentive to early treatment, and thereby invited neglect of conditions that would require more expensive free hospital treatment at a later date; these charges bore down particularly on groups with limited means, such as older people; and they created a precedent for extending charges to diagnosis rather than treatment.

Resource management

Also dating from the 1970s were a variety of initiatives designed to draw health professionals in hospitals into using financial and other management information to achieve more efficient and effective use of resources. These methods were designed to produce more exact costing of individual treatments, or hospital functions. In addition, availability of standardised information would enable costs to be compared within and between hospitals, and for costs to be assessed against health outcomes. Naturally, the full development of these techniques was dependent on advances in information technology. Further development of these methods in the 1980s was encouraged by the Griffiths Report (discussed below), after which the term **Resource Management Initiative** was adopted for the programme of further trials of these budgeting systems.

Very quickly it was appreciated that the Resource Management Initiative provided an information base requisite for a competitive system in which purchasers would contract for services on the basis of meeting particular cost and service requirements. The various components of the Resource Management Initiative were therefore regarded as one of the foundation stones for the *internal market in health care* of 1991 (described in Section 7.3.4) and, in the longer term, they became the corner-stone of the wider drive to improve the efficiency of hospital specialties.

In the course of the 1980s the Conservatives also introduced other significant management changes, many of them associated with the first **Griffiths Report** produced in 1983. Prime Minister Thatcher's use of Roy Griffiths to spearhead management reform in the NHS was itself significant and indicative of her government's general preference for guidance from the private sector. Instead of following the traditional course of remitting management reform to NHS professionals, Mrs Thatcher employed a small team headed by Griffiths, who was managing director of the powerful grocery chain, J. Sainsbury.

The Griffiths Report of 1983 recommended scrapping consensus management and replacing it by **general management**. This change was introduced in the late-1980s. It placed management responsibility at all levels within the hierarchy of NHS authorities in the hands of a single, accountable individual. These ranged from the NHS Chief Executive for each part of the UK, to Chief Executives in individual hospital units. The bias of recruitment into general management will be considered later in this chapter.

- What is the most striking difference between consensus management in the 1970s and general management in the 1980s?

- Under consensus management, medical, nursing and managerial personnel had a joint role in framing decisions, and agreement had to be reached within each management team and between local, district and regional levels in the NHS hierarchy. General management swept away all these arrangements and placed power in the hands of Chief Executives locally and nationally.

Beginning in the early 1980s, the Conservative government also introduced *performance reviews* and *performance indicators* to monitor increases in efficiency more effectively. It also introduced targets for efficiency gains. The government's efficiency programme attached particularly high priority to a form of 'self-policing' by doctors known as **clinical audit** (sometimes referred to as 'medical audit'), which embraces a variety of methods for analysing the quality of medical care, ranging from examination of specific procedures used for diagnosis and treatment to the more general examination of efficiency in the use of resources.

Trends towards privatisation

Health authorities also came increasingly under pressure to submit many of their non-clinical services to **competitive tendering**, which in practice rendered it likely that services previously provided within the health service would be contracted-out or privatised. This became one of the main means to meet efficiency targets because it offered the chance to reduce staff and therefore cut the massive staff bill of the NHS.

● Look back at Table 7.1. What functions were privatised and what was the impact of this change on overall numbers in the relevant staff group?

■ Privatisation embraced staff concerned with such functions as maintenance, catering, cleaning and laundry services. From the plateau of over a quarter of a million domestic and ancillary staff between 1978 and 1983, a huge decline to just under 99 000 had occurred by 1997.

Competitive tendering became a main avenue for privatisation, in line with the Thatcher government's more general drive to rein back the public sector. The drive towards privatisation culminated with the **Private Finance Initiative** (PFI), which was evolved in the 1990s by the Conservatives, but owing to a series of legal hitches, was not finally implemented on a substantial scale until after 1997 by the Labour government. PFI involves 'contracting-out' the building and supply of all non-clinical activity to private consortia under contracts of long duration.

You will recall from Chapter 1 that the new Norfolk and Norwich Hospital is one of the first and most ambitious of the hospitals to be built under the first phase of the PFI (Figure 7.7). It is anticipated that this development, which occupies a 63-acre site, will become designated as a new Teaching Hospital. It was originally envisaged that the new hospital would contain only 700 beds, but this has been revised upwards, and the intention is now to provide about 950 beds, which is still substantially below the number in the predecessor hospitals.

In the course of the 1980s changes in management in the NHS collectively brought about a substantial shift of culture. Indeed all public services were heading in the same direction. Public bodies increasingly imitated the private sector and in many

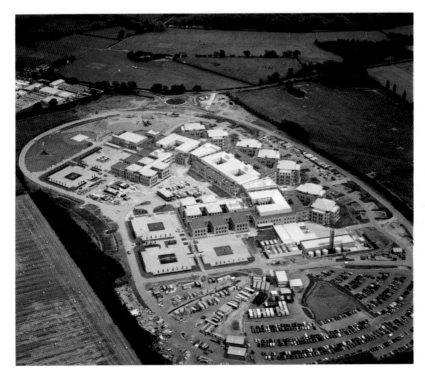

Figure 7.7 *The new Norfolk and Norwich Hospital is the response to a long-standing plan for a new District General Hospital mainly to supplant the Victorian Norfolk and Norwich Hospital, extended since 1948 under the NHS (Figure 1.3d), and the West Norwich Hospital (Figures 7.1 and 1.3g). It is due for completion in 2001. (Source: London Aerial Photo Library)*

cases the two were assimilated to an extent not contemplated earlier. This transformation within the public sector was called the **new public management** (see Box 7.1, to which we make several further references later in this chapter).

Box 7.1   Characteristics of 'new public management'

- Increased adoption of measures of *output*, indicating success in treatment of conditions, rather than reliance on input measurements such as levels of finance or numbers of personnel.

- Measures of performance and their adoption for purposes of pay and contracts, implying also a move from national to locally determined pay structures.

- Greater competition through the introduction of competitive tendering contracts and markets.

- Introduction of private sector styles of management practice such as general management and the Resource Management Initiative.

- Disaggregation of command and control bureaucracies into more independent, accountable units.

- Limitation of public bodies to being purchasers of services increasingly supplied by private providers.

- Increasing choice and influence of patients exercising their role as consumers, including creating effective machinery for facilitating and handling complaints.

- Expanding the role of clinical audit and regulation to monitor and control standards of work of professionals acting singly or jointly in a service context.

As the result of the importation of new public management, by the late 1980s the NHS was increasingly described among managers as an 'industry' rather than a service, while patients became designated as 'customers', whose exercise of choice was expected to ensure that performance was optimised.

Consistent with this new emphasis on consumer rights, in 1991 the Conservative government introduced *The Patient's Charter*, containing a set of new guarantees relating to standards of care in the NHS. *The Patient's Charter* was subsequently strengthened and the charter principle extended to facilitate the publication of 'league tables' showing the extent to which charter targets were being met. Application of the charter principle to the health service was yet a further small example of the growth of the new public management in the NHS.

A final stride in the same direction was represented by the internal market reforms, which represented the culmination of the Conservative government's efforts to recast the NHS in line with policies being applied elsewhere in the public sector.

7.3.3   Reorganisation

Given the severe restrictions on resources available to the NHS since 1974, successive governments have been forced to consider alternative means of supporting the expansion of services and increasing output. In particular, an urgent quest has taken place for a management structure that would bring about greater efficiency in the use of scarce material and human resources. This was extremely difficult due to the wide range of health services provided by the NHS in any one geographical area. Also the vast size of the NHS organisation necessitated some form of hierarchical structure, embodying an appropriate balance between centralisation and local devolution. The reorganisation project was also complicated by the need for collaboration with other services, especially the local authority social services.

Even in 1948 everyone appreciated that one of the main limits on efficiency was the hastily contrived *tripartite system* of organisation described in Chapter 6. Devising a new system that represented a genuine improvement on the 1948 model proved to be extremely difficult. The reorganisation of 1974, planned by the Conservative government under Edward Heath, was a hastily contrived compromise, which was radically altered in 1982. Shortage of space and the balance of priorities adopted for this book preclude consideration of the organisational arrangements in place between 1974 and 1991 — although it is worth noting that by the start of the new millennium very little trace of these reorganisations had survived.

However, before considering the radical reorganisations of the 1990s (Sections 7.3.4 and 7.3.5), it will be helpful to mention three of the main difficulties of principle that plagued successive efforts to reform the administration of the health service.

First, it has proved difficult to achieve an administrative structure that embraced all parts of the NHS. On account of their jealously guarded status as independent contractors, **family practitioners** (GPs, dentists, pharmacists, optometrists and ophthalmic medical practitioners), have been consistently hostile to incorporation within the rest of the health service. In the 1990s and into the new millennium, both the Conservatives' 'internal market' and Labour's 'primary care groups' further cemented the separate status of family practitioners (as you will see shortly).

Second, the divisions adopted in the NHS have always possessed an awkward alignment with respect to the boundaries of local government. This has of course added to the difficulty of creating a 'seamless' service, embracing health and social care. (Later in this chapter, in Section 7.4.1, we discuss one proposed solution to this problem — the creation of Primary Care Trusts.)

Third, the NHS has not arrived at a satisfactory arrangement for achieving a balance between executive power and local accountably at the regional and local level. The representative character of local and regional administrative bodies has been steadily eroded until, by the 1990s, they were constituted on the business model, with community interests being served by non-executive directors. This arrangement has been criticised for its amenability to political manipulation and lack of sensitivity to individual and local feeling.

At the time of writing (Spring 2001) these problems still have not been entirely resolved. The Conservatives wrestled with all three of these difficulties throughout the 1990s, during the period of the internal market in health care (Section 7.3.4); in the new millennium, Labour's integrated care policies faced the same struggle (Section 7.3.5). Successive UK governments have experimented with many different permutations, but it is still not evident that they have evolved a settled pattern of units of executive responsibility for the health service at either the regional or local level. The fact that the time interval between overhauls has tended to decrease suggests that stability is not within sight.

7.3.4 The internal market

The White Paper *Working for Patients* (Secretary of State for Health, 1989, implemented in April 1991) formally introduced the **internal market in health care**. With minor variations, this policy was implemented throughout the UK. Central to the internal market package, and consistent with the new public management changes (Box 7.1) already in train, was the **purchaser–provider split**. The internal market changes allowed suitably defined groups of service providers to 'opt out' from their local health authorities to become autonomous bodies, called **self-governing NHS Trusts**. These Trusts contracted to provide services for any purchaser satisfied that they were the most suitable suppliers of particular treatments or care. Instead of exercising direct management authority over health services, the Health Authorities were expected in future to act primarily as planners and purchasers of services on behalf of patients in their areas.

Even this purchasing role was not comprehensive, owing to the establishment of an alternative route to purchasing through **GP-fundholders**, who were given budgets with which to purchase a defined list of services on behalf of patients on their lists. The general characteristics of the internal market system in its final evolved form are indicated in Figure 7.8.

Figure 7.8 *The structure of the NHS in England in May 1997, the most developed expression of the internal market in health care. A similar structure was adopted in other parts of the UK. (Adapted from Wellard's NHS Handbook 2000/01, JMH Publishing, Wadhurst, East Sussex, Section 1.2, Figure 1)*

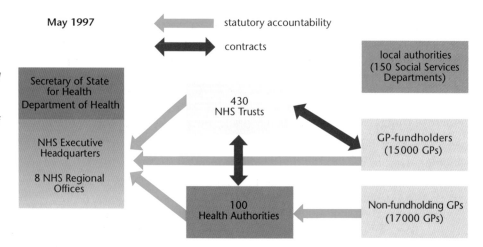

The internal market represented a substantial break with the past, so confirming the contention that 'taken together, the proposals represent the most far-reaching reform of the national health service in its forty year history' (*Working for Patients*, Foreword). The proposals aroused much greater opposition than other aspects of the new public management package. Labour politicians, the British Medical Association (BMA) and most bodies representing NHS staff believed that the internal market would fundamentally undermine the NHS and mark a return to the chaotic situation of the pre-war period.

● In comparison with the original ideals of the NHS (Chapter 6), what fears were aroused by the idea of an internal market?

■ 'Internal market' suggested rejection of the ideals of cooperation, rational planning, and protection of the most vulnerable, that were central to the aspirations of the founders of the NHS. The market suggested supremacy of the profit motive and competition, which would inevitably result in failures, closures, unemployment of health personnel, and irreversible loss of services, especially those needed by the vulnerable, according to the vagaries of the market.

Even within the Conservative government of the early 1990s there was some reticence about the internal market. At first it was not evident that the 'opting out' of hospitals to become NHS Trusts would extend beyond a few of the larger units, primarily the Teaching Hospitals. It was thought that GP-fundholding would be limited to a few large practices containing enthusiasts for this arrangement. In practice, generous financial inducements for opting out and fundholding were applied, with the result that by 1997 virtually the entire provider system was parcelled up into Trusts, while fundholding had extended to about half the number of GPs. (Non-fundholding GPs retained their traditional terms of employment.) The internal market changes were implemented in a broadly similar manner throughout the UK, but the pace of change differed, and many adaptations were introduced to reflect national circumstances.

Limiting the market

In the event, plunging purchasers and providers into an *unregulated* market was never seriously countenanced. The internal market scheme was modified to meet objections and the competitive system was developed only to a limited extent. Early fears that major Hospital Trusts would be bankrupted and closed down, or that 'expensive' patients (especially frail elderly or chronically sick people) would be rejected by GP-fundholders, turned out to be exaggerated.

Mitigation of the effects of competition was not limited to the Trust suppliers of services. Purchasers also took steps to avoid open competition with one another. Health Authorities increasingly involved non-fundholding GPs in their purchasing arrangements. A variety of collaborative schemes were evolved for purchasing within a locality — arrangements that were increasingly referred to as **locality commissioning** of health services. Indeed, in some cases locality commissioning involved collaboration between GP-fundholders and non-fundholders. Consequently, even before the 1997 general election, competitive purchasing was giving way to collaborative arrangements involving all GPs in an area.

In view of the above qualifications it is evident that the NHS evolved into an internal market only in the most restricted sense. In assessing the impact of the internal market experiment, it is also necessary to bear in mind that many of the changes taking place in health care in the 1990s were not the direct consequence of the internal market. For instance many improvements in performance related to a big injection of additional resources into the NHS in the early 1990s. Other changes were connected with policy initiatives that would have occurred regardless of the internal market, for example the new contract for GPs introduced in 1990, the community care reforms following the second Griffiths Report of 1988, and the Health of the Nation initiative of 1992 — all of which are discussed later in this chapter. These complications caused experts on the NHS to admit that the project of importing markets and related management innovations into the health service represented a problem of 'dark complexity' (Flynn and Williams, 1997, p. 157).

Bearing in mind the difficulty of making an assessment, it is possible to reach some provisional conclusions about the impact of the internal market changes. On the positive side it is evident that the purchaser–provider split made providers more conscious than before of the quality and costs of their services, while purchasers of all kinds questioned inherited patterns of providing services. Purchasers learned to use the new contractual system to obtain a better deal for their clients and secure more appropriate forms of treatment. The contractual system determined that purchasers and providers reached decisions about treatment on the basis of negotiation and with reference to the full body of relevant evidence. It is therefore arguable that the purchaser–provider system in principle represented a better basis for providing more economical and effective services, even if by 1997 these advantages had not been fully realised.

On the negative side the competitive system introduced a substantial rise in transaction costs owing to the complexity of contractual relations between purchasers and providers, and the high management costs of fundholding (Table 7.1 shows the increase in administrative and clerical staff). Strategic planning was sacrificed and big discrepancies in standards opened up between one place and another, exacerbating the 'postcode lottery' problem. It also increased the extent to which rationing was being applied without real reference to problems of equity in service provision.

Final judgement on the internal market system evolved by the Conservatives is not an easy matter, but it is clear that the strengths of the arrangements were insufficient for them to be preserved without modification, while the weaknesses were not so extreme as to justify scrapping the entire system.

7.3.5 Integrated care

In opposition Labour politicians were consistent critics of the internal market. Therefore dismantling the recently established system constituted one of Labour's main policy pledges prior to its landslide election victory in May 1997. Signifying the political importance of giving effect to this promise, the White Paper, *The New NHS Modern Dependable* was issued by the Department of Health in December 1997 (Department of Health, 1997). Similar policy documents were issued for Scotland, Wales and Northern Ireland. *The New NHS* outlined a broad package of measures designed to dismantle the internal market incrementally and establish the replacement system, for which the term **integrated care** was initially adopted.

'Integrated care' reflected the original spirit of Labour's reform programme for the NHS, but the concept was no longer prominent in *The NHS Plan* for England (and its counterparts for Scotland and Wales), issued by the Department of Health in July 2000, which set out the programme for the first 10 years of the new millennium.

The structure of the NHS in England in June 2001 is shown in Figure 7.9. The integrated care policy was adapted to the requirements of each part of the UK; for the most part, the differences relate to terminology of parallel administrative bodies, although, as mentioned in Chapter 1, devolution has accelerated the divergence of these arrangements.[2]

● What strikes you about the different terminology applied to the Conservative reforms of the NHS in the early 1990s, compared to the Labour reforms after 1997?

■ The Conservative emphasis on 'markets' is borrowed from economic theory and suggests competition between different parts of the health service, based on price.[3] The language of 'integrated care' represented a return to the ethos of cooperation and planning that were publicised as key features of the early NHS.

---

[2] Shortage of space precludes consideration of these differences, but the full detail is provided by references given in 'References and further sources' at the end of this book, for example *Wellard's NHS Handbook*.

[3] Dilemmas inherent in attempting to manage the NHS as though it were a conventional market are discussed in *Dilemmas in UK Health Care* (Open University Press, 3rd edn 2001), Chapter 2.

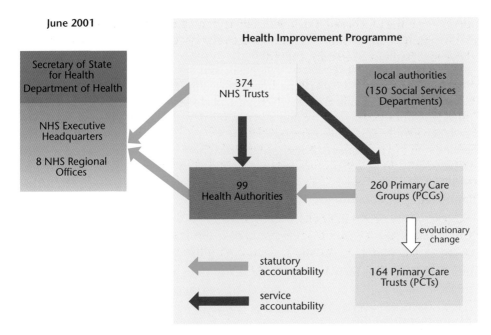

Figure 7.9   *The structure of the NHS in England in June 2001, showing contributors to the Health Improvement Programme. Owing to devolution, the structure applying in other parts of the UK is somewhat different, although the underlying principles were the same. By April 2004, all remaining PCGs had been converted into PCTs, and the 99 Health Authorities had been reorganised into 28 Strategic Health Authorities (SHAs). (Adapted from* Wellard's NHS Handbook 2000/01, *JMH Publishing, Wadhurst, East Sussex, Section 1.2, Figure 1)*

Labour promised that its reforms would be introduced on an evolutionary basis and only after thorough consultation and experimentation. In fact, as with the introduction of the internal market, New Labour has pushed forward rapidly and has arguably outpaced the Conservatives in the scope and range of its policy innovations. However, many of the plethora of changes introduced were firmly in the spirit of the new public management and therefore represented continuity with established trends. Even a large part of the structural framework established under the internal market has been maintained. Labour has therefore not interfered with the purchaser–provider split, the NHS Trusts, the Health Authority structure, or the central NHS Executive and its Regional Offices. Even the major changes affecting general practice could be regarded as the *universalisation* of fundholding and locality commissioning, as the following discussion suggests.

Primary care reforms

Labour's first priority for the health service, when elected in 1997, was the further development of locality commissioning. In England a two-stage process was adopted, commencing in April 1999, when all GPs were gathered into groups termed **Primary Care Groups** (PCGs, see Figure 7.9). Each PCG averaged about 50 GPs and *initially* about 480 such groups were formed in England. The PCGs were basically cooperatives of GPs, but with some input into decision-making by nurses working in general practices and social service professionals. PCGs were simultaneously providers of primary care and locality commissioners of secondary care (acute hospital services), guided by National Service Frameworks (explained below) drawn up by their local Health Authorities.

The second stage, commencing in April 2000 and to be completed by 2004, involved a development of PCGs into **Primary Care Trusts** (PCTs). This will establish PCTs as free-standing, statutory bodies, responsible for virtually the entire budget for hospital and community health services in their areas, and in some cases the whole mental health service. *The NHS Plan* (Department of Health, 2000a) contains proposals to further increase the scope of PCTs, which are expected to extend the range of directly-provided primary care services, and also commission all local health and social care for older people and other client groups with medical needs. PCTs will therefore extend into the territories of both hospital Trusts and local authority Social Services Departments. In an attempt to improve the coordination of service development, Health Authorities will be responsible for overseeing the production of **Health Improvement Programmes** (HImPs) for their areas. This represents the latest in a long line of attempts to induce greater cooperation between the NHS and local authority services.

When seen in context, even the flagship Labour plans for PCGs and PCTs emerge less as radical departures from previous policy than as further stages of the new public management programme, which has been unfolding for some twenty years.

Monitoring standards

Also consistent with the new public management, a whole battery of other innovations was introduced to coincide with the introduction of PCGs. Two important new statutory bodies, initiated under *The New NHS* White Paper are known by their acronyms: NICE and CHI (Box 7.2).

Also under *The New NHS* White Paper, a programme of **National Service Frameworks** (NSFs) was initiated to define national standards and to provide service models for the treatment of particular categories of patients. NSFs are produced on the advice of panels of specialists, called *expert reference groups*. The need for such guidance was suggested by persistence into the 1990s of inexplicable disparities in standards of treatment.

Box 7.2   NICE and CHI[4]

The **National Institute for Clinical Excellence** (NICE) is an independent body comprised of medical experts, NHS managers and patients' representatives. Its first chair was a professor of clinical pharmacology. Its main functions are to:

1   draw up clinical guidelines, which lay down the best medical practice for specific disease conditions. This involves the sensitive task of balancing considerations of clinical effectiveness and cost.

2   develop referral protocols to assist GPs in deciding about referral of patients to secondary care.

3   take a lead role in the exploitation of evidence-based medicine and in the development of clinical audit.

4   reduce the 'postcode lottery' in treatment which has long plagued the NHS.

The **Commission for Health Improvement** (CHI) is an independent body, chaired by a public health doctor and with a full time Director recruited from hospital administration. CHI will be comparable to Ofsted in education, but with a wider range of functions, and aims to prevent major failings in standards in health care. It will:

1   inspect all NHS Trusts and monitor standards of treatment, including compliance with National Service Frameworks, the Performance Assessment Framework and NICE recommendations.

2   oversee maintenance of clinical standards and the application of clinical audit.

---

4 NICE and CHI relate to England; equivalent organisations were set up in other parts of the UK.

The first efforts at evolving a national framework for care were the Calman–Hine review of cancer services, dating from 1994, and a plan for the development of paediatric intensive care services, published in 1997. (In Section 7.2.3, we have already noted Professor McVie's strictures about failure to implement the Calman–Hine review.) The 1997 Labour government adopted these two plans as models for its rolling programme of NSFs, the first of which related to mental health, the care of older people, coronary heart disease and diabetes. The NSFs lay down standards which constitute important guidelines for use in clinical audit. Indicative of the difficulties in obtaining even modest resources needed to begin the 'levelling up' of standards, the coronary heart disease NSF was not launched until March 2000, a year later than originally promised.

In July 2000 *The NHS Plan* established a further important central body, the Modernisation Agency, with a responsibility to drive forward the redesign of services at the local level. The degree of success of local health services in meeting modernisation targets in such key areas as health improvement or outcomes of health care, are measured by the **Performance Assessment Framework** (PAF). The PAF will, among other things, generate annual 'league tables' permitting comparisons of performance across the entire range of the health service. The PAF has also introduced a 'traffic light' classification of performance. Depending on classification as 'green', 'yellow' or 'red', service providers are subject to incentives or penalties with respect to specific functions. In the Spring of 2001 much publicity was attracted when forty hospitals were subjected to the 'red light' warning and attracted penalties on account of their filthy condition.

In addition to the above central regulatory agencies and frameworks, the Labour government has also launched a tide of other more local experimental schemes, such as Health Action Zones, NHS Direct (a telephone helpline staffed primarily by specially trained nurses), Walk-in Centres in key locations such as railway stations and shopping centres, and Healthy Living Centres.[5] These innovations reflect the new public management ethos through embodying such characteristics as direct appeal to the consumer, the targeting of areas in special need, competitive bidding, and partnership with the private sector. As further indicated in Section 7.5, in consideration of the changing role of health professionals, these new schemes also undermine traditional boundaries in their working practices, for instance by expanding the role of nurses and other health workers, or by employing nurses to undertake work traditionally done by doctors.

In summary

All of the above complicated changes have had important consequences for care. They reflect a gathering determination of governments in the course of the 1990s to increase the range of services offered by primary care teams and other agencies operating in the community. The aim of this development is to erode dependence on expensive acute services in hospitals, bring services closer to the patient and to ensure that more appropriate and prompt treatment is provided. Where recourse to secondary care in hospital is required, the above reforms aim to ensure that the services purchased are adapted precisely to the needs of the particular patient. This goal of providing a 'seamless' and effective service has proved more difficult to attain in practice than in theory, but governments from the 1990s onwards have been working to set in place structures more likely to improve services and patient satisfaction, while increasing efficiency and effectiveness in the use of resources available to the NHS.

[5] These initiatives are discussed further in *Dilemmas in UK Health Care* (Open University Press, 3rd edn 2001).

7.4 Care by the community

The previous section closely examined the structural and management reforms since the 1970s in sectors of the NHS concerned with primary and secondary care, i.e. mainly services concerned with disease management. These services account for the great majority of spending on the NHS. However, the strategy for health unfolding in the 1990s placed greater weight than ever before not only on the development of primary care, but also on *community care*. This term encompasses a range of services concerned with social support, aimed either at preventing the need for hospital care, or to achieve effective rehabilitation of those discharged from hospital.

Community care services are very disparate in character, thereby complicating the government's task of achieving a 'seamless' system of care. They fall partly within the NHS, but are also provided by local authority Social Services Departments, other local government departments, a multitude of voluntary agencies, and above all by family, neighbours and friends. Community care therefore embraces a shifting tide of functions. In the period since 1974, owing to persistent shortcomings of policy implementation and the undiminishing hold on resources by primary care and acute hospital services, the burden of community care has rested largely on the community itself. In this section of the chapter we look more closely at the attempt to increase the profile and effectiveness of community care in the period from 1974 to 2001.

7.4.1 Policy development

As already indicated in Chapter 6, ever since the beginning of the NHS, and especially from the 1960s onwards, there was an attempt to create more humane alternatives to long-term institutional hospital care. 'Community care', the term coined to describe this new thinking, was no more than a loose description of the many formal and informal alternatives to long-stay hospitals. The Ely Hospital enquiry of 1968, the first of many investigations into long-stay hospital scandals, made it clear that the old asylums and workhouses were no longer providing acceptable care for hundreds of thousands of people who were elderly, or judged to be mentally ill or classified as learning disabled.

Although the expansion of community care was uncontentious in principle, it provides one of the best examples of repeated delay in the implementation of policies, which supposedly occupy the highest priority. Over the last four decades many factors account for this embarrassing failure, including recalcitrance of professional vested interests, lack of resources and commitment among local authorities responsible for community care services, failure of cooperation across the inter-service divides, and instinctive inaction by central government on account of the resource implications.

The shortcomings of community care services provided by local government were at first disguised owing to the failure of the health service to implement its declared policy of closing down long-stay hospitals. The full extent of the defectiveness of the community care structure only became apparent in the 1980s, when the Conservative government imposed constraints on hospital expenditure. This prompted hospital authorities to embark on a headlong race to close down their long-stay hospitals and sell off their valuable sites for property development.

● Suggest why the demand for community care was accelerating in the 1980s.

■ There were several reasons, among them the growth in numbers of elderly people needing support to remain in their own homes; the rise in homelessness (Figure 7.10), partly consequent upon increases in unemployment; the reduction in hospital-bed numbers; and the emergence of AIDS as a new health problem requiring care in the community.

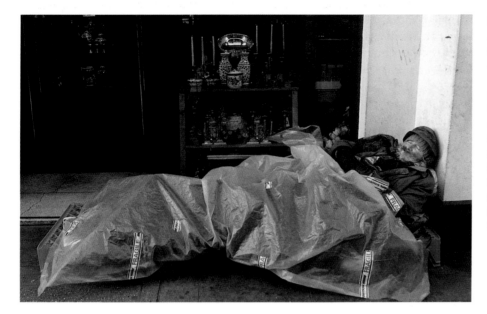

Figure 7.10 *A 'rough sleeper' lies in the doorway of an expensive shop in London. The 1980s saw rising homelessness and vagrancy, but appropriate health and social services were rarely available from the public sector. A variety of voluntary agencies attempted to remedy this shortfall. (Source: Roger Hutchings/Network)*

The perceived crisis in community care led to an intervention by the Audit Commission in 1986, a further report from Sir Roy Griffiths in 1988, and ultimately the NHS and Community Care Act of 1990.[6] As indicated in Table 7.2, the changes since the 1980s in the provision of residential care amount to a major revolution.

Table 7.2 Residential facilities for the main community care groups, England, 1985–1995.

Number of beds	1985 (thousands)	1995 (thousands)
Public sector		
NHS, elderly-care beds	55	37
NHS, mental-health-care beds	97	50
NHS, learning-disabled-care beds	50	18
Local Authority residential home beds	116	64
subtotal	*318*	*169*
Private/Voluntary sector		
residential home beds	117	213
nursing home beds	27	115
subtotal	*144*	*328*
total	**462**	**497**

Data compiled by the author from various Department of Health sources.

[6] These initiatives are considered in *Dilemmas in UK Health Care* (Open University Press, 3rd edn 2001), Chapter 4.

●   What conclusion about the balance of public and private provision can be reached from Table 7.2?

■   Public provision has decreased across the board, by approximately half over the period, while private provision has more than doubled. But the total number of residential places has not changed very much, increasing by just over 7 per cent.

Table 7.2 confirms the long-term trend in which the care of high-dependency patients has transferred from long-stay hospitals to nursing or residential homes. Those with a lower level of dependency have returned to their own homes after treatment, where they are dependent on domiciliary support, for instance from district nurses and home helps. As Figure 7.11 shows, as local authority and NHS residential places declined, services provided to people in their own homes expanded, but not in line with the steady build-up of demand. As noted below, this shift from public to private provision was driven by important changes in government policy concerning the financing of long-term care.

Publicity concerning community care policies has emphasised their constructive role in empowering the various classes of client, or 'consumer'. Governments of the 1990s claimed that as a result of recent policy changes, those in need of care were on a level with other citizens, having not only full access to appropriate care, but

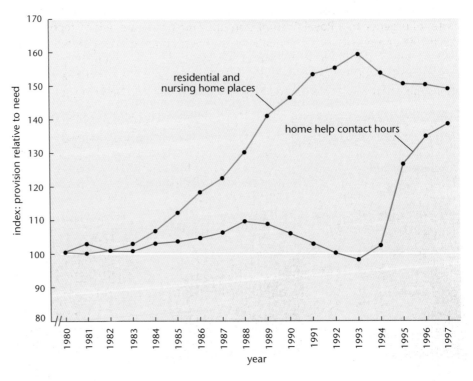

Figure 7.11 *Community health and social services provision for older people, England, 1980–1997. The data are expressed in the form of an index in which the provision in 1980 has been set as equal to 100. Changes in provision over time are then calculated in relation to this initial index number. Although local authority home-help services increased sharply from 1994, the policy of concentrating help on those in most need reduced the proportion of older people receiving the service. (Data from Department of Health, 2000,* Shaping the Future NHS: Long Term Planning for Hospitals and Related Services; *Consultation document on the findings of the National Beds Inquiry, Department of Health, London, Chart 5)*

also able to exercise an element of consumer choice. Great play is made about the 'seamlessness' of the new system, implying that the diverse agencies are mobilised in complete harmony. In reality, deficiencies in the system are suggested by the steady flow of adverse publicity attracting media attention. Fresh policy initiatives by the government indicate that previous official reassurances were over-optimistic.

For instance, at the launch of the National Service Framework (NSF) for mental health in November 1999, the minister concerned opened his speech by admitting that 'for too long, mental health services have been at the margins of the NHS'. The NSF was presented as a 'landmark' paving the way for 'more accessible services, more responsive services, services which support families, and services which work with the wider community to reduce stigma and discrimination'. Such admissions indicate how little progress had been made since ministers first made statements of this kind in the early 1960s.

A further aspect of the unresolved crisis in community care results from the shift in the type of provision for residential care since 1979 (Figure 7.12). As noted above, this has involved a run down of long-stay hospital provision, which is provided free under the NHS, and its substitution by alternatives provided mainly by the private sector, which necessitate substantial direct payments. For the poor these payments are covered by social security; for others *means testing* entails eventual loss of capital assets, including the family home.

The financial burden of long-term care, especially the impact on homeowners, has become a big political issue, the resolution of which was referred by Labour as a matter of urgency to a Royal Commission on Long Term Care, which reported in March 1999. Among its recommendations, the Royal Commission suggested various ways to reduce the financial burden of long-term care, including by providing personal and nursing care in nursing and residential homes without charge. This latter suggestion was implemented fully in Scotland, but *The NHS Plan*, July 2000,

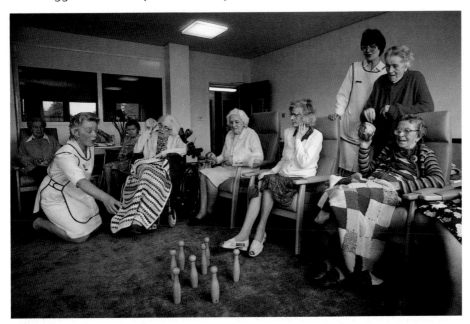

Figure 7.12   *Residents and staff in the recreation room of a private residential care home. Before 1980, costs were mainly met by local authorities; during the 1980s, social security financing increasingly took over; during the 1990s the costs were transferred to residents, with public subsidy being increasingly limited and subject to stringent means-testing. (Source: Barry Lewis/Network)*

allowed only for the provision of nursing care without charge. This arrangement applied in both England and Wales. *The NHS Plan* compensated to some extent by including some alternative proposals to reduce the financial burden on those requiring long-term care. The means-test limits will be slightly relaxed, and an entirely new Intermediate Care service will be provided free under the NHS. This is designed to reduce 'bed blocking' by patients no longer requiring hospital care, while also speeding up their rehabilitation. The impact in practice is likely to be small owing to the limited resources available for intermediate care, and the rigorous conditions attached to the funding.

7.4.2 Who cares?

The continued reliance on informal sources of care has remained a feature of government policy since 1979, but the focus has changed from supporting the person in need of care to supporting the informal carer.

> For many years it has been recognised that the main support for dependent people in the community is provided on an informal basis by their families and friends. The role of the statutory services is now seen as being to support the informal carers so that they can continue to look after their dependants in the community. (Department of Health, 1998, preface)

This reliance on informal carers has always been based on the assumption that a plentiful supply of female labour existed in the family and that women were somehow 'natural carers'. In 1979 the sociologist Hilary Graham wrote an article titled 'Prevention and health: every mother's business'. According to Graham, the burden of community care was placed primarily, if not exclusively, on women's shoulders. However, the balance shifted to some extent during the 1980s and 1990s. A study of informal carers conducted in 1995 as part of the General Household Survey (Department of Health, 1998) showed that among adults in Britain 3.3 million women and 2.4 million men were looking after, or providing regular care for a sick, physically or mentally disabled, or elderly person living with them or in another private household. One in eight adults in Britain was an informal carer, but in the age group 45–64 years the proportion rose to one in five.

Health promotion policy (discussed later in this chapter), with its emphasis on individual responsibility, also saw a pivotal role for women in relation to family health. In practice this was a function that women were increasingly unable or unwilling to fulfil. The prospects of turning to 'the community' and in particular its female members were more limited than ever before. The proportion of working married women rose sharply from the 1970s. Increasing mobility combined with decreasing family size meant that elderly people more often lived at a distance from relatives. For example in inner London, the proportion of elderly people who had a child living within five minutes' walk halved between the late 1950s and the late 1970s. Ties with neighbours were less close, more short-lived and also in some areas compounded by racial divisions.

Nevertheless, families tried to maintain their caring role. In one study of people over the age of 75, carried out in the late 1970s, over three-quarters of those with surviving children saw them at least once a week. Indeed, all studies show that these children are the predominant carers. However, the burdens on carers, often themselves elderly, are considerable. In the 1990s the sociologists Michael Young and Lesley Cullen studied the carers of people who were terminally ill with cancer and living in their own homes in the months before they died. Their article,

'The carer at home', focuses on the experience of carers and the difference they made to the lives of the people they looked after (Young and Cullen, 1996). (Open University students should read it now.[7])

● What does Young and Cullen's research demonstrate about 'who cares'?

■ Wherever there were close relatives living in the same household as the person in need of care, or living within a reasonable travelling distance, these family members took on the main responsibility. In the households discussed in the article, there were examples of wives looking after husbands and vice versa, and adult children looking after their parents; in one case, a woman in her seventies was the principal carer for her adult daughter during her final illness. Where relatives did not exist or were too far away, neighbours stepped into the breach, enabling the dying person to live independently in their own home for as long as possible.

The 1995 General Household Survey confirmed the earlier findings about the heavy burden on carers. This showed that a quarter had looked after their dependant for at least 10 years, nearly two-thirds spent at least 20 hours a week caring, while 855 000 carers spent more than 50 hours a week providing informal care (Figure 7.13). It also confirmed the limited extent of back-up services available. Over a third of carers reported that no-one else helped them look after their dependants, and 59 per cent said the person they looked after did not receive regular visits from health, voluntary or social services. Women were more likely to be caring unaided than men. In most respects the level of back-up actually fell between 1988 and 1993 (as Figure 7.11 illustrates), and it has not kept up with demand thereafter.

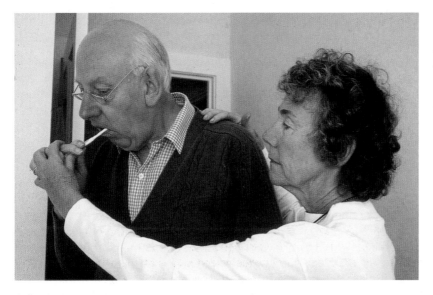

Figure 7.13 *Care in the community falls primarily on the shoulders of close family members, some providing 'round the clock' care, as this woman does for her husband who has Alzheimer's disease. (Source: Judy Harrison/ Format Photographers)*

It was not until 1986 that financial help was available for married women carers. In that year the European Court ruled that they were entitled to the Invalid Care Allowance. Previously this allowance was limited to relatives staying at home to care for a disabled person. The allowance was a specific concession for single women who were assumed to have sacrificed their career and pension opportunities, but

[7] This article appears in *Health and Disease: A Reader* (Open University Press, 3rd edn 2001) and is optional reading for Open University students during study of another book in this series, *Birth to Old Age: Health in Transition* (Open University Press, 2nd edn 1995; colour-enhanced 2nd edn 2001).

married women were excluded on the grounds that they were by definition available for caring in the home. As the Equal Opportunities Commission pointed out, this effectively excluded 99.5 per cent of those actually giving care. Although the Invalid Care Allowance is regarded as a 'wage for caring', it is set at a level much lower than either the basic pension or unemployment benefit, and it is liable to exclude carers from other benefits. Therefore the Invalid Care Allowance does little to ease either their financial problems or the strain of their situation.

The position of carers was marginally strengthened by the Carers' (Recognition and Services) Act, 1995, and to a greater extent by the Labour government's Caring about Carers strategy of 1999, which was backed up by legislation in the following year. Among other things, this established a fund to pay for carers to take short breaks from their responsibilities. In general, the strategy has strengthened the position of carers.[8]

7.4.3 Informal networks of care

With the decline of confidence in formal care, from the 1970s onwards there was a marked upsurge in the public profile of lay care and self-help. Perhaps its clearest manifestation in the 1980s came through the gay and lesbian community's response to AIDS. Informal 'buddies' provided lay care and support for people infected with HIV, or with AIDS, where, at least initially, formal statutory provision was non-existent. The power of lay groups to influence policy was demonstrated in 1987, when AIDS groups in the USA forced the pharmaceutical companies to abort their trials, and the government to speed up the regulatory process, in order to bring the drug AZT into immediate use as a palliative for AIDS. The same pattern was then repeated in the UK (Berridge, 1996, p. 184).[9] In Chapters 8 and 9, we consider the role of public protest in changing the marketing of anti-HIV drugs in developing countries.

The rise in popularity of complementary or alternative medicine (Section 7.4.4) was part of this trend. Use of these remedies has been backed by networks of lay information and advice, often in self-conscious opposition to the medical establishment, much as occurred with popular medicine in the nineteenth century. The widespread use of 'alternative' drugs without official approval by people with AIDS also caused difficulties during clinical trials of 'official' pharmaceuticals.

Other studies also showed how important lay beliefs about health remained in the 1970s and 1980s. For example the social anthropologist and general practitioner Cecil Helman demonstrated how what he called the 'folk model' of disease both differed from and resembled orthodox medicine.[10] Lay networks of information and advice also continued to operate. In the early 1970s, Christopher Elliott-Bins studied patients attending a general practice in Northampton. He found that 96 per cent of the patients had received some advice or treatment before consulting their GP (Elliott-Bins, 1973). One, a village shopkeeper with a persistent cough, had received advice from her husband, an ex-hospital matron, a doctor's receptionist, and five customers, three of whom recommended a particularly curious

[8] More discussion of the main issues affecting informal carers at the start of the new millennium occurs in *Dilemmas in UK Health Care* (Open University Press, 3rd edn 2001), Chapter 4.

[9] HIV infection and AIDS are discussed extensively in *Experiencing and Explaining Disease* (Open University Press; 2nd edn 1996; colour-enhanced 2nd edn 2001) Chapter 4.

[10] The article by Cecil Helman, 'Feed a cold, starve a fever', appears in *Health and Disease: A Reader* (Open University Press, 2nd edn 1995; 3rd edn 2001) and is set reading for Open University students during study of *Medical Knowledge: Doubt and Certainty* (Open University Press, 2nd edn 1994; colour-enhanced 2nd edn 2001).

remedy: Golden Syrup, a boiled onion gruel, and the application of a hot brick to the chest. Elliott-Bins repeated this study thirteen years later in the same general practice; the pattern of self-care and lay health advice had remained largely unchanged (Elliott-Bins, 1986).

A wide range of **self-help groups** has flourished since World War II. *Alcoholics Anonymous* (AA) was one of the first, arriving in the UK from the USA in the late 1940s. 'AA' has remained a 'non-political' organisation, avoiding input into alcohol policy. Its model of encouraging heavy drinkers (or alcoholics) to develop the will-power to cease drinking through mutual self-help, was widely copied by other self-help groups. This type of self-help group is called 'inner-focused' since it is primarily concerned with mutual support among people united by a particular health problem (Katz and Bender 1976; see Figure 7.14).

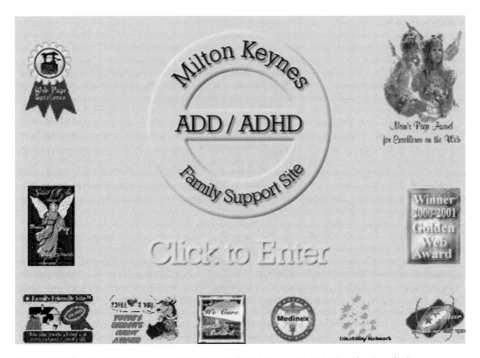

Figure 7.14   *The Milton Keynes Attention Deficit (Hyperactivity) Disorder Family Support Group, established in 1996, is one example of the increasingly well-organised self-help groups that flourished in the 1990s. The use of the Internet has greatly extended the effectiveness of such groups. (Source: Courtesy of Milton Keynes ADHD; Photo: Andy Noble)*

● Can you suggest other inner-focused health-related groups?

■ The range is enormous, but includes Narcotics Anonymous, Weight Watchers, Tranx (for tranquiliser users), National Association for Colitis and Crohn's Disease, Arthritis Care, Cancerlink and Body Positive (for HIV-positive people).

Many self-help groups have evolved to perform an additional 'outer-focused' role, acting as a pressure group on behalf of sufferers and their carers, using their influence to heighten policy awareness, attracting resources and conducting or funding research. The British Diabetic Association, founded in 1934, illustrates this type of development, and the National Ankylosing Spondylitis Society, founded in 1976 is a more recent example of the same type (Kelleher, 1994). Campaigning self-help groups have attracted a big following, including support from celebrities, and they

Figure 7.15 *Campaigns by particular groups to raise awareness of their needs in the community have sometimes involved direct action, as in this protest by wheelchair users in Nottingham against lack of access to public transport. (Source: John Birdsall Photography)*

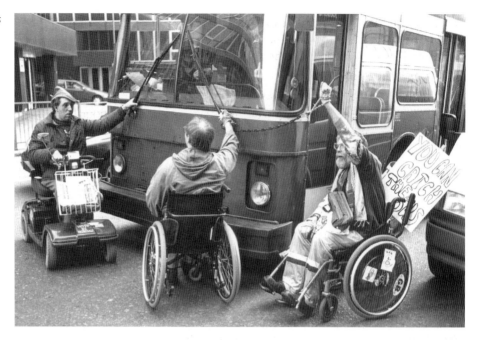

are adept at gaining media coverage (Figure 7.15). Their importance extends beyond fund-raising into acting as a vehicle for educating and influencing public opinion. Their influence is reinforced by the existence of radio and television programmes, such as the BBC Radio 4 'In Touch' and its associated Action Line. The Internet has acted as a further boost to the proliferation and effectiveness of self-help groups.

Just occasionally the pressure groups come into conflict with the professional establishment, as for instance in 1996 when the myalgic encephalomyelitis (ME) groups contested the Royal Colleges' report, which sought to reascribe their condition as Chronic Fatigue Syndrome (Royal Colleges of Physicians, Psychiatrists and General Practitioners, 1996). Overall, self-help and lay care and advice remained the major source of health and social care in the UK in the 1990s, with no sign of diminishing participation in this informal sector of the health-care system.

7.4.4 Complementary and alternative medicine

Complementary and **alternative medicine** have become increasingly important components of health care in the UK. The meaning of these terms has shifted since the 1960s, when any therapeutic technique that fell outside orthodox medical practice was considered 'alternative' and suspect by most Western doctors. However, techniques such as osteopathy and chiropractic gradually gained acceptance from the medical establishment and were among the first to be referred to as 'complementary' to orthodox medicine. The term gained ground until most practitioners in the 1990s referred to themselves as offering therapy that complements (or is at least not in conflict with) orthodox medicine, although some still see themselves as providing an alternative to it. We use the acronym CAM here to cover all forms of complementary and alternative medicine.

The sources of inspiration for the CAM movement are diverse: for example, acupuncture draws on systems of belief and practice from the East rooted in antiquity; homeopathy is a Western system based on earlier ideas, but developed in the nineteenth century; Bach flower remedies, the Alexander technique and the Hay diet were invented between the two World Wars. CAM techniques are most used for chronic health problems such as arthritis, back pain, eczema or stress, which the NHS finds difficult to treat effectively. CAM also appeals on account of its holistic approach, the generous time given to consultations, and its empowerment of the patient — all features that tend to be missing in Western medicine as experienced in the busy NHS.

Confidence in CAM is also reinforced when the evidence of randomised controlled trials (RCTs) demonstrates its efficacy, as for instance when the ancient traditional remedy St John's Wort (*Hypericum*) was shown to be superior to the modern drug imipramine as an anti-depressant (Woelk, 2000).

By any standards CAM techniques have experienced spectacular growth in popularity, benefiting from the 1960s onwards from the increasing mood of dissatisfaction with orthodox medicine described at the start of this chapter. Estimates suggest that there were 12 million CAM consultations in 1993, rising to 15 million in 1997 (Zollman and Vickers, 1999), although this still only represents about 5 per cent of the number of GP consultations. The most rigorous survey to date (Thomas *et al.*, 1995) concluded that 33 per cent of the UK population had, at some time, consulted a CAM therapist or used a complementary medicine bought over-the-counter, and over 10 per cent had done so in the previous year.

Table 7.3 reports the situation for the UK and for some other Western countries in 1985–1992. These comparative data are difficult to interpret because in some European countries access to such therapies is covered to some extent under national health insurance schemes, but they confirm the widespread popularity of complementary medicine. (We compare systems of funding health care in Chapter 9.)

● From the data in Table 7.3, what strikes you about the balance of take-up of complementary therapies in different countries?

■ There are big variations. For example, homeopathy is very popular in Belgium and is often used in France, Denmark and the Netherlands, but in Sweden, the UK and the USA the manipulative therapies have a greater following. (Legal prohibitions limit these manipulations to registered doctors in France, hence their low level of use.)

Table 7.3 Percentage of population reporting use of complementary medicine, compiled from public opinion surveys in various Western countries, 1985–1992.

	Unspecified forms of complementary medicine	Acupuncture	Homeopathy	Manipulation (including osteopathy and chiropractic)
Belgium	31	19	56	19
Denmark	23	12	28	23
France	49	21	32	7
Germany	46	n/a	n/a	n/a
Netherlands	20	16	31	n/a
Sweden	25	12	15	48
UK	26	16	16	36
USA	34	3	3	30

n/a = not asked for

Source: Fisher, P. and Ward, A. (1994) Medicine in Europe: Complementary Medicine in Europe, *British Medical Journal*, **309**, pp. 107–111.

Consistent with the growth in demand, the number of CAM practitioners has steadily increased, from an estimated 30 000 CAM therapists in the UK in 1982 who were not qualified in orthodox Western medicine, to about 40 000 in 1999 (Zollman and Vickers, 1999). Numbers are predicted to be rising in the new millennium by about 10 per cent each year.

The rise of CAM has induced a change of attitude on the part of the BMA. From the beginning of the twentieth century to 1980, the BMA consistently denounced alternative practitioners as quacks. Prompted by an intervention from HRH Charles, Prince of Wales, who called for a more open-minded approach, the BMA produced a report on *Alternative Medicine* in 1986, which was predictably sceptical. However, in 1993 the BMA revised its ideas and issued a further report entitled *Complementary Medicine: New Approaches to Good Practice*, which, as the title suggests, was more conciliatory.

The practitioner status of complementary therapists was rising. In 1996 the Prince of Wales made a further significant intervention by setting up his 'Initiative on Integrated Medicine', which published its first report in 1997 (Foundation for Integrated Medicine, 1997). The report drew on the deliberations of four working groups on research, regulation, education and training, and the delivery of integrated health care.

The Initiative also laid down guidelines for the professional development of CAM, and for the systematic familiarisation of other health professionals in CAM procedures. With the growing legitimacy of complementary medicine, an increasing number of registered medical practitioners, nurses, physiotherapists and midwives opted for training in these techniques. By the millennium nearly 4 000 orthodox health-care professionals were also registered as CAM therapists, around 40 per cent of GP surgeries referred patients for CAM treatments (Figure 7.16), and over 70 per cent of these treatments were paid for by the NHS (Zollman and Vickers, 1999). Some sectors were quicker than others to adopt CAM techniques; for instance, by 1995, over 95 per cent of hospices were using them as part of palliative care.

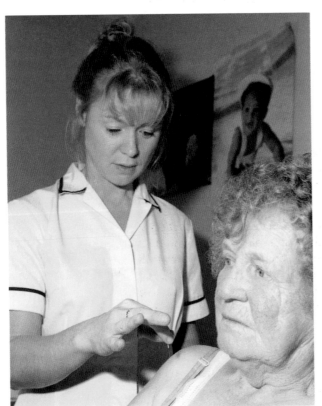

Figure 7.16 *From the 1990s onwards, general practitioners in the UK began to approve the training of conventional practice staff in complementary and alternative medical techniques and therapies. A practice nurse uses acupuncture to treat a 'frozen shoulder' in a GP's premises. (Source: Tony Woodcock)*

7.5   Upheavals in the health-worker hierarchy

We have already fully considered the major policy developments that took place in the NHS and in community care since 1974, and also briefly touched upon quantitative changes from 1973 to 1997 in the main staff categories working in NHS hospitals (Table 7.1). It is now necessary to consider more closely the impact of big policy changes on the individual professions and how these have affected the balance of relations between the main professional groups.

In the decades since 1974, health-care occupations have continued the shifts of boundary and of status that we described in Chapter 6. From the 1970s onwards the entrenched power of the medical profession became threatened by an alliance of left-wing radicals and right-wing governments. The former sought the 'end of medical hegemony' in order to emancipate other health workers and give genuine empowerment to patients. Ultimately, this radical programme made very little mark. More far-reaching were the reforms initiated by the Conservative governments of the 1980s in the effort to improve efficiency and give better value for money in health care. The professions in general came under suspicion for obstructing these goals, but the medical profession was perhaps the most targeted.

7.5.1   Hospital clinicians

As you know from previous chapters, hospital clinicians represented the elite of the medical profession. However, since 1979 their power and influence has been constantly under threat. The new public management and internal market programmes described earlier were not specifically aimed at reducing the power of clinicians, but strong management certainly undermined the virtually unrestricted influence that clinicians had exercised since the beginning of the NHS. For instance, the Griffiths 'general management' reforms of the late 1980s swept away many channels of influence effectively controlled by clinicians under the 1974 reorganisation.

From this point onwards the authority of clinicians within hospitals was no longer supreme; indeed it was actively challenged by general managers and their increasingly numerous administrative staffs, many of whom were drawn from outside the health-care professions. It was managers rather than clinicians who spearheaded application of the new public management throughout the hospital system. Progressively under the 1983 Griffiths Report and Resource Management Initiative, clinicians were grouped into *clinical directorates*, dispensing rigidly defined budgets, and accountable to the Trust general manager as the main budget holder. Managers also assumed a new degree of involvement in the appointment of hospital clinicians and also in determining their level of income.

The dominance of hospital clinicians was also adversely affected by introduction of the internal market in 1991. Prior to the market they determined the ground rules for dealing with patients referred by GPs. Under the internal market these referrals were controlled by contracts negotiated between purchasers and providers. Hospital clinicians were not in a position to dictate the outcome. In order for the hospital to secure contracts, clinicians were answerable to managers for delivering services of acceptable standard and cost. The contracts limited the discretion of consultants to dictate programmes of care and they arguably inhibited their clinical freedom.

● What effect do you think the internal market system had on the balance of relations between hospital consultants and those GPs who became fundholders?

■ GP-fundholders were at liberty to take their custom elsewhere if consultants failed to offer services of attractive specification, or complete the quota of referrals agreed in the contract, so the balance shifted towards greater power for the primary care sector.

Introduction of the internal market was also associated with the introduction of *clinical audit*, which (as described in Section 7.3.3) relied on a variety of measures to evaluate the quality of clinical care. Clinical audit was essentially a 'self-policing' mechanism, controlled by the Royal Colleges and applying to all branches of medical practice. This was in principle a welcome invitation to confirm the quality of the work of individual hospital clinicians. However, it also served the broader purpose of bringing individuals into line with defined standards, thereby reducing variations in practice and limiting the autonomy of individual practitioners.

In the 1990s hospital clinicians also had to adjust to a new system of training and career structure. With the rising professional standing of nurses and others within hospitals, clinicians have been forced to work to a greater degree with others as equals (Figure 7.17a). Also, as noted above, resource constraints prevented much-needed modernisation of their services. Low pay and shortages among junior doctors and support staff constituted an additional strain (Figure 7.17b). In the light of these factors, hospital clinicians are not quite the autonomous elite that once they were. But they still preserve a generous pay system, the right to undertake private practice and limited hours of duty. Accordingly, controls and restrictions over their traditional freedoms and work have not gone as deep as they sometimes complain.

Indicative of the power exercised by hospital clinicians, although *The NHS Plan* declared a radical attitude towards renegotiation of their contract, the actual proposals for curtailment of their privileges amount to insignificant changes. Even these modest proposals have been rejected with vehemence by the consultant leadership. In many respects the management changes of the 1990s enhanced the authority of clinicians by bringing them into the centre of decision-making and budgetary control.

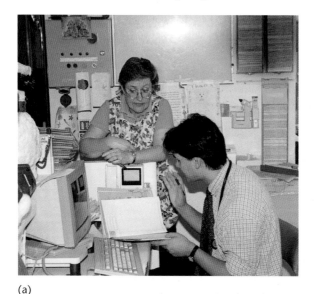

(a)

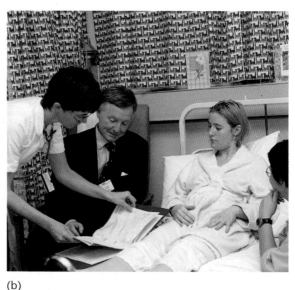

(b)

Figure 7.17 *(a) The shortage of junior hospital doctors came to a head during the 1990s when steps were taken to reduce their long hours and to improve their relatively low pay and adverse conditions of service. (b) Hospital consultants remain the elite of the medical profession, despite the trend in the 1990s towards working with other health professionals on a more equal basis. (Source (a) and (b): Mike Levers)*

Clinical governance

The centrality of clinicians is emphasised by the concept of **clinical governance**, which occupies a prominent place in the Labour government's new management philosophy. Clinical governance aims at 'creating an environment in which excellence in clinical care will flourish' (NHS Executive, 1999). Every unit of operation of the health service is required to set up a framework to take action on such things as clinical audit, evidence-based medicine, professional self-regulation and continuing education. Clinicians are expected to play a lead role in these local programmes.

Within the medical profession, responses to clinical governance have ranged from applause to derision. In the fiftieth anniversary issue of the *British Medical Journal*, clinical governance was single out as the 'Big Idea' of the Labour government (Scally and Donaldson, 1998). Clinicians in general were less enthusiastic; clinical governance was ridiculed as rhetorical nonsense and the government's proposals for its implementation were criticised for heaping yet further bureaucratic burdens on already hard-pressed clinicians. Given this unenthusiastic response, it is not surprising that, in the hospital sector, clinical governance has not in practice assumed anything like the prominence anticipated at the outset. Indeed, the concept is hardly mentioned in the July 2000 *NHS Plan* (Department of Health, 2000a).

Finally, it is important to note that, since the late 1990s, the reputation of the entire medical profession, but especially hospital clinicians, has been seriously undermined by a series of highly-publicised cases of criminal action, incompetence and unprofessional conduct. The scale of these lapses reached such proportions that, at the turn of the millennium, the government was forced to take action to restore public confidence in the medical profession. Within the NHS many measures were introduced to improve the monitoring of standards. Also, the General Medical Council (GMC), the body that for 150 years had exercised the statutory responsibility for 'protecting patients', was forced for the first time in its history to contemplate serious reform. Proposals for an overhaul of the GMC were published in November 2000. It remains to be seen whether these reforms will be significant enough to restore public confidence in the credibility of these arrangements for regulating medical practice.

7.5.2 GPs and the primary health care team

You have seen in the previous chapter that the new contract of 1966 reversed the decline in general practice. As a result of improving GP recruitment, the average list size in the UK for a general practitioner fell from 2 500 in 1952 to 1 800 in 1995. This inevitably brought about an improvement in working conditions. Women have been particularly prominent among new entrants, increasing their stake in general practice from 10 per cent in 1952 to 31 per cent in 1995, and they have come to play a more dominant part in general practice than in any other medical specialty.

- Table 7.4 (overleaf) reveals another trend in general practice. Briefly summarise the main points.

- The proportion of doctors working single-handedly has steadily declined from its dominant position at the outset of the NHS. Small-group practice established itself as the norm in the 1980s, but the largest groups are dominant in the 1990s. This trend suggests that in future GPs are likely to work in ever-larger groups.

Successive changes in the GP's contract and conditions under the various reforms of the 1990s created financial inducements to form larger practices. Besides being

Table 7.4   Percentage distribution of partnerships of general practitioners, England, 1952–1999.

Data complied by the author from Ministry of Health, *Annual Report 1953; Health and Personal Social Services Statistics for England* (various years); *Statistics for General Medical Practitioners in England, 1989–1999.*

Year	1 GP	2 GPs	Partnerships of 3 GPs	4 GPs	5 GPs	6 or more GPs
1952	44	33	14	6	2	1
1980	14	18	24	20	12	12
1995	10	13	16	18	17	26
1999	9	12	14	17	16	31

financially attractive, group practice has held out the possibility of gains for both GPs and their patients. The largest practices facilitate the greatest improvements connected with economies in scale, such as employment of larger numbers of practice staff, fuller opportunities for multi-professional teamwork, for training and for audit, more highly equipped medical centres, more effective use of information technology, and therefore a greater range and quality of services to patients. By contrast, primary health care for remote rural areas of the UK, such as the Highlands and Islands of Scotland (Figure 7.18), are inevitably provided by the staff of small general practices, often employed by a single-handed GP.

In describing this acceleration towards larger partnerships, two leading experts in this field conclude that the 1990s represented the phase of most rapid change experienced in general practice since the beginning of the NHS (Bosanquet and Salisbury, 1998). As a consequence of the changes described above, it is arguable that general practitioners have improved their professional status to the point where they can no longer be compared adversely with other medical specialties.

Important for maintenance of their public credibility has been the GPs' alignment with the concept of primary health care (PHC). This doctrine, enshrined in the 1978 *Alma Ata Declaration* of the WHO, was elaborated initially as a reaction against the application of inappropriate high-technology medicine in developing countries (this is discussed in detail in Chapter 8). What was needed, it was argued, were

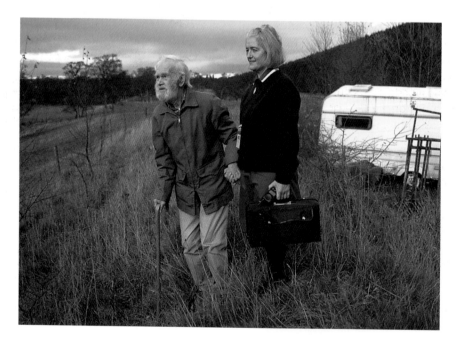

Figure 7.18   *A practice nurse visits a patient living in a caravan in a remote location in the Scottish Highlands. (Source: John Paul Agency, Inverness)*

simple dispensaries, basic health advice and personnel with a limited but specific training. The same arguments were then applied to industrialised countries: GPs in Europe were effective in adapting the PHC concept to serve as the basis for their own professional legitimisation. In 1977, an influential European Working Group defined the role of the general practitioner as giving:

> ... personal, primary and continuing care to individuals, families and a practice population, irrespective of age, sex and illness. It is the synthesis of these functions which is unique ... it will include and integrate physical, psychological and social factors in its considerations about health and illness. (Leeuwenhorst Working Party Report, *The general practitioner in Europe,* quoted from Horder, 1998, p. 258).

● The above definition highlighted the term 'primary'. What connotations does this carry?

■ 'Primary' indicates the first point of contact in seeking medical assistance, but it also carries the connotation of being of the first order of importance, as emphasised by stress on the *comprehensiveness* of the credentials of GPs and their 'unique' role.

It is therefore understandable why primary health care came to the forefront of the professional development of GPs, instead of their being regarded as inferior 'generalists'. Central to the idea of primary care, and inevitable from its broad-ranging functions, was the idea that GPs would work in teams, and that these would involve other health workers. The days when a GP's wife acted as receptionist, chaperone, nurse, and accountant (in addition to the domestic role) were ended.

Between 1964 and 1977, the proportion of practices with an attached nurse increased from 12 to 84 per cent. Only 1 per cent of GPs did not have a receptionist in 1977, compared with 25 per cent in 1964. The (often male) GP was joined by members of middle-stratum occupational groups: nurses, health visitors, receptionists — occupations that had a predominantly female workforce. By the 1990s it was common for the largest practices to employ some 50 staff and there were many more female GPs (Figure 7.19).

It is noticeable that clinical governance is being taken up with greater alacrity in primary care than in the hospital sector. Clinical governance is strengthening the hand of GPs committed to improving standards; these innovators appreciate that it provides a further incentive for the promotion of teamwork within primary care (Pringle, 2000).

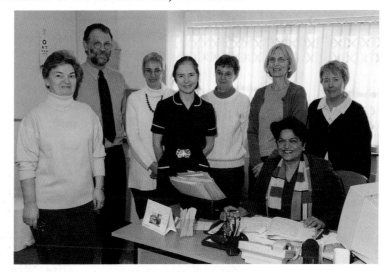

Figure 7.19 *Some of the 28 members of a primary health care team in a large group general practice in Milton Keynes, 2001. From left to right: medical receptionist, practice manager, medical receptionist, senior practice nurse, medical receptionist, medical secretary, (seated) the GP and senior partner in the group practice, and the counsellor. Not shown: four more GPs, two more practice nurses, three district nurses, two physiotherapists, two health visitors, one midwife, one dietician, one more medical secretary and four more receptionists. (Compare this photograph with Figures 6.10 and 6.11, images of GPs in the 1950s and the 1970s.) (Source: Tony Woodcock)*

7.5.3 Nurses

As noted in earlier chapters, the nursing, midwifery and health visiting professions have separate histories, but they have in the course of time become more closely interconnected. Since 1980 they have been regulated by the United Kingdom Central Council for Nursing, Midwifery and Health Visiting (UKCC), and a single Review Body determines their pay. All nurses qualify via the same general nurse training before specialisation, and many who work as midwives or health visitors possess all three qualifications. The great majority of nurses work in NHS hospitals; a much smaller number work in private sector hospitals and nursing homes.

As already noted with respect to Table 7.1, about one-quarter of the NHS hospital nursing workforce are not qualified Registered Nurses. There is no standardised training for these staff, known variously as health care assistants, nursing assistants or nursing auxiliaries. Midwives work partly in hospital, partly in the community. An increasing number of Registered Nurses, as well as nurses with special district nursing training and health visitors work in the community, in association with general practitioner groups.

Since the 1960s nurses have enhanced their professional status, although they have enjoyed nothing like the ascendancy of the GPs with whom they work in primary care. Gains by the nursing profession tend to be secured with great difficulty over a long period of time, and then prove hard to sustain. Two examples, nurse management and nurse education, usefully illustrate this conclusion.

Nurses in management

The 1974 NHS reorganisation (building on the Salmon reforms discussed in Chapter 6) gave *nurse managers* enhanced status as part of the *consensus management teams* in all tiers of the NHS regional administration. In practice senior nurses lacked the training, support, or even inclination to establish their reputation as managers in the decade before the Griffiths Report of 1983 (Robinson and Strong, 1987).

Under the Griffiths management changes, consensus management was abandoned and nurses lost some of their hard-won managerial authority and their representation on key management boards. Nurses lacked the embedded foothold in health service administration at all levels that doctors had secured for themselves. Indeed the Griffiths Report made no mention at all of nurses, although they were (and remain) numerically the single largest component of the health-care labour force. A few nurses have subsequently enjoyed successful careers at the various levels of general management, but nursing has not in general acted as a viable entry route to NHS management.

Responding to public concern over the perceived weakness of senior nurses in the hospital ward, *The NHS Plan* promised to restore confidence by reinstating a 'modern matron' figure, who will be 'a strong clinical leader with clear authority at ward level' (Department of Health, 2000a, paragraph 9.21). (You may wish to reflect on the image of the 'hospital matron' of the past, by looking back at Figure 6.9.)

Nurse education and registration

Nurse education has been a similarly difficult struggle to attain greater parity with the position enjoyed by doctors. By 1974 nurses had been trying for a century to secure an academic education separate from their training on the wards. This reform was regarded as fundamental for securing parity with other professions, including on matters of remuneration. Without this change the nursing profession would neither attract sufficient recruits nor avoid loss from wastage.

However, employers resisted the academic training of nurses on the grounds that it would reduce the already inadequate nursing presence on the wards. The Briggs Report of 1972 provided new impetus to the reform of nurse education and training, but implementation of its recommendations was delayed until the 1980s. In 1980, as a first stage, the UKCC was established, together with four subsidiary National Boards for each part of the UK. The UKCC gave nursing an equivalent to the General Medical Council. Between them, the UKCC and the National Boards exercised comprehensive responsibility for education, training and professional regulation in nursing, midwifery and health visiting.

It took until 1987 for the UKCC to amend the original version of its Project 2000 report (UKCC, 1986), which called for a fresh approach to nurse education in line with new thinking on the professional structure within nursing. It specified a detailed pattern for a three-year period of academic education and training, and limited the ward service contribution of trainees to 20 per cent, compared with the traditional diploma system, which involved about half the training being spent on the wards. The first Project 2000 pilot schemes were not established until 1989.

The graduate path to nursing has been popular and it looks likely to supplant the traditional diploma training, but academic institutions still lack the capacity to produce an all-graduate profession. This is an outcome that medical critics of Project 2000 resisted, contending that graduate nurses are inappropriately educated and lack essential practical skills (Rivett, 1998, pp. 342–3, 446–7). Celia Davies, who was Project Officer to Project 2000, notes the dilemma for the 'new nursing', which runs the risk of devaluing caring in the pursuit of an elite status for nurses, with the aim of securing greater parity with doctors (Davies, 1995).[11]

Responding to criticisms about nurse education, both the Labour government and the UKCC investigated this problem. As a result the UKCC introduced a package of reforms in basic education designed to improve the practical skills of nurses. Also, reflecting general concern over regulation in other health professions, the UKCC came under scrutiny, and in April 2002 it is being replaced by the Nursing and Midwifery Council, a body possessing strengthened powers to protect the public from shortcomings in nursing practice.

Specialisation and professional status

Within the hospitals, nurses have become more highly qualified and specialised in line with the demands of advanced treatment. Many nurses are no longer generalists, but specialists working in such fields as cancer or geriatric care, or even narrower sub-specialisms such as intensive care for which particular post-registration qualifications are ideally required. Given the shortage of nurses and increasing labour intensity of hospital work, the supply of specialist nurses is outstripped by demand.

For example, surveys undertaken in 1996 and 1997 found that 15 per cent of nurses working in paediatric intensive care lacked the basic qualification in children's nursing, while 59 per cent possessed no paediatric intensive care post-registration qualifications. Of even greater concern, nurses fully trained for this work ranged from 19 per cent to 80 per cent across paediatric intensive care centres in England (Paediatric Intensive Care Taskforce, 1997). The shortage of many groups of specialist nurses has been profoundly damaging. For instance it has reduced the efficiency of

[11] An article by Celia Davies in *Health and Disease: A Reader* (Open University Press, 3rd edn 2001) entitled 'Professionalism and the conundrum of care', is set reading for Open University students during study of *Dilemmas in UK Health Care* (Open University Press, 3rd edn 2001); it could usefully be previewed now if you have time.

cancer care and limited bed availability in strategically important fields such as intensive care, and thereby it has impaired the capacity of the NHS to react to life-threatening emergencies.

In an attempt to improve recruitment to specialised hospital nursing, in 2000 the government launched a new senior grade, the Nurse Consultant (Figure 7.20a). *The NHS Plan* contained further proposals for expanding this grade, which it is anticipated will achieve greater parity for nursing staff with senior hospital doctors.

Renewed emphasis on primary and community care and generous funding made available for the development of GP-fundholding in the 1990s created new avenues for the professional advancement of nurses outside the hospital sphere. As GPs became more preoccupied with management, other practice staff absorbed many of their routine functions, increasingly including clinical activities. After a slow start in the 1980s, specially trained *nurse practitioners* established themselves in primary care, where they often provide the first point of contact for specific groups of patients and determine the course of their treatment. Nurse practitioners are required to possess an accredited training qualifying them to make professionally autonomous decisions. By the year 2000 there were about 3 000 nurse practitioners, two-thirds of whom were located in primary care; the others were established in hospital settings such as accident and emergency departments.

In primary care *practice nurses* are more numerous than nurse practitioners and exercise less independence (Figure 7.20b). By the year 2000 there were about 11 000 of these practice nurses, which represented an increase of about a third since 1990. Practice nurses undertake a wide variety of quasi-medical functions, such as taking charge of health promotion clinics, the care of chronic disease, and they are now delegated an important role in the treatment of problems such as asthma, diabetes and high blood pressure. In addition to the nurse members of the 'Practice Team' employed by the general practitioner (e.g. in Figure 7.19), health centres, and more recently medical centres, also house health visitors, home nurses and midwives employed by the local Health Authority.

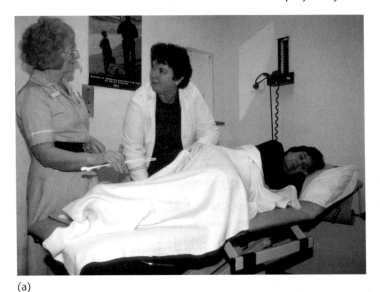

(a)

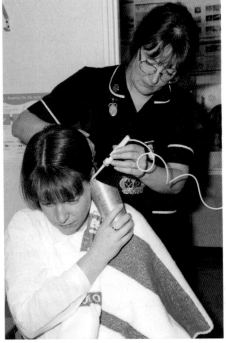

(b)

Figure 7.20 *Two examples of the take-over by nurses of health-care work that was formerly carried out by doctors. (a) A Nurse Consultant, assisted by a nurse, prepares to perform an examination on a patient in a 'day-case' ward. (Source: John Callan/Shout) (b) A practice nurse syringes wax from a patient's ear in a health centre. (Source: Tony Woodcock)*

Changing professional boundaries

It is evident that various of the initiatives of the 1997 Labour government in the field of nurse training and primary care will lead to further changes in the boundaries between the health professionals, and quite likely further career options for nursing groups (Figure 7.21). For instance, a wide range of functions has been proposed for 'linkworkers' in primary care, professionals who provide a bridge between defined classes of patients, such as minority ethnic groups, and the practices serving them (Gillam, 1999, p. 1215). The government has determined that nurses and health visitors will play a lead role in the development of NHS Direct, Walk-in Centres and Healthy Living Centres.

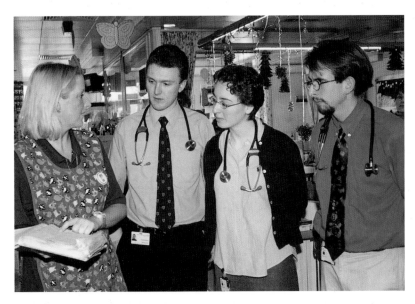

Figure 7.21 *Professional boundaries between doctors and nurses began to blur in the 1990s. A paediatric nurse briefs three junior hospital doctors about a patient's case-notes. The doctors are identified by their stethoscopes, but the nurse is in charge of the case conference. (Source: Mike Levers)*

Some of the instances of blurring of professional boundaries have been contentious. For instance the response of successive governments in the course of the 1990s to the campaign by junior doctors to reduce their working hours has led to greater pressure on nurses to take over tasks formerly performed by doctors, such as intravenous injection of drugs. The agreement announced in May 2000 to reduce the maximum average working week for junior doctors to 56 hours (to be phased in from August 2001) is likely to increase the workload of nurses still further. The government has pledged to create an additional 1 000 places in medical schools by 2005, but it will take until 2008 for the first of these new junior doctors to reach the wards. The receding corps of qualified nurses has also come under increased pressure owing to the need to supervise the growing numbers of health care assistants and other subordinate staff on hospital wards. These pressures have eroded the opportunity to engage in the holistic form of nursing care central to recent nursing ideology.

As Table 7.1 demonstrated, reforms in nurse education and expanding professional opportunities in the 1980s proved insufficient to offset the deterrents of uncompetitive pay, the stressful nature of nursing work and a generally adverse climate in NHS hospitals. As a consequence, the incoming Labour government faced a severe crisis of nurse recruitment. In 1997 it responded by introducing a wide variety of emergency measures, including improved pay, increasing the management authority of ward sisters and creating a new top clinical grade of Nurse Consultant for nurses, midwives and health visitors.[12]

[12] Contemporary issues facing the NHS workforce in general and nurses in particular are the subject of *Dilemmas in UK Health Care* (Open University Press, 3rd edn 2001), Chapter 6.

These initiatives and active recruitment campaigns from 1999 onwards reversed the decline in new entrants and 'returning' nurses. A striking feature of this revival was increased reliance on recruitment of nurses from abroad, mainly from the European Union, South Africa, Australia, the Philippines and New Zealand (Gunning, 2000). This trend was a cause of embarrassment to the UK government, which had given assurances that nurses would not be recruited from poor countries where their services were needed. We return to this issue in Chapter 9.

7.6   Promoting the public health

7.6.1 Fragmentation of public health

In considering the public health strand of the recent history of health care it is now necessary once again to revert back to 1974. As noted in Chapter 6, the status of the Medical Officer of Health (MOH) was severely diminished under the NHS. The policy changes associated with implementation of the recommendations of the Seebohm Report of 1968, and the local government and NHS reorganisations of 1974, carried this policy trend to its logical conclusion. The post of MOH was abolished and the functions of public health departments of local authorities were redistributed.

The former MOH and his medical and nursing staff were transferred to the newly established area and district health authorities of the NHS; the MOH social-service staff became one of the main elements in the new Social Services Departments of local government; former sanitary inspectors, renamed environmental health officers, became the nucleus of environmental health departments of local government. The former MOH medical staff were now rechristened *community physicians*. Their profession retained control over medical aspects of public health, but this was a minority interest as community physicians were increasingly absorbed into the labyrinthine machinery of health-service management created in 1974.

As a consequence of the 1974 changes, environmental health officers exploited the community physicians' declining stake in public health to enhance their own role. Through their statutory duties concerning environmental protection, food safety and control, health and safety at work, housing, and communicable disease control, environmental health officers moved without difficulty into a key strategic position in public health. It is evident that after 1974 public health lost its unified character and indeed risked becoming territory contested between two professions: medically-qualified community physicians and non-medical environmental health officers.

The fragmentation of public health was in fact more complex owing to the new concern in the late 1970s with disease prevention, health education and health promotion, which had all traditionally been pursued within the framework of public health. This broader context meant that aspects of public health also became the business of other agencies, including primary health-care teams, designated health education personnel, local education authority and social work staff. This wider participation resulted in a new concern for public health issues, but it also exposed the lack of coherent arrangements for mobilising these forces to the best effect.

The Acheson report 1988

A succession of public health scandals in the 1980s, beginning with a *Salmonella* outbreak at the Stanley Royd Hospital, Wakefield, and 'legionnaire's' disease at Stafford, both of which resulted in fatalities, shook public confidence and prompted an inquiry into the future of the public health function, chaired by Sir Donald Acheson, the Chief Medical Officer. The Acheson Report of 1988 made a determined effort to reinstate 'public health medicine' and this title was again adopted for medical professionals engaged in this field (Department of Health and Social Security, 1988).

This first Acheson Report (there was another in 1998) made wide-ranging recommendations. Particularly important was its proposal for the appointment of assigned Directors of Public Health at all levels in the health service, to assume management responsibility for the public health effort within the NHS. These Directors of Public Health were to some extent reincarnations of the MOH, and indeed the revival of an MOH duty was proposed — the production of annual public health reports as expressions of their professional guidance. The Acheson Report also recommended that health authorities should be given a formal public health role. In the attainment of these objectives the authors recognised that it was necessary to achieve more effective collaboration between the NHS and local government services such as environmental health, education and social services.

Public health and the internal market

The Acheson recommendations were adopted by the Conservative government in 1988 and were broadly implemented in the changed structural environment of the internal market. In some respects the internal market assisted the attempt to provide more coherent leadership in public health because, for the first time in the history of the NHS, public health doctors had the capacity to influence the strategic development of the entire health service, including primary care — an area where they had previously exercised no influence.

However, in other respects the internal market and its successor, integrated care, have perpetuated divisions within public health. Throughout the 1990s public health specialists within health authorities[13] have faced exactly the same ambiguity about their role that arose in the context of the 1974 reorganisation. Management considerations have again taken precedence over public health, which was neglected because the energies of the small public health specialism have been almost totally absorbed by endlessly-changing management systems. Also, while in theory public health specialists were at least able to shift resources in accordance with the objective needs of populations in their area, in practice this was sacrificed to 'crisis management' or pacifying powerful vested interests in the medical specialties (Jewell, 1999, p. 164).

Experts in the field anticipate that dismantling the internal market will assist the reassertion of public health priorities, but they still need to contend with the structural and professional divisions that sprang up in 1974. There is no single figure of authority for public health in any one area, and responsibility for public health remains fragmented between all the separate professional groups listed above. As indicated in the following section, many initiatives have been taken to advance public health, but their effectiveness is handicapped by the fragmentation of professional responsibility and the lack of coherent frameworks for collaboration between the competing stakeholders.

[13] The Health Authorities created within the NHS in 1991 are capitalised (as in Figures 7.8 and 7.9); prior to that date we have used 'health authorities' as a generic term for all providers of health services, including local authorities.

7.6.2 Prevention and inequality

As already noted in the previous section, the 1970s were marked by a new level of concern about the *prevention of ill health.* This was certainly not the initiative of community physicians, who were preoccupied with their new managerial role in the reorganised NHS. The impetus came from abroad. A key document setting out an individualistic 'lifestyle' approach to health promotion was the Lalonde Report (called after the Canadian Minister of Health), *A New Perspective on the Health of Canadians*, published in 1974. Lalonde was influenced by the work of Thomas McKeown who argued that the overall health of the population bore less relationship to medical advances than to overall standards of living and of nutrition.[14]

Many countries followed in publishing similar lifestyle-oriented documents and there was a rapid growth of interest in preventive medicine. In Britain, the Department of Health and Social Security's policy document, published in 1976, was entitled *Prevention and Health: Everybody's Business.*

● What do you think is the significance of this title?

■ It appears to imply that prevention of illness is a personal matter, not primarily the business of governments, nor of industry, nor does it bear much relation to structural and economic factors.

The Royal Commission on the NHS, reporting in 1979, concluded that a significant improvement in health required more active disease prevention policies, and **health education** was part of this resurgence. The emphasis in health education (like other forms of prevention) at this date was on the *individual's* responsibility for his or her own health, rather than on *structural* causes of ill health. The focus was therefore on *single-issue campaigns*, in particular those giving advice on smoking, alcohol and healthy eating in relation to heart disease (Figure 7.22a), but presented in terms that left action to the discretion of the individual. Especially after 1979 this approach was justified by libertarian arguments, and it was consistent with the growing distaste for the 'Nanny State'. This conveniently allowed the government to keep questions of health education at arm's length and thereby prevent clashes with powerful vested interests.

The pioneering epidemiological research of Richard Doll and Austin Bradford Hill, published in the 1950s, had established the link between smoking and lung cancer.[15] The massive revenues that the government derived from tobacco ensured that, until the 1990s, government policies focused on exhortation to consumers rather than enforced controls on the tobacco companies (Figure 7.22b). In the absence of convinced leadership from successive governments, campaigning was left to 'outsider' bodies, such as the Royal College of Physicians, and ASH (Action on Smoking and Health). The Royal College of Physicians' first report, *Smoking and Health*, appeared in 1962. Thereafter governments were forced to take the tobacco issue more seriously, but progress was painfully slow. By the 1980s governments faced overwhelming demand to take action, but still there was an unwillingness to confront the tobacco interests. In September 1981, Sir George Young, then a junior

[14] McKeown's ideas were mentioned earlier, in Chapter 4 of this book, and are extensively discussed in *World Health and Disease* (Open University Press, 3rd edn 2001), Chapter 6.

[15] Sir Richard Doll is the principal speaker on an audiotape for Open University students, 'Smoking: A Global Health Problem', associated with *World Health and Disease* (Open University Press, 3rd edn 2001).

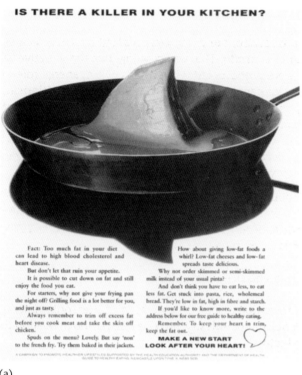

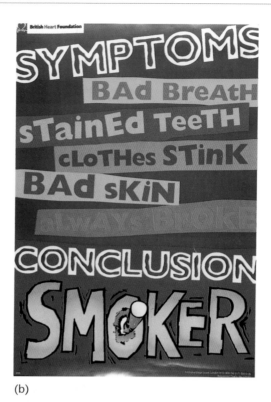

(a)   (b)

Figure 7.22   *(a) 'Is there a killer in your kitchen?' Poster produced by the Health Education Authority in the late 1980s as part of their 'Look after your heart' campaign. The target for most health education initiatives of this period was to persuade individuals to change 'unhealthy' behaviours such as eating fatty food or smoking cigarettes. (Source: Health Promotion England) (b) Modern health education messages, like this anti-smoking poster aimed at teenagers, are less concerned with threats to health than with threats to self-image. (Source: The British Heart Foundation)*

health minister and a determined promoter of a stronger line against the tobacco companies, was moved to the Department of the Environment. This was widely seen as a helpful gesture to the tobacco industry (Taylor, 1984, p. 128–50).

Similar pressures affected other areas of concern to health educators. A report on alcohol, produced by the government's own 'Think Tank' in the 1970s, which recommended a more determined action to achieve reduction of alcohol consumption, was never officially published. Instead of a strong lead from the government in the form of a White Paper, the issue was remitted to the Department of Health and Social Security, which in 1981 produced an anodyne document, *Drinking Sensibly*. This avoided any direct challenge to the alcohol industry. The food industry was also influential in structuring the discussion of problems affecting nutrition and the food supply. Nutritionists such as John Yudkin attacked the power of the sugar industry. The resignation of the Conservative Health Minister, Edwina Currie, in 1988 over the '*Salmonella* in eggs' furore was another demonstration of the power of the farming lobby in nutrition questions.[16]

● What do you consider to be the main limitations of single-issue, health education campaigns aimed at changing individual behaviour?

■ They suffer from an inability to present health problems as at least partly the result of broader structural factors in society, and hence to develop policies

---

[16] Public reactions to food safety scandals in the UK are discussed in *World Health and Disease* (Open University Press, 3rd edn 2001), Chapter 11.

aimed at social change. They are also likely to be obstructed by interests exercising powerful political influence. (The extent to which health education can be successful at changing personal behaviour is another contentious issue.[17])

In the 1980s, attempts to break out of the single-issue framework and broaden the health debate ran into determined government opposition. A crucial episode was the attempt by the Thatcher government in 1980 to restrict circulation of *Inequalities in Health* (Department of Health and Social Security, 1980, or the Black Report as it was known, after Sir Douglas Black, Chairman of the Working Group), the first government-funded document to point out economic and structural causes of inequalities in health. Clumsy attempts at suppression merely provoked greater media interest, and then the publication of a successful paperback edition, with the result that the report's conclusions about the widening 'health divide' between the better-off and those in relative poverty became better known than they otherwise might have been.

Attempts by successive Conservative administrations to deflect attention away from the problem of inequalities in health were unsuccessful. Indeed, the escalation of unemployment and related problems of poverty merely increased concern about the health consequences. In response to growing public concern, and at the risk of confronting government susceptibilities, Margaret Whitehead produced a follow-up to the Black Report in 1987, called *The Health Divide*, which also achieved widespread publicity.

These two reports inspired further investigations of inequalities in health. One of the main researchers was Professor Peter Townsend, a member of Black's team. Labour in opposition made much of this issue, and it was even elevated into a general election manifesto commitment. Signifying readoption of inequality as a major policy priority for the first time in nearly twenty years, in 1997 the new Labour government commissioned Sir Donald Acheson to produce a further follow-up to the Black Report. This second Acheson Report, *Independent Inquiry into Inequalities in Health*, was published in November 1998.

● What did the report find had happened to the 'social gradient in health' in the years since the Black Report first identified it?[18]

■ It confirmed that inequality in health remained a problem of undiminishing importance; indeed, the gap in health experience between the most affluent classes and manual workers or long-term unemployed had widened during the 1980s and 1990s. Areas of social deprivation and high unemployment continued to have morbidity and mortality rates significantly above the national average (Figure 7.23).

Consistent with the Labour government's commitment to tackle inequalities in health, it responded positively to the 1998 Acheson Report and highlighted the issue in many of its policy documents. In June 2000 it launched the Health Development Agency (HDA) with the explicit aim of providing evidence to professionals and local communities about projects that prevent ill health and reduce

---

[17] The constraints on health education and other health promotion or disease prevention strategies are discussed in *Dilemmas in UK Health Care*, (Open University Press, 3rd edn 2001), Chapter 8.

[18] Competing explanations for inequalities in health in the UK are discussed in *World Health and Disease* (Open University Press, 2nd edn 1993; 3rd edn 2001), Chapters 9 and 10.

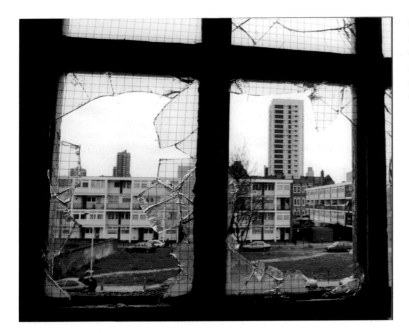

Figure 7.23   *Tower Hamlets in East London. The residents of deprived inner-city environments are consistently found to have higher than average rates of mortality and morbidity from almost all causes. (Source: Mike Levers)*

the health divide. The HDA was described by the Department of Health as the public health 'sister' to NICE (Box 7.2), both organisations emphasising the need for evidence of effectiveness.

7.6.3   Health promotion and the 'new public health'

The limitations of the lifestyle approach to public health was underlined by escalating problems of unemployment and poverty throughout the world and by a growing recognition of threats to health posed by environmental pollution and food safety, which were not capable of resolution by adjustments in personal behaviour. These problems existed on a global scale and required confrontation by the concerted action of governments and the international community.

Public health professionals responded by reformulating their thinking about public health, which was re-branded as the **'new public health'**. Through emphasising the importance of confronting health hazards in the physical environment, the new public health represented a conscious reference to the priorities of the Victorian sanitarians. This is indicated by the widely cited definition of the new public health contained in the *Health Promotion Glossary* commissioned by WHO Europe:

> The terms build on the old (especially 19th century) public health which struggled to tackle health hazards in the physical environment (for example, by building sewers). It now includes the socio-economic environment (for example, high unemployment). (Quoted in Draper, 1991, p. 10)

● In what way does this definition revise Victorian thinking about public health?

■ It introduces an additional factor, control of the socio-economic environment.

By citing high unemployment as its example, the definition indicates that the new public health adopted a broad framework for its thinking about the socio-economic environment. It implied the need to confront the full diversity of factors that contributed to inequalities in health. The same trend of thinking was evident in the field of **health promotion**, which developed alongside the new public health and represented a major refinement of health education. Whereas health education had traditionally dispensed paternalistic advice to individuals on changing their lifestyle, health promotion focused on the empowerment of citizens and local communities, with the goal of giving them full control over factors that affect their health. You will notice that the above definition of the new public health derives from *Health Promotion Glossary*, an indication of the close proximity of these two revisionist movements.

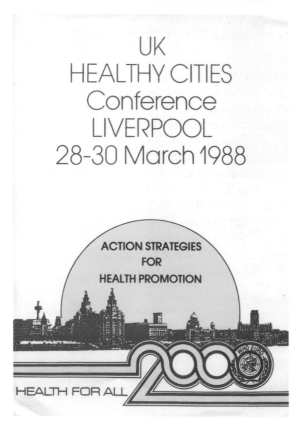

Figure 7.24   *A 'Healthy Cities' campaign poster from a conference in Liverpool, 28–30 March 1988. Liverpool was one of the municipalities in the UK most active in promoting WHO Europe's Healthy Cities initiative; others included Glasgow and Sheffield. (Source: Courtesy of Professor John Ashton)*

Health promotion and the new public health largely originated within the WHO. These concepts were embodied in the WHO's strategy of Health for All by the Year 2000 (Mahler, 1975), adopted by the World Health Assembly in 1981. The full framework for health promotion was confirmed in the WHO *Ottawa Charter for Health Promotion*, dating from 1986. In Europe the strategy of Health for All was taken further through adoption of an ambitious set of WHO targets for the improvement of health.

The WHO Healthy Cities project was an additional source for practical action in the field of health promotion and the new public health. It is notable that in Britain, the initiative for promoting WHO objectives came primarily from local government rather than the NHS. Many local authorities in Britain established local strategies for promoting health, which went beyond supplying educational information to individuals and addressed such issues as industrial pollution, traffic congestion and facilities for leisure. For example, the first book on the new discipline to be published in the UK, *The New Public Health* by John Ashton and Howard Seymour, 1988, grew out of health promotion work in Merseyside (Figure 7.24).

The limited and selective manner in which the new public health approach was taken up indicated that its advocacy was politically sensitive and risked offending powerful vested interests. This paralleled the situation facing those researching inequalities in health, described above. Consequently, the various groups of professionals engaged in the new public health soon discovered that they faced a major conflict of interests in squaring the radical advocacy role of the new philosophy with the constraints imposed on them by the political framework in which they were employed.

The focus on local action embodied in the new public health philosophy was taken forward by the Labour government elected in 1997 in the form of Health Improvement Plans (or HImPs), to be developed for local populations. HImPs are intended to identify the specific health needs of their population and the actions needed to achieve clear targets for health improvement within nationally-determined health priorities. The action plan is developed collaboratively, integrating inputs from health and local authority services, but with the Primary Care Groups taking a major role. This represents another way in which GPs have moved to centre stage in determining the character of the entire range of local services.

7.6.4 Communicable diseases

The years during which the specialty of public health medicine was being reformed and the new public health was emerging, coincided with the build-up of anxiety about escalating threats to health from environmental sources. After the long period during which chronic and degenerative diseases had dominated policy discussions relating to mortality and morbidity, **communicable diseases** came back on the political agenda. Starting in the 1970s there emerged concerns about the safety of vaccines used to protect young children from infectious disease. As referred to earlier, outbreaks of food poisoning due to *Salmonella*, *Listeria* and *E. coli* became an increasingly common occurrence and they highlighted the shortage of public health specialists in this field.

In the public mind these old public health enemies were eclipsed by the new threats from AIDS and BSE. The advent of AIDS as a potentially epidemic disease began to dominate the health agenda in the mid-1980s. Bovine spongiform encephalopathy (BSE) emerged as a more general threat in the 1990s. Moreover, owing to difficulties in obtaining compliance with complex therapeutic regimes, homeless people 'sleeping rough' in the community began to act as a reservoir for the revival of tuberculosis. TB was just one of the instances where misuse of antibiotics risked once-treatable infectious diseases again running out of control.[19] The rise of antibiotic resistance grew into a problem of major importance during the 1990s, complicated still further by the excessive use of antibiotics in agriculture. These major threats to health highlighted the massive importance of the public health function and also the scale of the dangers that would emerge unless multidisciplinary effort in this field was accorded the highest priority.

7.6.5 Health of the Nation

Under the heading, **Health of the Nation,** or later variants, this has been one of the central themes of public health throughout the 1990s and into the new millennium. Indicative of the power of historical precedent, the title of this initiative draws attention to its affiliation with the great sanitarian tradition. Benjamin Ward Richardson's exposition of the ideas of Edwin Chadwick (as described in Chapter 4) was titled 'The Health of Nations', and this in turn echoed the 'One Nation' philosophy of Benjamin Disraeli, which itself possessed an important sanitarian ingredient.

The immediate occasion for the Health of the Nation initiative in the 1990s was the imperative for the UK to contribute its share to the health promotion and public health programmes of the WHO. The first definitive presentation of the new policy was the White Paper, *The Health of the Nation,* 1992, which provided a strategic framework for achieving tangible improvement in key areas of public health. For the first time the UK government adopted specific targets for health improvements. Action was promised in five key areas: coronary heart disease and stroke; four types of cancer; mental illness and suicide; sexual health (sexually transmitted disease and rates of conception among under-16s); and accidents in various age groups. The White Paper accepted that the programme required close collaboration between public bodies and voluntary agencies. It also laid down guidelines using cost-benefit analysis to improve efficiency in the use of resources devoted to the new programme.

[19] Tuberculosis is the subject of Chapter 4 in *Medical Knowledge: Doubt and Certainty* (Open University Press, 2nd edn 1994; colour-enhanced 2nd edn 2001); antibiotic resistance is discussed in *Human Biology and Health: An Evolutionary Approach* (Open University Press, 3rd edn 2001).

Over the next five years the Conservative government dutifully pursued the Health of the Nation programme. Although by no means regarded as a comprehensive solution, it was generally welcomed as a constructive and positive contribution. However, it was also censured by some experts for concentrating on 'easy' targets, which represented no more than an extrapolation of existing trends. Even then some assumptions proved to be over-optimistic. For instance, given the Conservative government's unwillingness to take a firm line against the tobacco companies, even on advertising, it was not surprising that the target to reduce smoking among eleven to fifteen-year olds by at least 33 per cent by 1994 was not met. In general, among proponents of the new public health there was frustration that the procedures of the internal market prevented sufficient priority being given to Health of the Nation targets.

Some other important areas where health improvement was needed and could readily be attained were not considered for reasons of political expediency. For example, by not adopting targets for dentistry, the government deflected criticism over its charges for dental checks, introduced in 1989. It did not act on the long-standing proposal to fluoridate water, despite this being regarded as the cheapest and most effective preventive measure in the field of public health, thereby evading confrontation with the anti-fluoridation lobby.

In practice the White Paper still placed the main burden for health improvement on the individual, while only modest expectations were adopted for government agencies. But the major limitation of the Health of the Nation initiative was its continuing neglect of the problem of inequality in health between social groups, and avoidance of reference to such problems of environmental degradation and inferior housing that undisputedly make such a big contribution to health inequality. Indeed, the White Paper explicitly accepted that the UK was likely to fall short of the WHO target of reducing health inequalities by 25 per cent by the year 2000, and indeed this proved to be the case.

7.6.6 Our Healthier Nation

The Labour government returned in 1997 was alert to the weaknesses of the Health of the Nation programme and it adopted a high-profile commitment to public health. This was a political necessity considering the shock to public confidence of the long-running BSE saga when, in 1997, it was conceded that BSE was in all probability implicated in human deaths from vCJD.[20] Also, the winter before the general election witnessed a fatal *E. coli* outbreak in Scotland, in which 27 elderly people died. Labour appointed the first ever Minister of Public Health; it conceded the case for an independent Food Standards Agency; it introduced Health Action Zones to improve health in selected areas afflicted by high levels of poverty and poor health; and it made plans for improving on the Health of the Nation policies, which included giving more explicit attention to the health inequality issue. Labour's public health programme was called Our Healthier Nation, and was outlined in a White Paper (Department of Health, 1999), with suitable variant White Papers for other parts of the UK.

Labour also promised more decisive leadership against tobacco advertising and in favour of water fluoridation. Many other aspects of Labour's plans for modernising the health service possessed positive implications for public health and inequality issues. In practice, however, improvements on the public health front in their first

---

[20] Prion diseases, which include BSE in cattle and vCJD in humans, are discussed in *Human Biology and Health: An Evolutionary Approach* (Open University Press, 3rd edn 2001), Chapter 5.

term of office were more modest than might have been expected. By the turn of the millennium, no action had been taken on water fluoridation. Labour earned scorn from the anti-smoking lobby through its decision to phase in the ban on tobacco advertising over a long period and its reluctance to confront tobacco sponsorship of certain sports (Figure 7.25). A survey of smoking trends among teenagers in England in 1998 (Department of Health, 1999a) reported a slight downward trend since 1996, but 12 per cent of girls and 9 per cent of boys aged 11–15 years were regular smokers (the targets for the campaign shown in Figure 7.22b).

Our Healthier Nation and the second Acheson Report of 1998 on inequalities in health were only moderately well received. In particular they were not regarded as adequate responses to health inequalities connected with poverty. The scale of this problem was underlined by a major survey, *The Widening Gap*, published by researchers from Bristol University in December 1999 (Shaw *et al.*, 1999). As with all other recent public health initiatives, it seems that Our Healthier Nation is unlikely to constitute a major breakthrough. *The Guardian* summed up the mood of reservation on the eve of the millennium:

> Labour has a disappointing record on public health. Neither its green paper nor its marginally improved white paper set out targets for reducing health inequalities. Too much was left to the discretion of health authorities. Even the Tories had more targets … In the last reshuffle, the status of its public health minister was downgraded. (*The Guardian* editorial, 3 December 1999)

Even if Our Healthier Nation represents only a modest step forward, at least in the 1990s, in response to some serious crises and spurred on by WHO, the UK has displayed more serious concern with public health than in any previous decade since World War II.

In the next chapter we return to the developing world, where the role of doctors in public health was being eroded by a revolution in health care. You will notice some similarities with developments in the UK in the same period: the importance of volunteers, the focus on primary care at the expense of high-technology medicine, as well as reversion to privatised and market-oriented mechanisms of health care.

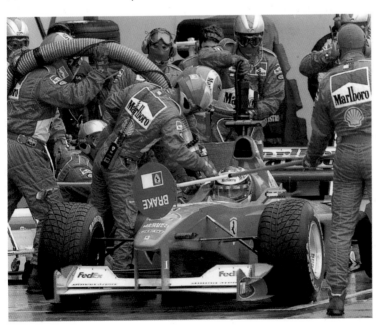

Figure 7.25 *Successive UK governments from the 1970s (when the health risks of smoking were finally accepted) onwards, failed to honour their promises to legislate to curb cigarette advertising in association with sports, despite the likely association with the rise in teenage smoking. (Source: Reuters/Popperfoto)*

OBJECTIVES FOR CHAPTER 7

When you have studied this chapter, you should be able to:

7.1 Define and use, or recognise definitions and applications of, each of the terms printed in **bold** in the text.

7.2 Explain why it has proved difficult to reduce reliance on secondary acute-hospital services and expand the scope of primary care in the UK.

7.3 Discuss ways in which the major reorganisations of the NHS since 1974 have reflected the influence of the 'new public management', and comment on factors that have counteracted this influence.

7.4 Explain why, in recent decades, client groups in need of community care have experienced particular difficulties in achieving an adequate level of support and a sustainable balance between formal and informal care.

7.5 Assess the shifting balance in the hierarchy of health-care occupations in the UK since 1974, and discuss the underlying causes and consequences of the drive towards professionalisation.

7.6 Evaluate the strengths and weaknesses of the various initiatives designed to restore general confidence in public health in the period covered by this chapter.

QUESTIONS FOR CHAPTER 7

1   (*Objective 7.2*)

To what extent is the following description of the change in character, and shift in balance, between primary and secondary health care a reflection of actual trends in the UK since 1974? Give reasons for your answer.

> ... improvements in medical technology mean that patients will spend fewer days occupying hospital beds and there will be a corresponding increase in the treatment of patients as out-patients, and in the community, by GPs and nurses. The concept of the 'general' hospital, with a broad range of services designed to cater for the needs of most patients, will decline. Instead there will be a smaller number of specialist units which maximise the use made of expensive equipment. This implies a movement from secondary to primary care and an increase in the power of GPs both in terms of the numbers of patients they treat and their influence over the distribution of health service resources. Their role as passive partners in the enterprise of health, removed from the reality of hard decisions about costs and benefits, will be eroded. Inevitably, they will be drawn into the debate about priorities in health care. (Newdick, 1995, p. 273)

2   (*Objective 7.3*)

Michael Power argues that:

> ... [a major] reason for the rise of the NPM [new public management] has been the success of political discourses which have demanded improved accountability of public service, not

simply in terms of their conformity to legally acceptable process but also in terms of performance. It has been argued that taxpayers have rights to know that their money is being spent economically, efficiently, and effectively — the three Es — and that citizens as consumers of public services are entitled to monitor and demand certain minimum standards of performance, as embodied in Citizens' Charters. Whatever the reality of popular pressure for these changes, the NPM claims to speak on behalf of taxpayers and consumers and against cosy cultures of professional self-regulation. Taxpayers and citizens, rather like shareholders, are the mythical reference points which give the NPM its whole purpose. (Power, 1997, p. 45)

In what ways has the new public management, and other factors operating within the NHS, served to make health-care professionals more responsive to the interests of patients as consumers? What evidence is there that consumer interests are not yet being met?

3   (*Objective 7.4*)

Writing in 1987, Martin Bulmer described the gulf between rhetoric and practice with respect to the attempt to evolve a 'seamless' service of community care.

> Despite the rhetoric of 'interweaving', sharing care and complementarity, there are relatively few examples of successful combinations of the two which endure for any length of time. Truism though it is, one of the first targets must be intra- and inter-organizational boundaries in the personal caring fields. Within social services departments, home-help services and social work teams are too insulated from each other. Within local health services, district nurses, health visitors and general practitioner services are run too much in parallel, without adequate co-ordination. Social services as a whole, and health services as a whole, are largely ineffective in co-ordinating their activities, a proposition which is being demonstrated once again in the closure of large mental institutions. (Bulmer, 1987, p. 220)

In the period since 1974 , why has so little progress been made to establish the kind of multidisciplinary partnerships between the NHS and local government services that are required for a viable system of community care? What policy initiatives have aimed at overcoming these difficulties?

4   (*Objective 7.5*)

Read the following passage in which Pamela Abbott and Elizabeth Meerabeau sum up in favour of the contentions made in Jane Salvage's book, *The Politics of Nursing*, published in 1985.

> Both groups [Nursing and social work professions] have justified their strategies for achieving professional status by arguing that this would improve client/patient care. However, it is not clear that achieving professional status would necessarily do this. The strategies successfully used to achieve professional status by the medical profession seem as much about protecting and enhancing the status of doctors as about protecting the public and providing a higher level of service. Jane Salvage (1985) has argued that, if nursing became professionalized, this would lead to nurses

identifying with doctors rather than with care assistants and ancillary staff, relatives and the friends of the patients. This, she suggests, could strengthen barriers between nurses and patients, and also create barriers between workers, rather than encouraging them to work as a team to meet the needs of patients. She concludes by arguing that strategies of professionalization are less about meeting the needs of patients/clients than about an occupational group pursuing its own narrow interests. (Abbott and Meerabeau, 1998, p. 15)

Discuss the extent to which increasing professionalisation within health-service occupations (not only in nursing) show signs of protecting the 'narrow interests' of the relevant professions, as the authors of the above quotation claim, rather than meeting the needs of patients. Your answer should address aspects that counteract the claim as well as points that support it.

5   (*Objective 7.6*)

The following assessment is by David Hunter, a leading analyst of health and public policy:

A re-engagement of public health practitioners with the social and environmental determinants of health is therefore both long overdue and welcome. There are signs that countries, including the UK, are beginning to address the core business of public health, namely, improving the health of populations for which its practitioners, wherever they are located, are responsible. Growing public awareness of, and concern over, public health issues in response, *inter alia*, to a series of crises affecting food safety (i.e. BSE and the *E. coli* tragedy) and the environment (e.g. transport policies and road traffic accidents) is forcing governments to take public health policy seriously and put it higher up the political agenda. (Quoted in Griffiths and Hunter, 1999, pp. 12–13)

What support can you find for this positive assessment, and what signs suggest that it may be unduly optimistic?

CHAPTER 8

Health care in the developing world, 1974 to 2001

8.1 Introduction   254

   8.1.1 Variation in health profiles in low- and middle-income countries   255

8.2 The evolution of health policy in low- and middle-income countries, 1970–8   257

   8.2.1 Experiments with basic health services   257

   8.2.2 Changing ideas about poverty, health and development   262

   8.2.3 Concern about population growth   262

   8.2.4 Activities and policies of international organisations   263

8.3 Implementing primary health care in poor countries, 1978 to the mid-1980s   267

   8.3.1 Building on lay care: community health-worker programmes   267

   8.3.2 Implementing community health-worker programmes   269

   8.3.3 Traditional midwife training   271

8.4 Primary health care: comprehensive or selective?   274

   8.4.1 Selective PHC in practice: a fading dream?   276

   8.4.2 Immunisation — a successful programme   278

   8.4.3 PHC: 'our sacred cow, their white elephant?'   280

8.5 Changing agendas in the 1990s: decline of PHC and the rise of health sector reform   280

   8.5.1 Economic and political factors undermine PHC   280

   8.5.2 The health-sector reform movement   282

8.6 The impact of AIDS and other infectious diseases   285

8.7 Emerging and re-emerging infectious diseases   287

8.8 Ecological deterioration: polluting the land   289

8.9 PHC or health sector reform: rhetoric and reality   291

Objectives for Chapter 8   293

Questions for Chapter 8   293

Study notes for OU students

This chapter builds upon your knowledge and understanding of health and disease in low- and middle-income countries, as presented in *World Health and Disease* (Open University Press, third edition 2001), Chapters 2–4 and 8. In particular, we suggest that you refresh your memory of the diversity of health experience between and within low- and middle-income countries and the complex connections between economic development, population growth and social inequality. During your study of Section 8.3.1 of the present chapter, you will be asked to read an article by David Werner, 'The village health worker: lackey or liberator?' in *Health and Disease: A Reader* (Open University Press, second edition 1995; third edition 2001). A second reader article, by Bloom and Xingyuan, on health sector reform in China is set reading for Section 8.5.2 (it is only in the third edition 2001). A television programme about health care in South Africa, 'Catching the good health train', relates to this chapter; before you watch it, we strongly suggest that you view Video 1 again, 'South Africa: health at the crossroads'.

8.1   Introduction

This chapter continues the discussion of contemporary diversity in health care by providing a broad overview of health and health-care systems in low- and middle-income countries and the way in which health policies have changed. It covers the period from the 1970s to 2000 and focuses on major shifts in health policy — from the *primary health care approach* at the beginning of the period (Sections 8.2–8.4), to the *health sector reform movement* towards the end (Section 8.5 onwards).

Although the trend towards greater emphasis on primary health care was by no means limited to low- and middle-income countries, (its counterpart in the industrialised world, as you have seen in Chapter 7, was in the expansion of primary health care teams, health promotion and the new public health), this chapter focuses on developing countries. The main questions addressed are:

* Why was the introduction of the primary health care approach a significant change in health policy?
* How was primary health care interpreted when ministries of health in low- and middle-income countries tried to put policy into practice?
* Why did attention shift from primary health care to an emphasis on health sector reforms?
* What have been the main problems in the implementation of both these policies in low- and middle-income countries?

8.1.1 Variation in health profiles in low- and middle-income countries

Although it used to be common to use the term 'Third World' as shorthand, after the break up of the Soviet Union (then perceived as the 'Second World') at the end of the 1980s, it became more usual to refer to this very heterogeneous grouping of nations as low- or middle-income countries rather than a bloc.

● Summarise some of the main dimensions of diversity within and between low- and middle-income countries at the end of the 1990s.[1]

■ You might have thought of some of the following categories (to which we have added examples in brackets):

1 *GNP per capita* (ranges from 80 US$ in low-income Mozambique to 1 050 US$ in the Philippines).

2 *Under-five mortality rates* (297 per 1 000 population in that age-group in Mozambique, 80 per 1 000 in the Philippines).

3 *Population size* (Nigeria has a population of over 100 million; Botswana, which is almost the same geographical area, has just over 1 million people).

4 *Rural-urban differentials* (infant mortality rates in Mozambique's capital, Maputo, are about 90 per 1 000 live births, but in some rural areas are 173 per 1 000 live births).

5 *Intra-urban differentials* (in Manila the infant mortality rate in the urban slums is three times higher than in other parts of the city).

Infant and under-five mortality rates declined in the great majority of developing countries in the first decades after World War II, and continued decreasing into the 1990s. However, from the late 1980s, economic stagnation and recession led to deteriorating living standards and health conditions in many countries, and — especially in those countries affected by the AIDS epidemic, such as Zambia — there was an increase in child mortality among the poorest groups in the 1990s. Consequently, when we look at indicators of health in low- and middle-income countries, we see a world of huge contrasts. And those differences are reflected in many other ways. A worker in Benin described two faces of Africa, but he could just as well have been writing about Asia or Latin America:

> There is the educated, literate, charming and welcoming Africa where the tourists go, where the business people trade and where project coordinators hatch their schemes. There the five star hotels, exotic cuisine, swimming pools and safari clubs with telexes, telephones and faxes. There the ministries of health or development, there the besuited people with power and influence. But there is the second Africa, usually beyond the city boundaries, beyond the tarmac and neon lights, perhaps 50 km away along dusty or muddy tracks where there are no banks or telephones and children are taught in crumbling mud brick shelters that pass for schools ... where English or French is hardly spoken ... (Potter, 1991, p. 1 558)

[1] As discussed in *World Health and Disease* (Open University Press; 3rd edn 2001), Chapters 2, 3 and 8.

Figure 8.1 *At the beginning of 2000, the WHO reported that one-sixth of the world's population (1.1 billion people) lacked access to a treated water supply and two-fifths (2.4 billion people) lacked access to adequate sanitation (WHO–UNICEF, 2000) — as in this shanty district of Recife, North Eastern Brazil (Source: Julio Etchart)*

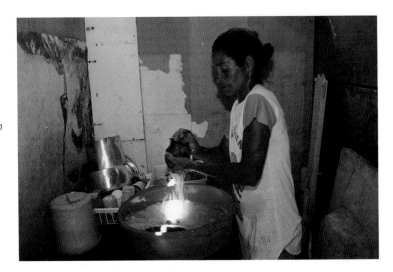

Differences between rural and urban populations persist. But it is *urbanisation* that has increased over the past decades, and which demands attention because of the huge inequalities between groups within cities. For many urban dwellers in slum areas, environmental conditions are damaging to health — overcrowded housing, squalid roads and thoroughways, inadequate sanitation and water supply (Figure 8.1).

Rapid industrialisation has created high levels of environmental pollution. In Mexico City schools are occasionally closed for a day because of the poor quality of air. Access to the existing health services, medicines, doctors and nurses may be limited. Not only do poor urban dwellers have to cope with violence and injury in cities (both major causes of death), but they also suffer from infectious diseases and malnutrition as well as the chronic cardiovascular diseases and cancers typical of modern Western societies.

Data from many countries suggest a single explanation: access to the conditions that improve people's health is highly inequitable. Both rural and poor urban populations lack sufficient and clean water supplies and sanitation. Education, although widespread, is seldom available beyond primary school, and its quality is variable; employment opportunities are few, especially in rural areas. Shortage of food adds to people's vulnerability. And health care is patchy: in cities even very poor people sometimes go to private medical practitioners rather than use public health services. In the countryside, people continue to turn to traditional or folk medicine for help when ill, sometimes because formal 'Western' care is not easily available, sometimes because they prefer, or have more confidence in, the traditional sector.

● Can you think why even poor people will pay for health services rather than get them free?

■ Your answers might include the following: private practitioners may practice closer to where people live, and may be open for consultation in the evenings when people return from work; they may provide more privacy in consultations, and be perceived to give a more personal service. They often have drugs on hand, to sell to patients. Public services, on the other hand, are often very crowded, queues for consultation are long, privacy may be restricted, staff are sometimes perceived to be abrupt and to have little time for clients or patients. Stocks of drugs are often unreliable.

8.2 The evolution of health policy in low- and middle-income countries, 1970–8

Although there had been many reports about developing comprehensive health services based on health centres during and after World War II, what was actually implemented during the following decades were *centres of excellence* in many developing countries: the university hospitals emulating the teaching hospitals of the industrialised world. As you will recall from Chapter 6, these were all in urban areas, usually in the capital, and absorbed a high percentage of the health budget. By the late 1960s, however, a real shift in thinking about medicine was occurring, although it was only in the 1970s that widespread dissemination of new ideas occurred.

Four areas of influence and changing ideas that laid the basis for the primary health care approach, particularly in the developing world, are discernible in this period, although any such division is to some extent arbitrary and overlapping. Policy change occurs as the result of a complex series of events and ideas not easily distinguishable over time. However, it is possible to focus on four areas; we will look at each in turn.

1 Experiments in particular countries to find alternative means for improving health;

2 Changing ideas about poverty, health and development;

3 Concern about population growth;

4 Activities and policies of international organisations such as WHO and the United Nations Children's Fund (UNICEF).

8.2.1 Experiments with basic health services

By the late 1960s and early 1970s, there was considerable disillusion in both the industrialised world and the developing world with the role of medicine and the way in which health services were organised. The commonly held assumption that disease could be fully accounted for by a model based on molecular and cellular biology as its basic scientific discipline was increasingly challenged.

Anthropologists, sociologists, and psychologists interested in the medical area, showed the importance of socio-economic, cultural and life-history factors in explaining ill-health. They also researched and wrote about the popularity of non-Western systems of health care. As in the West, people predominantly treated themselves or sought care from friends and relatives or indigenous practitioners. In the poor countries of the world, lay care networks were even more extensive than in the industrialised world, partly because of well-established indigenous systems of care, partly because of the limited concentration of Western medical systems.

Although sulphonamides and antibiotics had greatly increased medical effectiveness in the treatment of infectious disease, some medicines had damaging effects, some were costly but useless, and some multi-national drug companies used dubious means to promote their products, especially in poor countries (we return to this subject in Chapter 9). There were also immense problems caused by side-effects and unintended consequences of prescribed and over-the-counter drugs (e.g. thalidomide could be bought from pharmacies in some developing countries for years after it had been withdrawn in most industrialised countries).

Much of the debate centred around the diffusion of medical technology: how and why independent developing countries retained the health infrastructures inherited from their colonial past and aspired to ideas that were inappropriate to the health situations in their own countries. For example, an Indian doctor, Debabar Banerji, suggested that the colonial inheritance had had damaging effects on health services. The inappropriateness of selection and training, he suggested, had alienated health workers from the people they served. The costly emigration of newly graduated doctors to the Western developed world was indicative of a professional identification reinforced by irrelevant training (the scale of emigration is assessed in Chapter 9).

The inappropriateness of aspects of Western-type medical training and service delivery was increasingly recognised. Maurice King's *Medical Care in Developing Countries* (1966, reprinted seven times between 1967 and 1973) became the bible for English-speaking health workers in developing countries. The book was the result of a symposium held in East Africa, at which a number of doctors argued that health services were not reaching those in need, for several reasons.

● Do you recall David Morley's 'three-quarter's rule' (Chapter 6)?

■ Three-quarters of the health budget was spent on hospitals that served less than one-quarter of the population (Morley *et al.*, 1983).

In *Medical Care in Developing Countries* another concern was that health services were attempting to treat illnesses that were preventable. There were no 'medical' solutions for malnutrition, a major complicating condition in many children's illnesses. The underlying cause of much disease was poverty, and other solutions — social, educational, economic and political — had to be sought. King's book therefore emphasised the need for more *preventive health measures* (such as immunisation or ante-natal care), and to move health services nearer to the population by building health centres and clinics in rural areas. In order to increase access to health services, the use of *medical auxiliaries* was strongly advocated. This laid the first step towards accepting lay care, by acknowledging that biomedical training for doctors was not necessarily the only, or even the best, way to provide health services.

In Tanzania, such ideas were actually implemented in the late 1960s. The *Arusha Declaration* of 1967, which set the framework for social and economic policy for the whole country, emphasised the need to give priority to rural areas. Tanzania introduced a comprehensive system of rural health posts, dispensaries, health centres and hospitals, emphasised the need for preventive services, and began to train a variety of health workers for different levels of services: for example, the village health workers and medical assistants.

The **village health workers** were expected to cater for basic health needs in the villages: their dominant focus was on preventive and promotive skills: advising mothers on what foods were nutritional for children, how to make or give salt-sugar solutions during episodes of diarrhoea, encouraging them to take children for immunisation, build latrines or home gardens. (Figure 8.2 shows that initiatives of this kind continue to the present day.) But they were also taught to treat a number of ailments, for which they had some simple drugs such as aspirin, chloroquine (for malaria) or tetracycline eye ointment.

Medical assistants were trained to do more curative care — diagnose and treat a much greater variety of illnesses, prescribe more drugs, do simple operations — as well as undertake preventive tasks such as immunisation. They were also expected to support and supervise the village health workers, who could refer patients to them.

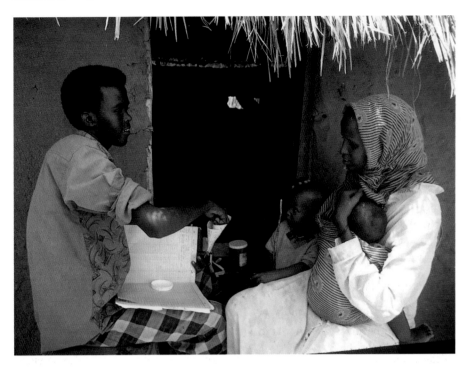

Figure 8.2 *The training of village health workers to cater for basic health needs began in the later 1960s, and was a prominent feature of the primary health care approach in developing countries in the 1970s and early 1980s; despite being overtaken by other developments in the 1990s, it still goes on – as here in a Kenyan village in 1999. (Source: Giacomo Pirozzi/Panos Pictures)*

Although there were shortfalls in Tanzania's innovative approach, it was for many a shining example of what a developing country could do to try to meet its people's basic health needs. In 1972 the government health expenditure ratio between urban and rural areas was 80 : 20 — by 1980 it was 60 : 40. This shift reflected a real improvement in the rural health infrastructure, as shown in Table 8.1.

Table 8.1 Growth in rural health-care infrastructure in Tanzania, 1972 and 1980.

Facilities and health workers	1972	1980
health centres	99	239
dispensaries	1 501	2 600
medical assistants	335	1 400
rural medical aides	578	2 310
maternal and child health aides/midwives	700	2 070
health assistants	290	681

Data cited in Heggenhougen, K., *et al.* (1987) *Community Health Workers: the Tanzanian Experience*, Oxford University Press, Oxford, p. 28.

● What else does Table 8.1 tell you?

■ While the number of *facilities* roughly doubled, the number of health *workers* increased between three and five times.

China too, inspired many to look for alternatives to existing health services. The Cultural Revolution of 1966–9 placed emphasis on developing the rural areas, and information about the mass mobilisation of the Chinese people against endemic diseases was beginning to be disseminated by the early 1970s. Doctors such as Joshua Horn, who worked in China for many years after Mao TseTung's revolution, described the system of **barefoot doctors** — health workers in their time off from the fields.[2] The symbiotic relationship between the community and its barefoot doctors caught the imagination of many concerned about how to increase the rural populations' access to health care. Although China was a low-income country (GNP per capita in 1980 was US$290), life expectancy had improved from 47 years in 1960 to 67 years in 1980, infant mortality rates were similar to those in the industrialised countries, and preventive programmes had greatly decreased the prevalence of diseases such as schistosomiasis (bilharzia).[3]

For many the Soviet Union was another source of inspiration. The *feldshers*, who had been introduced in the nineteenth century in Russia, were school leavers who were trained to provide care to rural populations. Popular images included them riding off on horseback into the bleak and thinly populated steppes. Borrowing from this example, Venezuela introduced a system of auxiliary health workers to extend health care to remote areas of the country, where it was difficult to attract doctors. In Guatemala, in the hub of the Indian highlands, an American doctor — Carroll Behrhorst — helped to train ordinary villagers to provide basic health care to their own communities.

Although admired by many, such schemes were not without their critics, and the conservative medical establishment took a decade to be convinced that health care could be provided by any other than a doctor trained over six or seven years. Behrhorst describes one such medical specialist taken to see the health promoters in Chimaltenango, Guatemala.

> He was sceptical that men with so little formal education could dispense adequate medical care, but as the day wore on and he found the promoters dealing knowledgeably with one ailment after another, his scepticism wilted. Finally, he thought he had caught one of the promoters giving incorrect treatment. 'You have the right disease but the wrong remedy,' he said to the promoter. 'The specific indicated here is penicillin.' The Indian promoter shook his head 'Ah,' he replied, 'but this patient is allergic to penicillin'. (Quoted in Newell, 1975, p. 36)

A handful of countries made radical shifts in health policy and, by the 1970s, were receiving international attention for the resulting improvements in health status.[4] Cuba, which lost one-third of its doctors after the revolution, reconstructed its basic health services, building up a network of polyclinics or health centres, and brought down its infant mortality rate to the lowest in Latin America. Costa Rica was another exception in Central America, with health status levels comparable to those in the developed world. Sri Lanka had much lower infant mortality rates than neighbouring India. In all these countries there was some involvement of the community in tackling its own health problems, whether through local organisations or education campaigns. It seemed that even relatively poor countries could improve the health of their people, through a redistribution of resources that emphasised access to education and health services and food security.

---

[2] An article in *Health and Disease: A Reader* (Open University Press, 3rd edn 2001) by Gerald Bloom and Gu Xingyuan, 'Health sector reform: lessons from China' begins by describing the period up to the late 1970s when village health workers became a dominant feature of health care in China. Open University students will read the whole article later in this chapter.

[3] Schistosomiasis and its impact on health in low-income countries is discussed in *World Health and Disease* (Open University Press, 3rd edn 2001), Chapter 3.

[4] These countries have become known as the 'superior health achievers' because they have been able to achieve health improvements throughout their populations, despite being low-income countries; see *World Health and Disease* (Open University Press, 3rd edn 2001), Chapter 8.

However, a *caveat* is in order here. The reasons why health improves (or mortality declines) are extremely complex. The countries mentioned above also had some, or all, of the following features: a substantial degree of autonomy for the female population; a dedication to education; an open political system; a largely civilian society, without rigid class structures; a history of some egalitarianism. Other countries that did not apparently introduce radical political or social changes in the 1960s and 1970s also experienced improvements in health, probably because they displayed some of the features mentioned above. In contrast, countries in which mortality remained high during the 1970s lacked the above characteristics.

Table 8.2 is a reminder of the relationship between infant mortality rate (IMR) and female education.[5]

Table 8.2   Infant mortality rates per 1 000 live births relative to income and female education in selected developing countries, 1988.

Country	GNP per capita /US$	IMR /1 000 live births	% female age group in primary school
low mortality			
Sri Lanka	420	32	102[1]
China	330	31	124[1]
Jamaica	1 070	11	106[1]
Thailand	1 000	30	(94)[2]
high mortality			
Saudi Arabia	6 200	70	65
Algeria	2 680	73	35
Ivory Coast	740	95	58
Morocco	610	80	56

[1] Figures are expressed as the ratio of female pupils to the population of female school-age children. Countries differ in what they consider primary school age. For some countries, school enrolment ratios exceed 100 per cent because some pupils are younger or older than the country's standard primary school age (usually 6–11 years, but not always).

[2] In lieu of numbers of females enrolled in primary school (not given for Thailand) the figure in brackets refers to the percentage of adult females who are literate. (Adapted from Caldwell, J. C., 1986, Routes to low mortality in poor countries, *Population and Development Review*, **12**, p. 174, using data from World Bank (1990) *World Development Report* and UNICEF (1990) *The State of the World's Children*, Oxford University Press, Oxford)

The high IMR countries are largely Muslim, or have large Muslim minorities, and are characterised by the separate and distinctive position of women. By the late 1990s, the percentage of females enrolled in primary schools in Saudi Arabia and Algeria were reported to have increased from the 1980s figures (to around 73 per cent and 96 per cent respectively), and infant mortality rates had fallen to 21 and 34 respectively (World Development Report, 1997, p. 226).

[5] For a full discussion, see *World Health and Disease* (Open University Press 3rd edn 2001), Chapter 3.

8.2.2 Changing ideas about poverty, health and development

Soon after World War II, development theories had stressed the over-riding importance of investment in the physical elements of national growth — industry, roads and dams — and saw health and other social services such as education as non-productive consumption sectors. Thus government money expended on such services was perceived as a dissipation of national savings.

By the late 1960s these theories were increasingly challenged. There was growing scepticism about who was benefiting from development. In many countries with high rates of economic growth, the rapid rise in income per capita was firmly concentrated in the hands of fairly small numbers in the population, and many groups were worse off than they had been in the previous decade.

In the 1970s, experiences of low-income countries like China and Sri Lanka, as well as middle-income countries like Cuba and Costa Rica, suggested that it was possible to have reasonable rates of growth *and* to redistribute some of the benefits to the poor. It was not necessary to wait for the benefits of growth to 'trickle down' from richer to lower income groups.

In 1976, a conference held at the *International Labor Organization* (ILO) — one of the specialised agencies of the United Nations — most clearly rejected past strategies for development, which had focused on improving the infrastructure, and identified a new priority based on the eradication of poverty, the provision of basic needs and productive employment for the whole population. The ILO conference turned from a narrow focus on industrialisation to setting minimum targets for *basic needs*: food consumption, clothing, housing and the provision of essential services in the areas of water, sanitation, education, health and public transport. People's health would improve if their basic needs were met: one of these needs was health care, and it was apparent that there were gross inequalities in access to health services (the scale of which is assessed in Chapter 9).

8.2.3 Concern about population growth

During the 1960s, one of the common explanations for poor countries' slow rates of development was that economic growth was being dissipated because it had to be divided among ever more people. The growth in population was seen by many as a fundamental brake on development.[6]

Concern was expressed that the world's resources were finite, and that pollution, misuse of existing resources, and consumption demands were all increasing. Robert McNamara, then President of the *World Bank*, also noted in 1979 that uncontrolled population growth could lead to high levels of poverty, stress and overcrowding which would threaten social and military stability. The developing world's view of the population 'explosion' did not always coincide with the developed world's view, but by 1970 many billions of dollars were being spent on population control activities by international, national and private bodies. Three-quarters of the funds went into **family planning** activities, often employing lay women for information and promotion of family planning methods among their neighbours. By the mid-1980s, family planning (or family spacing) was seen as an essential element of primary health care services, although it was not always fully integrated into such services, but delivered separately (for example in Bangladesh).

[6] For a full discussion of population growth and the measures by which countries have attempted to control it, see *World Health and Disease* (Open University Press, 3rd edn 2001), Chapters 4 and 8.

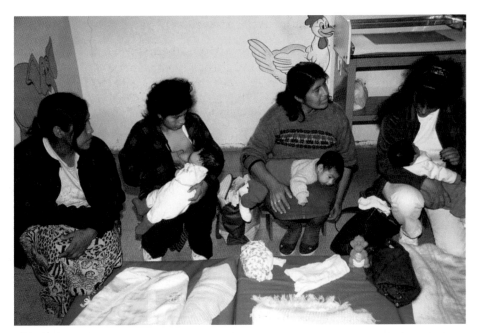

Figure 8.3 *Mothers attend a 'Children's workshop' with their babies on the outskirts of Lima, Peru, to discuss and learn about child-rearing, breastfeeding, and contraception and to give each other mutual support. (Source: WHO/HPR/TDR/Crump)*

In the decade of the 1990s there was again a sea-change in policies related to family planning, and at the *International Conference on Population and Development*, held in Cairo in 1994, women's groups in particular argued that family planning should be linked to a much broader concept of reproductive health – which would include a focus on sexual health and reproductive tract infections as well as family planning (Figure 8.3).

8.2.4 Activities and policies of international organisations

The ideas and experiences described above were brought together by two international agencies that played a particular role in promoting what came to be known as the 'primary health care approach' (defined below). Both are agencies of the United Nations: the WHO (the specialised agency for health) and UNICEF (the United Nation's Children's Fund) which often played a supportive role to the health professionals in the WHO. These organisations played an important part in developing and disseminating health policy, in offering technical assistance to low- and middle-income countries to implement health programmes and in funding such programmes. How did these two organisations take a critical part in the shift of health policy?

In the early 1970s, WHO experts were trying to explain apparent failures in the malaria eradication programme. Technical reasons for the difficulties in malaria eradication were acknowledged, but the dominating cause of failure was the lack of a complete and continuing health-service infrastructure which could reach every household *and* remain in place. Malaria eradication had been introduced as a **vertical programme** — that is, a programme with its own funds, workers, vehicles and supplies, which worked separately from all other health services. When the campaign had finished in one area, it moved on to another and, because it was not integrated into the basic health service, there was no continuing activity – so the mosquitoes returned.

One of the WHO instigators of the primary health care movement, Ken Newell, writing in 1988, argued that the primary health care approach owed its genesis to this failure. A special working group set up within WHO to look at problems in basic health services reported in 1973 that not only was access to health services very uneven, especially between urban and rural areas, but also:

> ... there appears to be widespread dissatisfaction of populations with their health services ... Such dissatisfaction occurs in the developed as well as in the third world. (WHO, 1973, p. 106)

The report went on to enumerate the reasons for such dissatisfactions, which included failure of health services to meet people's expectations, inadequate coverage, great differentials in health status within and between countries, rising costs and:

> ... a feeling of helplessness on the part of the consumer who feels (rightly or wrongly) that the health services and the personnel within them are progressing along an uncontrollable path of their own which may be satisfying to the health professions, but which is not what is most wanted by the consumer. (WHO, 1973, p. 106)

The 1973 WHO report had two important effects: first, it defined the **primary health care approach**, which — for the first time — clearly brought together features which had been developing for over a decade. Although the report concentrated almost totally on health services and the health sector, it emphasised the need to involve the consumer, to tap local resources, to 'make medicine 'belong' to those it should serve' and called for a 'national will' as well as 'international will' for positive health. Second, the report legitimised WHO's leadership role in changing health policy. The report drew attention to WHO's role as 'world health conscience':

> It is possible to use WHO not only as a forum to express ideas or dissatisfactions, but also as a mechanism which can point to directions in which member states should go. (WHO, 1973, p. 108)

As part of the search for new solutions in health services, a joint WHO–UNICEF committee commissioned a study of successful programmes using alternative strategies for providing health care. As you have seen, a number of countries (Tanzania, the Soviet Union, Guatemala, Cuba) and many non-governmental organisations had experimented with innovations in health services, through expanded use of auxiliaries, health centres and community involvement. Some of these radical approaches were disseminated in two books widely publicised by WHO — both published in 1975: *Alternative approaches to meeting basic health needs* (Djukanovic and Mach, 1975) and *Health by the people* (Newell, 1975).

In the meantime, WHO began to take a much more active role in persuasion and promotion of a particular health message, firmly orchestrated by Halfdan Mahler, who became Director-General in 1973. In 1975 he launched the idea of 'Health for All by the Year 2000' as WHO's contribution to the UN's 'New International Economic Order', proposing urgent action now to achieve 'in the twenty-five years of a generation what has not hitherto been achieved at all' (Mahler, 1975). Health had to be considered in the broader context of its contribution to, and as a lever for, social development.

This climate of ideas provided the context for the *International Conference on Primary Health Care*, held at Alma Ata in 1978, and sponsored by the WHO and UNICEF, with a substantial financial contribution from the host country, the Soviet Union. A report on *primary health care* was prepared for the meeting, which was attended by representatives of 134 governments and 67 international organisations.

The **Declaration of Alma Ata** outlined the role of primary health care in 'Health For All by the Year 2000':

> A main social target of governments, international organisations and the world community in the coming decades should be the attainment by all the peoples of the world by the year 2000 of a level of health that will permit them to lead a socially and economically productive life. Primary health care is the key to attaining this target as part of development in the spirit of social justice. (WHO–UNICEF, 1978, p. 3)

Primary health care itself was defined as

> ... essential health care based on practical, scientifically sound and socially acceptable methods and technology made universally accessible to individuals and families in the community through their full participation and at a cost that the community and country can afford to maintain at every stage of their development in the spirit of self-reliance and self-determination. It forms an integral part both of the country's health system, of which it is the central function and main focus, and of the overall social and economic development of the community. It is the first level of contact of individuals, the family and the community with the national health system, bringing health care as close as possible to where people live and work and constitutes the first element of a continuing health care process. (WHO–UNICEF, 1978, p. 3; for example, see Figure 8.4)

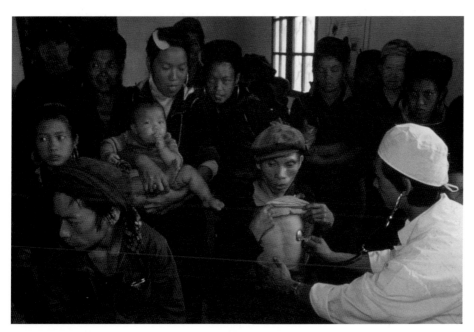

Figure 8.4 *Tuberculosis and malaria are common in the Nung population of Viet Nam; here a travelling doctor visits the Luc-Ngan district to conduct health checks and give treatment. Bringing health care as close as possible to where people live and work was the 'first element' in WHO–UNICEF's original vision of primary health care in developing countries. (Source: WHO/TDR/Martel)*

Primary health care was understood to include (at least) the components in Box 8.1:

Box 8.1   The main elements of primary health care, as envisaged in 1978

promotion of food supply and proper nutrition;

an adequate supply of safe water and basic sanitation;

education concerning prevailing health problems and ways to prevent and control them;

maternal and child health, including family planning;

immunisation against the major infectious diseases;

prevention and control of locally endemic diseases;

appropriate treatment of common diseases and injuries;

provision of essential drugs.

Behind the rhetoric was a serious shift in ideology — at the centre of which was a concern with *equity*, *community participation*, and a changing emphasis on *prevention* and *health* rather than on treatment and disease. It was by no means only applicable to poor countries — industrialised countries were also signatories to the Alma Ata Declaration. But it is difficult to translate an ideology into practical reality, and as you will see, in the late 1980s and 1990s the primary health care approach came up against problems in implementation, and was also challenged by a competing health care reform ideology, championed by the World Bank — one of many different organisations that play an international role in health (Box 8.2).

Box 8.2   International organisations with a role in global health issues

The World Bank is an international financial institution founded in 1944 with the aim of assisting member states with reconstruction and development; among many other activities, including health data collection, it provides loans to countries for their health sector programmes.

United Nations agencies with a role in health include WHO (the World Health Organisation), UNICEF (the United Nations Children's Fund), ILO (the International Labor Organization), and UNFPA (the United Nations Population Fund).

Bilateral agencies such as the UK's Department for International Development, the Swedish Development Agency, or the United States Agency for International Development, all play a role in WHO as members of the organisation; they also give aid to low- and middle-income countries through government-to-government agreements. Both UN agencies and bilateral agencies are often referred to as 'donors'.

Non-governmental organisations (NGOs), such as Save the Children or Oxfam, also make critical contributions to health development at both the international and the domestic level.

8.3   Implementing primary health care in poor countries, 1978 to the mid-1980s

Primary health care endorsed at Alma Ata gave the concept of public health an international boost. It was believed that reaching 'Health for All by the Year 2000' could only be achieved if new approaches were taken to deal with health problems which stemmed from socio-economic and environmental, as well as biological causes. The broad, equity- and community-based primary health-care strategy emphasised the need for *multi-sectoral action*, that is, collaboration between different government sectors such as health care, education and agriculture. But it was difficult to translate this aim into practical activities.

In the industrialised world the call came for a *new public health movement* — reorienting attention *away* from health services, and *towards* the environment, promotion of good health and community participation. (The gap between the rhetoric and the reality in Britain was discussed in Chapter 7). In low- and middle-income countries, the concept of primary health care focused attention *more* on health services and people's participation in them — an approach that soon became known by its acronym (PHC) in the agencies promoting it.

In the search for practical programmes of activity in the developing world, the broad concept of PHC was gradually narrowed down and focused on two assumptions, outlined in Box 8.3.

Box 8.3   Assumptions underlying the concept of PHC in low- and middle-income countries

1   Conventional medical resources were not available in rural areas — doctors and nurses were unwilling to work outside urban health facilities and their numbers were insufficient. Therefore it was essential to train members of rural communities to deliver basic health care to their own people. The Chinese barefoot doctor and similar village health-worker schemes could be universally applied all over the developing world.

2   Most of the health problems in low- and middle-income countries were preventable and susceptible to elementary methods of care and simple drugs, which could be provided by community health workers. Improving environmental conditions and hygiene, raising awareness about health behaviour, and providing preventive care, such as immunisations against childhood infections, were the most effective means for improving health, but real gains could only be achieved with significant participation of communities. Selecting which of all these activities to undertake was initially assumed to be simple.

Let us look at the practical consequences of these assumptions in turn.

8.3.1   Building on lay care: community health-worker programmes

Many low- and middle-income countries confronted their shortages of professionally trained health staff by shifting the boundaries between lay and formal care. Acknowledging that people within communities were *already* giving care, they argued that, with relatively short training, villagers could both prevent and treat common complaints that had been the remit of health professionals. They would become the link between the formal health services and the community, and stimulate action to involve people in their own health care. These villagers were expected to deal with common problems which could be managed with limited training and supplies – thereby relieving higher-level health centres or hospitals from routine problems so that they could focus on providing services which required more sophisticated training and resources.

The 'catch-all' term **community health worker** (or **CHW**) only came into general use in the 1980s. Community health workers were given different names: 'village health workers' in Tanzania, 'community health aides' in Jamaica, 'village health guides' in India. Some countries introduced a *new* cadre of community health worker while others extended programmes initiated long before Alma Ata. There was an important difference between the programmes that employed community health workers in the 1960s and early 1970s, and those that were introduced after Alma Ata. The earlier programmes were *indigenous* efforts to meet local needs, whereas later initiatives were often motivated more by a government's desire to show a commitment to PHC and were *imposed* on health workers and communities. However, in most programmes, the tasks of CHWs were similar.

● Can you list some of the health activities CHWs were trained to do?

■ Your answers might include the following: to encourage mothers to breastfeed; to educate villagers on nutrition — food production, storage and preparation; to encourage households to take children to be immunised and to be aware of hygienic practices around water and latrines; to treat common ailments with simple drugs such as aspirin or cough medicines, or to refer patients to the next level of health facility.

On what models did countries base their CHW programmes? Two had by then received significant publicity: *national government programmes* such as the Chinese barefoot doctor scheme, and small, *non-government projects*. These models differed in style and ideology. In his article, 'The village health worker: lackey or liberator?', David Werner describes a number of these programmes in Latin America. This article has become a classic in the literature on PHC. (It is reproduced in *Health and Disease: A Reader*, Open University Press, 3rd edn 2001. Open University students should read it now, and then answer the following question.)

● Werner contrasts the appropriateness of professional auxiliaries and village health workers. What does he consider are the benefits of the latter?

■ They are trained for short periods, therefore their training is not expensive; they are selected from the community in which they live, and this predisposes the community to both support and accept them; furthermore they are often already accepted by the community because of their standing as traditional healers or midwives.

Note that Werner saw such workers as having an important political role, as agents of change. However, it is one thing to nurture a small-scale community health-worker programme with committed, dynamic and charismatic leadership such as that of Werner (and there are many other examples all over the developing world), but it is quite another to provide the same level of support and enthusiasm in a large, national, community health-worker programme that depends on the existing health infrastructure and professionals.

By the mid-1980s many countries had national community health-worker programmes. Many were composed of *unpaid volunteers* with a fairly narrow range of largely educative tasks. For example, Thailand had trained both village health volunteers as well as village health communicators for every village in the country, and other countries had very large numbers of CHWs: 100 000 in Sri Lanka, 40 000 in Zambia, 1 million in Indonesia. Other countries trained fewer community health workers, but paid them a salary or honorarium: by the mid-1980s Botswana had over 600 in place, Colombia 5 000, Jamaica over 1 200.

8.3.2 Implementing community health-worker programmes

It soon became apparent that CHWs working in national programmes in the 1980s were faced with particular difficulties not always anticipated from previous experience. First, it was clear that very few CHWs were actually chosen in an open way by their *communities*. In many countries, it was the community *leaders* or *health workers* who chose the CHW. Debbie Taylor, a writer on development issues, provides a vivid profile of a village volunteer, Samchai, in Thailand, which is mirrored the world over:

> He had hoped that being trained as a health volunteer would give him more opportunities to help the other villagers. He had been disappointed not to have been selected when the *puyaiban* first chose people for training three years ago. It was only to be expected, he supposed, that the *puyaiban* would choose his relatives and friends first. But it made him feel so frustrated to see them all pocketing their *per diems* and stowing away their piles of training manuals unread — knowing that they had neither the time nor the inclination to use their training properly. What was even worse, the son of the *puyaiban*'s best friend — who had gone for the longer 15 day training to be a health volunteer — did not live in the village any more. He had gone off to work in Bangkok ... (Taylor, 1986, p. 38)

Gradually it was acknowledged that communities were not homogeneous, and that local politics could affect which community health workers were chosen to 'serve the community'. This raised questions of suitability, commitment and loyalty, with huge variations within and between community health-worker programmes.

Second, it was soon realised that community health-worker programmes were *not cheap*. Although training was short, and community health workers received only basic supplies, large numbers had to be trained. While savings could be made by using unpaid volunteers, drop-out rates were high. This was hardly surprising in those places where all community health workers were women — the group most heavily burdened with daily tasks.

In some countries *volunteer programmes* seemed to work better than others: religion, among other factors seemed to play a part. For example, in Buddhism, voluntarism is a positive value and countries with large Buddhist populations such as Thailand, Burma and Sri Lanka had large volunteer programmes. However, religion was seldom the whole story. In Sri Lanka, health volunteers were largely young, well-educated women, who had few job opportunities. When asked, the majority said they volunteered in order to give service, but also because they hoped that voluntary work would lead to future employment.

In those national programmes where community health workers were paid a salary by the ministry of health (Botswana and Colombia, for example), the cost of running the programme was much higher, and fewer were trained. Paid community health workers tended to be committed to their job, especially given the paucity of employment opportunities in rural areas. However, research showed that many felt allegiance to the ministry of health and preferred to work in health centres or dispensaries, rather than visiting people in their homes.

● Can you think why working in the health centre rather than visiting homes may be a problem?

■ For all sorts of complex reasons, not everyone attends the health facility, even when they are ill; the community health worker was not necessarily reaching the whole community.

By the end of the 1980s, questions were being asked about the *effectiveness* of community health workers. Many argued that community health workers were captured by the health service professionals and used as 'extra pairs of hands':

> The journey from the nearest town took five hours, half of it on a sandy road past nothing but salt pans, baobab trees and the odd fleeting glimpse of a springbok. We arrived at the health clinic in Maun — a large village of about 70 000 people — just before noon. The morning's work was almost over. A nurse was taking a woman's blood pressure, a few mothers and babies were waiting patiently to see another nurse. Outside a small group was sitting under a tree, receiving nutrition education. The chief nurse was welcoming, and when we explained why we had come her enthusiasm was uninhibited. 'Family welfare educators?' she exclaimed, indicating the woman who was sweeping the clinic floor. 'We couldn't do without them! It's wonderful to have extra pairs of hands in a busy clinic like this!' (Walt *et al.,* 1990, p. vii)

Others argued that community health workers could not support communities who wanted *drugs* and *emergency services* when they were ill. One writer described the frustration of a community health worker in Tanzania:

> On one of our walks we stopped by a crumbling hut of an elderly couple. The wife was sick, ashen looking, lying on her cot with pain in her right leg, terribly thin and anaemic. No latrine, disorder all around. The man was busy building a small spirit house where food would be placed to placate the spirits so that his wife would get better. The CHW suggested to the husband that he take his wife to the health centre — but how, when she could not walk? Under the circumstances, the CHW could offer no other advice ... (Heggenhougen *et al.,* 1987, p. 76)

The problem was that, by the mid-1980s, many low-income countries were beginning to cut back on services because of diminishing resources and debt repayments. This situation worsened in the 1990s. For example, expenditure on health care in Zimbabwe fell by a third, and Niger, in common with many other Sub-Saharan African countries, was spending more on debt repayments than on health and education combined.

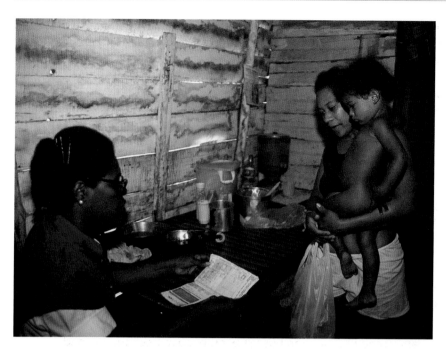

Figure 8.5 *The conditions in which primary health care is often conducted in poor districts is apparent in this health clinic in Recife, North Eastern Brazil. (Source: Julio Etchart)*

The first level of care to be affected by the squeeze on available resources was the one furthest away from the capital (Figure 8.5). Drugs and other supplies became increasingly erratic; in some countries salaries for health workers were not paid for months; fuel and spare parts for transport were increasingly unavailable; visits to peripheral health posts or communities became rare. Staff became demoralised as support or supervision for community health workers became minimal. People soon learned that their health facilities often ran out of drugs and vaccines and the general quality of care was low, so they stopped attending.

8.3.3 Traditional midwife training

The other group who were given training through the 1970s and 1980s were the **traditional midwives**, who were the main source of help in childbirth in many developing world countries. A sociologist, Jacqueline Vincent-Priya, who lived and worked in Malaysia for four years, made a special study of traditional midwives:

> Without exception they all had a tremendous range of experience; most had borne children of their own and served a long apprenticeship before they began practising. One of their big advantages is that they share the same ideas and the spiritual and practical life of the mothers for whom they give their services so freely, and they usually know these mothers well. Whatever help the traditional midwife gives is always given according to what the mother feels she needs, and her autonomy is rarely questioned or compromised. Traditional midwives usually have some spiritual calling for their work, which gives them and their clients confidence in their ability to deal with both normal and abnormal births. They use techniques which are appropriate to their situation: bamboo is a good thing to use for cutting the umbilical cord in communities which neither understand nor have the facilities for sterilising instruments. In every group I visited there were simple, cheap and easily available remedies for most of the common problems associated with pregnancy and birth. (Vincent-Priya, 1991, p. 199)

The rationale for training traditional midwives in elements of *Western obstetric practice* was obvious — some were known to use unsterile, inferior, and occasionally, harmful practices. But there were, in some countries, underlying tensions between traditional and government practitioners. For example, Vincent-Priya pointed out that, according to the local Malaysian newspapers, traditional midwives were 'a bad thing'. Malaysia had trained many government midwives, who were perceived to have a superior training (general nursing followed by midwifery) and therefore to provide safer conditions for mother and child.

● Can you suggest why there was so much emphasis on training large numbers of *traditional* midwives?

■ In many countries it was simply not possible to train sufficient government midwives or to persuade women in rural areas to go to maternity clinics to give birth. Even in urban areas women sometimes preferred delivery by a traditional midwife rather than go to the clinical surroundings of a city hospital or health centre; traditional midwives were less expensive and would go to the women's homes, so mothers were not parted from their other children.[7]

Many countries, with assistance from WHO and UNICEF, introduced short training courses for traditional midwives, typically lasting one to three weeks (Figure 8.6). Women learned about family planning methods, antiseptic techniques and detection of high-risk pregnancies. They were often rewarded at the end with a simple maternity kit (for example, a pair of scissors or razor blade, rubber gloves, soap). By the mid-1980s considerable experience with training programmes had been recorded, but increasing scepticism about their value was being expressed.

The sociologist Patricia Jeffery and co-workers, writing about northern India in 1988, observed that *dai* training programmes (*dai* is the Hindu name for traditional midwife) had failed to take into account the complex cultural constraints on Indian women. They were valued essentially for their childbearing capacity, but they did not control any of the decisions that affect pregnancy, such as the use of antenatal services, acceptance of tetanus toxoid, or the need for rest and adequate nutrition. Local understanding about childbearing — which included strong notions of shame and

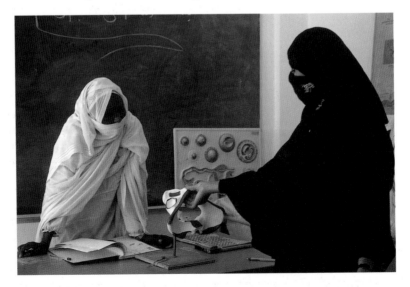

Figure 8.6 *Midwives in Ibb, a town in the Yemen, receive a short training in basic anatomy and obstetric procedures. (Source: Sheldur Netocny/Panos Pictures)*

[7] Note the striking parallels with the United Kingdom debate about the benefits and limitations of home vs. hospital births — discussed in *Birth to Old Age: Health in Transition* (Open University Press, 2nd edn 1995; colour-enhanced edn 2001), Chapter 3.

pollution — were not considered in the training. Even if *dais* had been trained by health professionals, and retained and used their new knowledge (which was difficult to ascertain) they were limited in where they could help:

> The Harijan dai is welcome only while the new mother is herself unclean: the Caste Hindu *dai* is tainted by her work. Only for a Muslim among Muslims or a Harijan among Harijans, and then not always, are the barriers between a *dai* and her client at a minimum. Government health staff, as urban superiors, are socially distant in one direction, while the *dai*, as a polluted menial, is socially distant in the other. (Jeffery *et al.*, 1989, p. 219)

Drawing on experience from years of fieldwork with Maya midwives in Yucatan, Mexico, and on participation in government-sponsored training courses for indigenous midwives, the anthropologist Brigid Jordan was scathing in her criticism of the training programmes. In her analysis of instructional methods she drew attention to inappropriate modes of teaching that put emphasis on definitions and irrelevant messages:

> In Yucatan, as in many parts of the world, women believe that the most fertile time is immediately before and after menstruation, because at that time 'the uterus is open'. Women who want to avoid pregnancy will have intercourse at midcycle when they believe the uterus to be closed — exactly at the most fertile time. The medical staff, however, were not aware of this belief, and anyway, there was no space for discussing it in the lesson plan. So the family planning course failed to impart the single piece of information which could be expected to have significant impact on contraceptive behaviour. (Jordan, 1989, p. 297)

Jordan did not gloss over the difficulties of imparting knowledge that challenged traditional views but argued that, at the end of the course, midwives graduated successfully because they had learned to give their trainers the 'right' answers, although these bore little resemblance to how they would later practise.

However, there were differences between training programmes, and some may have been more successful than others. One report from Zimbabwe described a programme as highly successful because of the positive relationship between the formally trained maternity assistants at health clinics and the traditional midwives, or *vanambuya*, who were trained once a fortnight over a five- or six-month period.

> The great advantage of the programme is that it is locally administered. The maternity assistants get to know the traditional midwives well, and in many of the clinics collaboration between them has been enthusiastic. Maternity assistants noted that many traditional midwives have been encouraging women to go to antenatal clinics, and to take children for immunisations. (B. Booker quoted in WHO, 1984, p. 21)

By the 1990s, with maternal mortality rates still very high (for example, in many low-income countries, including Mozambique, Nepal, Rwanda, Sierre Leone, Yemen, Ethiopia – up to three in every 200 women died in pregnancy or childbirth), there was no clear evidence that such training had resulted in improved maternal or perinatal outcomes. There was a growing acknowledgement among researchers and practitioners that while training traditional midwives was still important, much more needed to be done to improve formal emergency care services and the skills of those providing it.

8.4 Primary health care: comprehensive or selective?

From its beginning in 1978 there was a divergence of opinion on how far PHC could be implemented.

● Can you think of one major hurdle to overcome if PHC was to be implemented equally across a whole population?

■ The cost of meeting the basic health needs of the whole population would be immense.

In 1979, just one year after the Alma Ata meeting, two specialists in tropical medicine, Julia Walsh and Kenneth Warren, argued that PHC was idealistic and that it would cost too much to guarantee basic primary health care to all. They suggested that countries should identify their most common diseases, ascertain what low-cost or cost-effective technologies existed to deal with them, and then concentrate resources on these. They gave an example by comparing lassa fever, *Ascaris* (round worm) and malaria (Walsh and Warren, 1979).

Lassa fever, they argued, would be a low priority because it was fairly rare, and although often fatal, there was little that could be done about it. On the other hand, although *Ascaris* was extremely common, people suffered little direct morbidity, and it would need such continuous treatment and improvements in basic hygiene, that it too, was of low priority. However malaria was very common, did cause significant morbidity and sometimes mortality, and was preventable or treatable through a number of different methods. Therefore, countries should give priority to activities in malaria control programmes. Walsh and Warren called this **selective primary health care**.

However, many argued that *selective* PHC diverted attention away from the original all-encompassing concept of primary health care. One of PHC's early protagonists, Ken Newell, said that it represented a revolutionary change, which highlighted the environmental and social aspects of health, removed health care from the dominance of the medical profession, and encouraged people's participation (Newell, 1988). In this sense of PHC — later called **comprehensive primary health care** — health and development were closely aligned.

● How did selective PHC contrast with comprehensive PHC?

■ The principles of equity, prevention, multi-sectoral collaboration and community involvement underpinned comprehensive PHC and yet were hardly mentioned by those in favour of selective PHC. The selective approach to PHC was much more focused. It concentrated upon specific diseases or interventions and special groups (children under five, mothers, the poor). It was medically oriented.

Selective PHC also had the advantage of being relatively easy to implement. Within a few years of the Alma Ata meeting, many international donors were re-defining PHC as a *package of low-cost interventions*, which were based on assumptions about the most effective methods of improving the health of young children. The four most widely adopted assumptions are shown in Box 8.4. The activities that flow from these four assumptions were called the **GOBI interventions** (growth monitoring, oral rehydration, breast-feeding, immunisation).

Box 8.4 Assumptions about low-cost interventions to improve children's health

1 If children were *weighed* regularly during their vulnerable first years, those who were not growing as they should (because of illness or poor nutrition), could be identified at an early stage, and preventive action could be taken. Weighing a child, and marking its progress on a growth chart was not difficult (see Figure 8.7).

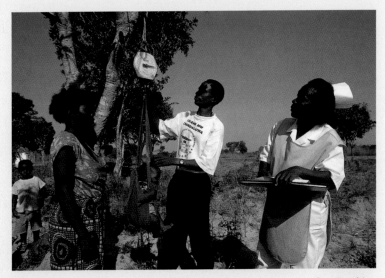

Figure 8.7 *Growth monitoring in a rural community near Lusaka, Zambia. (Source: Giacomo Pirozzi/Panos Pictures)*

2 As many as one-half of the deaths from diarrhoea among infants and children could be averted if *dehydration* was prevented or treated. This could be achieved by giving them oral rehydration solution (ORS), a relatively simple mixture of water, salt and sugar. ORS could be mixed at home or distributed in sachets by community health workers or volunteers; mothers could be taught how to make it, and when to administer it.

3 There was a clear link between *breast-feeding* and health. Those children who were exclusively breastfed for at least 4–6 months were protected from contracting diarrhoeal diseases and some other illnesses. In some countries, especially in Latin America, mothers were only breast-feeding for very short periods (a few weeks) and they had to be encouraged to lengthen this.

4 *Vaccines* were increasingly efficient, especially against the infectious diseases of childhood (measles, diphtheria, tuberculosis, tetanus, polio and whooping cough), and these killing or maiming diseases could be prevented if significant numbers of children could be immunised against them (Figure 8.8).

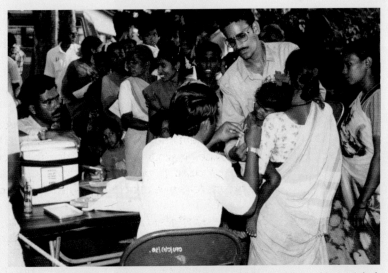

Figure 8.8 *Mothers wait in line to have their children vaccinated in a trial of a new leprosy vaccine, India, 1990. (Source: WHO/TDR/Gupte)*

The GOBI interventions were imaginatively and energetically promoted by UNICEF in particular, but also by many other aid donors who supported health programmes in developing countries. Later, other factors that had a link with health were added to the list: family spacing, female education and food supplementation.

Many donors of financial and technical assistance favoured *selective* PHC programmes.

● Can you think why?

■ Limiting activities to a core set of vertically directed deliverables made it easier to set and then achieve targets, and achieve them relatively quickly. Numbers of immunisations or oral rehydration sachets given could be counted, growth charts examined. It was more satisfying for aid donors (who had to persuade their constituents at home that their money was being sensibly spent) to focus on a specific disease and intervention than try to take account of all the common problems presented at health clinics.

8.4.1 Selective PHC in practice: a fading dream?

For many countries, such selective interventions were equated with PHC, and were implemented widely through training community members to undertake them. However, enthusiasm for selective PHC was faltering in the late 1980s, partly — as you will see later — because the international community of organisations such as WHO and UNICEF, and bilateral agencies who were providing advice and financial resources to poor countries, were shifting their priorities from PHC to health sector reform. But the change also came about partly as a result of negative experiences: for example, the four 'pillars' of the GOBI interventions were starting to collapse.

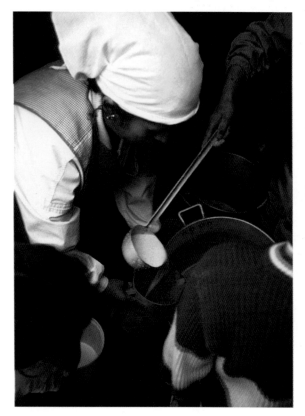

Growth monitoring was increasingly criticised as being seen as an end in itself, rather than as a means of identifying vulnerable children and acting to improve their nutrition. Screening requires accuracy in several sequential steps: reading the weight, plotting it on the child's growth chart, and interpreting the child's growth pattern. Establishing the *reasons* for growth faltering is usually done by talking to the mother. A number of studies suggested that none of these things was being done very well, and indeed, some health workers expressed a helplessness in knowing how to intervene, even if they did recognise that a child was malnourished. A health education talk was not always particularly helpful when families simply lacked food (Figure 8.9).

A similar anxiety was growing about *oral rehydration*. Initial euphoria at the ease with which women learned to make oral rehydration solutions at home safely and effectively, was later challenged because knowledge

Figure 8.9   *Villa El Salvador, Peru; local women dispense fortified milk to children — under the* Ley del Vaso de Leche *(Law of the Glass of Milk) passed in the early 1990s, to improve the nutrition of Peruvian children. (Source: WHO/ HPR/TDR/Crump)*

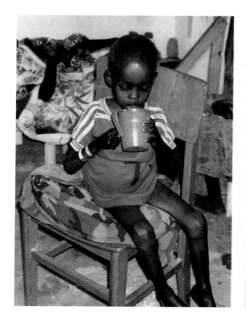

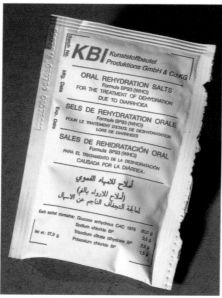

Figure 8.10   *Left: This child is drinking oral rehydration solution (ORS), mixed by her mother from sugar, salt and water. (Source: Manjit Kaur) Right: A low-cost ORS sachet of a type often distributed in primary health-care programmes. (Source: courtesy of ECHO International Health Services, Ltd)*

did not necessarily lead to use. Even if mothers used oral solutions, it was often used only for specific *sorts* of diarrhoea. Chowdhury and Vaughan (1988) showed that the terms that health workers used for diarrhoea meant: 'very severe diarrhoea' to mothers. Women believed that *less* severe diarrhoea could best be cured with traditional remedies. So ORS was only given in a small percentage of cases.

A study in Bangladesh after ten years of a well-supervised oral rehydration programme, showed that most mothers thought oral rehydration solution would *stop* diarrhoea, whereas ORS prevents dehydration, but may make diarrhoea *worse* initially. This may have discouraged mothers from giving it to their children; it is also extremely time-consuming to feed a sick infant with oral rehydration solution, which does not taste particularly good (Figure 8.10). Commercial companies also saw an opportunity to market fruit-flavoured sachets of ready-mixed ORS powder, which was often unsuitable and expensive.

Concerns about the decline in the number of women *breast-feeding* in middle-income countries — especially in Latin America — and the resulting increase in infant morbidity and mortality — led some countries to introduce health education campaigns to encourage women to continue breast-feeding for longer periods (see Figure 8.11).

But, however attractive, television, radio and poster campaigns were pitted against the powerful influences of the multinational food industries. In the 1980s 30 per cent of the revenue of Bangladesh television came from baby food adverts. One such advertisement

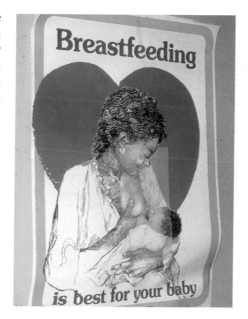

Figure 8.11   *Posters exhorting mothers to feed their babies with infant formula milks are being replaced in many low- and middle-income countries by posters encouraging mothers to breastfeed. This one is from Belize. (Source: Sean Sprague/Panos Pictures)*

was described as follows:

> The chubby baby on the television screen is heading for the plate of food on the table by his mother's chair. Glancing up from her newspaper, she smiles indulgently. 'No, this isn't for you. For you, Cerelac'. Cut to the same baby, grinning happily, with the remains of his meal smeared around his mouth. Cut to tins of Nestle's Cerelac. (Burgess, 1990, p. 45)

Other, more subtle promotion methods were used by the infant food industries, by, for example, providing maternity services with free samples for all recent mothers:

> Mothers coerced into bottle feeding in this way leave hospital with a tin of formula and a dwindling supply of breast milk. If they persist in bottle feeding, their babies are 25 times more likely to die of a gastrointestinal, respiratory, or other infection. The cost of purchasing further formula poses an enormous financial strain and puts the nutritional status of whole families at risk. Typically, artificial milk consumes around 50 per cent of the household income. (*The Lancet*, 1990, p. 1151)

Although WHO passed an *International Code on Breastmilk Substitutes* in 1981, countries found it difficult to implement in its entirety. Throughout the 1980s and 1990s non-governmental organisations, WHO and UNICEF monitored violations of the Code (for example, poor labelling or advertising practices, free samples for professionals or new mothers), and campaigned to get countries to introduce legislation incorporating the provisions of the Code instead of depending on voluntary agreements. After 1992, when the joint WHO–UNICEF *Baby Friendly Hospital Initiative* was launched (among other things, to prevent infant formulas being given free in maternity services) three countries — China, India and Brazil — enacted strong laws to put the Code into practice.

Even in 2000, infant feeding remained a controversial issue. At a meeting in Geneva a group of specialists accused WHO of stifling their criticisms of the babyfood manufacturers' marketing and other practices; they claimed that WHO was establishing partnerships with private industry and did not want to appear too critical.

8.4.2 Immunisation — a successful programme

The fourth 'pillar' of GOBI, immunisation, raises even more complex issues. The huge effort and resources put into immunisation campaigns in many of the developing countries may well deserve to be seen as the *public health revolution* of the less developed world. In the mid-1970s nearly 5 million children globally were dying every year of six infectious diseases: measles, tetanus, whooping cough, diphtheria, tuberculosis, and polio. Millions more were permanently disabled. In 1980, only about 5 per cent of children in *low-* and middle-income countries were immunised against these six diseases. By the end of the 1980s, well over 80 per cent were fully immunised by the time they were one year old (see Figure 8.12). Indeed, some countries had coverage figures that were better than those in the United Kingdom.

The great drive to immunise children was spearheaded throughout the 1980s and 1990s by the Task Force for Child Survival, which brought together the efforts of the WHO, UNICEF, the World Bank, the United Nations Development Programme (UNDP), the Rockefeller Foundation and many bilateral aid agencies. A typical

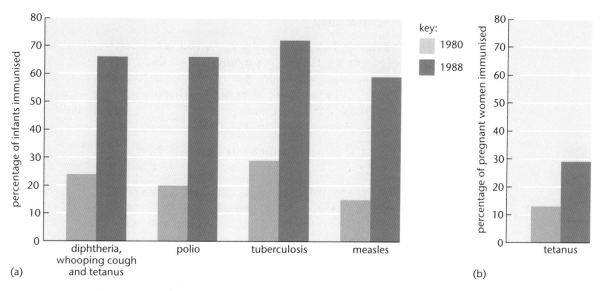

(a)   (b)

Figure 8.12   *During the 1980s aggregate world figures showed dramatic increases in coverage of immunisation against the main diseases of childhood for which vaccines exist. (Source: WHO/UNICEF: UCI Reports, cited in UNICEF, 1990,* The State of the World's Children, *Oxford University Press, Oxford, Figure 3, p. 15)*

campaign showed the President of the country on the front page of the national newspaper, 'giving the first shot' in a national two- or three-day campaign, which involved teachers, policemen and priests, as well as health workers. Posters promoting immunisation were widely distributed (see Figure 8.13). As we said earlier, in some countries the results were spectacular.

● Such campaigns also have their drawbacks — can you suggest the main pitfalls?

■ Children missed by a three-day annual campaign, or born just after it, have to receive their immunisations elsewhere. If immunisations are not part of the basic health services, then campaigns may have only transient

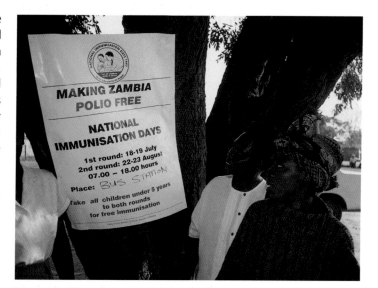

Figure 8.13   *Immunisation campaigns pass on, but the posters reminding mothers to have their children immunised remain on the walls of clinics and other public places, as here, in Zambia. (Source: Philip Wolmuth/Panos Pictures)*

effects; the energy expended on immunisation may divert resources from other important services; infections for which no vaccine exists may be neglected.

Nevertheless, there were major successes. By the end of the 1990s the number of cases of polio world-wide had fallen by almost 90 per cent to 5 000 a year. The Americas were declared polio-free, and the disease had disappeared from Europe and China. Transmission was restricted to a number of countries, such as Afghanistan, Democratic Republic of Congo, India, Nigeria and Pakistan. There was a world-wide push to eradicate polio from these countries, and rid the world of polio (as was accomplished for smallpox in 1976). If polio is eradicated, savings on vaccination costs world-wide will amount to US$1.5 billion a year.

Although the immunisation campaigns of the 1980s and 1990s could boast considerable success, there was no room for complacency. In 1999 WHO reported that, in spite of the great advances, one in five children were still not fully immunised against the six major killer diseases (WHO, 1999).

8.4.3 PHC: 'our sacred cow, their white elephant?'

We have focused on PHC in the 1970s and 1980s because it was promoted as a radical change in health policy, even if it was not always understood or was implemented as if it meant simply introducing a community health worker programme, training a few traditional midwives, or selecting a few health activities. But does this suggest that the concept was flawed? Was PHC 'our sacred cow, their white elephant'? (Reidy and Kitching, 1986).

Many would concur that PHC was adopted with much enthusiasm and haste, but with insufficient attention to planning and management; that the complexity of delivering even simple services and interventions was underestimated; that it was often imposed in a 'top-down' manner where what was needed was extensive dialogue with health workers and communities in order to change attitudes; that the real costs of implementation were not sufficiently considered, and that some issues, such as the role of the private health sector were ignored

But for most, the basic concept of PHC retained its moral imperative. However, PHC was introduced into a fast-changing world, which threatened many of its premises. As you will see, by the end of the 1980s, the *health-sector reform movement* was being strongly advocated, and it shifted attention away from PHC to consider issues of financing and organisation of health systems. In the final part of this chapter, we look at what happened to PHC in the last decade of the twentieth century as it was displaced and repackaged by the health-sector reform movement.

8.5 Changing agendas in the 1990s: decline of PHC and the rise of health sector reform

When PHC was launched in 1978 the prevailing climate was hopeful and optimistic. Its architects could hardly have imagined the negative trends in economic growth, the extent of borrowing and the changing ideology which would reinforce political thinking in the capitalist world, and bring about the demise of the communist bloc. Many ministries of health (especially in the newly independent developing countries) had enjoyed increases in resources during the 1970s and thought (erroneously) that PHC would be inexpensive.[8] At the international level, donor agencies accorded health more attention than ever before. The two UN agencies that promoted PHC had committed directors who pushed for change decisively and forcefully. Other key professionals in international agencies, non-governmental organisations, and ministries of health soon accepted the persuasive arguments in favour of PHC in low- and middle-income countries.

8.5.1 Economic and political factors undermine PHC

Within a few years of the endorsement of PHC, however, the global economic, political, and social environment had changed dramatically. By the mid-1980s

---

[8] There are echoes here in the policy of community care in the United Kingdom — see *Dilemmas in UK Health Care* (Open University Press, 3rd edn 2001), Chapter 4.

economic growth had slowed or even reversed. Of course the effect was not uniform: growth continued in most of East and South-east Asia, but recession hit many poor countries in Africa and Latin America particularly hard.

Heavy debts and falling incomes led countries to try to reschedule their repayments in the 1980s, and this in turn meant that the financial institutions such as the World Bank and International Monetary Fund (IMF) insisted on **structural adjustment policies** as a condition for rescheduling repayments and getting new loans. Structural adjustment took the form of dampening down demand, devaluation of currency, withdrawal of subsidies on fuel and staple foodstuffs, and deep cuts in government expenditure. Structural adjustment loans were made conditional on organisational and policy reforms. In many countries, governments were (among other things) required to reduce the number of civil servants in ministries, and to introduce charges for education and health services previously provided free.

At the level of households, such economic effects were devastating. In the 1980s, average incomes in Africa fell by between 10 and 35 per cent. The slow progress that had been occurring, for example, by increasing access to clean water, education and medical care in the previous decades came to a halt. For many households, living standards slipped back to what they were in the 1970s.

As governments had less to spend, so budgets for different sectors requiring public funding were cut. Tanzania's health budget went from 15 per cent of government expenditure in 1980, to 4 per cent in 1998. With fewer internal resources for health, health ministries found themselves highly dependent on external aid for even basic equipment and essential drugs. By the late 1990s, for example, Mozambique's ministry of health received 50 per cent of recurrent expenditure and over 90 per cent of capital expenditure from external sources.

Economic recession was accompanied by *political changes* of huge import. On the one hand, instability, low intensity warfare, an unprecedented increase in refugees, and the migration of displaced persons, affected numerous countries all over the world. During the 1980s, major armed conflict took place in eleven countries in Africa, six in Latin America, thirteen in Asia and six in the Middle East (Zwi and Ugalde, 1991). In Mozambique, Sudan, Uganda and Ethiopia alone, there were a million deaths and five million people displaced. There were also violent protests at the results of structural adjustment policies — removals of subsidies, increasing costs, rising inflation. In many poor countries people took to the streets to protest against the rising cost of living.

At the same time, structural adjustment fitted well with the ideological shift to neo-liberal economic policies that emphasised *individual* over *collective* choice, and *private* sector, *market* provision over *public* sector, *state* provision. This was heightened with the break-up of the Soviet Union in 1991, and the widespread disillusion expressed with communist regimes and centrally planned economic policies. While there are still debates about the impact of the structural adjustment programmes, evidence from a number of countries suggested that malnutrition increased, especially among the poorest groups. School enrolment fell and more people were homeless. Fewer people were utilising health services, or they were attending for treatment later in their illness, because they could not afford to pay higher charges.[9]

---

[9] A project to bring affordable health services to rural areas of South Africa by railway is illustrated in a television programme for OU students 'Catching the good health train'; but the train can only visit each of its scheduled stops around this vast country once every two years.

8.5.2 The health-sector reform movement

Until the late 1970s, the main UN organisations involved in health were WHO and UNICEF. However, in 1980 the World Bank began direct lending for health projects, and playing a more proactive role in deciding health policy. This was clearly signalled by its 1987 and 1993 publications *Financing Health Care: an agenda for reform,* and *Investing in health* which advocated a diminished role for the state in the provision and financing of health services, and a greater reliance on the market. This was part of the broad neo-liberal ideology of the time, which affected all sectors, and which emphasised liberalisation, privatisation and the reduction of the role of the state in service-provision.

As the World Bank's expenditure on health grew (Figure 8.14) and WHO's fell during the 1990s, so leadership in health policy shifted from WHO to the Bank. The World Bank was able to put conditions on health loans, and so insist that governments wanting to borrow money, had to follow the health reforms being advocated. What were these health reform measures?

Health sector reforms have been defined as 'a package of policy measures affecting the organisation, funding and management of health systems' (Zwi and Mills, 1995). These measures included increased privatisation of provision (contracting out services from public to private providers, encouraging private practice); compulsory health insurance schemes, introducing *direct charges* paid by users for previously free services; and making health service providers more accountable to consumers (Box 8.5).

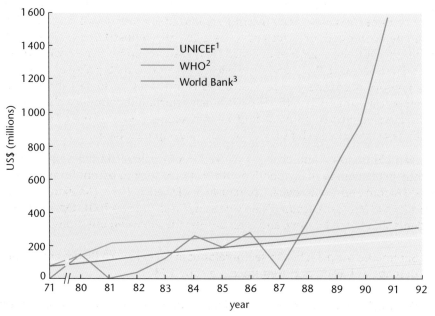

[1] UNICEF's 'Basic Health', 'Water & Sanitation' and 'Child Nutrition' programmes.

[2] WHO regular budget only

[3] World Bank PHN Sector approvals

Figure 8.14   *Trends in multilateral health sector expenditure, 1971–1992. (Source: Buse, K. 1994, Spotlight on international organizations...The World Bank,* Health and Policy Planning, *9, pp.95–9; derived from data in IRBD, 1971–1991,* Annual Reports; *UNICEF, 1986–1992,* Annual Reports; *WHO, 1971–1992,* The Work of WHO; *WHO, 1985,* Handbook of Resolutions and Decisions.)

Box 8.5 Components of health sector reform (adapted from Cassels, 1995)

Improving the performance of the civil service	Reducing staff numbers, new pay and grading schemes, better job descriptions etc.
Decentralisation	Decentralising responsibility for the management and/or provision of health care to local government or other agencies
Improving the functions of national ministries of health	Organisational restructuring, improving resource management, strengthening policy and planning functions
Broadening health financing options	Introduction of user fees, community finance, voucher systems, social or private insurance schemes
Introducing managed competition	Promoting competition between providers of clinical care and/or support services
Working with the private sector	Establishing systems for regulating, contracting with or franchising providers in the private sector (for example hiring outside contractors to provide a clean linen service for a public hospital)

The range and scope of reforms differed from country to country, but in both rich and poor countries, there was significant discussion about what changes should be made to existing health systems. Some countries, such as Zambia, embraced health sector reforms enthusiastically, and re-modelled their entire health systems, while other countries (many in Latin America) introduced only marginal changes. Reforms were often contested, or perceived to be externally imposed. For example, in the former socialist bloc countries of central and Eastern Europe some groups tried to defend free access to PHC services, while others argued that quality of care would only improve if providers were allowed to charge fees. In some Latin American countries, ministries of health were extremely reluctant to introduce changes they anticipated would be unpopular, and felt that reforms had been forced on them by multilateral agencies such as the American Development Bank.

An example of how these changes worked out in practice in the most populous country in the world can be found in 'Health sector reform: lessons from China', by Gerald Bloom and Gu Xingyuan, originally published in 1997. (An extract appears in *Health and Disease: A Reader,* Open University Press, 3rd edn 2001; Open University students should read it now, and then answer the following questions.)

● Summarise the main health sector reforms in China, which Bloom and Xinguan describe as having occurred since the early 1980s.

■ You might have noted the following: funding of the health service became increasingly reliant on out-of-pocket payments by service users; health services were decentralised, with considerable autonomy given to the local level; health facilities became semi-autonomous, generating their own revenue and using profits to pay bonuses to staff or buy new equipment; health workers were given greater freedom, for example to set up in private practice; political mobilisation for public health campaigns decreased.

● According to Bloom and Xingyuan, what have been the main effects of these reforms on the provision of health services in China? What aspects of the reforms are at the root of these effects?

■ Inequalities between rural and urban areas in access to health care have grown, and so too has the inequality in access *within* the countryside, with poor rural areas unable to fund services comparable to those in richer counties. Preventive programmes have also been weakened and are less successful in the poorer areas. The deterioration is due to a combination of factors: the abolition of most controls over health workers, many of whom have gone into private practice and moved to urban or richer rural areas to earn more; as the costs of providing health care have risen with the growth in expenditure on new drugs and medical technologies, resources have been diverted from poorer areas and from preventive programmes, and experienced staff have left inferior facilities.

The health-sector reform movement did not entirely dismiss the lessons learned from the PHC approach. For example, many accepted that CHW programmes had failed because formal health systems were unable to provide necessary support — such as drugs and other supplies. Research had shown declines in the utilisation of health clinics that ran out of drugs, and also that some communities were apparently willing to pay for drugs. As a result, attempts were made to strengthen PHC through the sale of essential drugs.

In 1987 a meeting of African Ministers of Health at Bamako in Mali — announced what was later referred to as the *Bamako Initiative*, focused on the principle of direct charges to users for essential drugs, to be implemented through a 'revolving' drug fund, managed at community level. While donors such as UNICEF would still supply essential drugs in the first instance, health workers could make small charges for such drugs, and then use the resulting funds to re-stock drugs. Although widely criticised at the time, Bamako Initiative programmes were adapted to different circumstances in different countries, and created a link between PHC and health reforms through their focus on community financing, community participation and local management (McPake *et al.,* 1993).

Another of the health sector reforms, **decentralisation**, also built on the foundations laid by PHC, by emphasising the need to improve formal health systems at the local level, and by making them more responsive to local conditions and accountable to local communities. Thus aspects of PHC were re-packaged under the decentralisation policy, which emphasised the pivotal role of district health systems for supporting community level health care through improved supervision, ongoing training, guaranteeing supplies and responding to referrals of patients from local communities.

However, the health-sector reform movement did, on the whole, lead to a completely different emphasis on financing and organisational issues in the health sector, based on the economic concerns about efficiency and effectiveness. The emphasis on health sector reforms was also fuelled by the need to find new resources and new ways of coping with the appearance of a new disease — HIV/AIDS; the increase in other familiar re-emerging infectious diseases, such as TB, spreading through the increase in migration and international travel; and the pressures on people's health from ecological deterioration.

8.6 The impact of AIDS and other infectious diseases

Added to the bleak economic outlook from the mid-1980s, was the spectre of *AIDS* (*Acquired Immune Deficiency Syndrome*).[10] At first it was not clear how many people would be affected, but it soon became apparent that the disease would touch all countries in the world. By the turn of the new millenium, more than 95 per cent of all HIV-infected people were living in the developing countries, and the epidemic was most advanced in some parts of Sub-Saharan Africa.

By the end of the 1990s studies reported that between 20–50 per cent of pregnant women in some areas were HIV-positive, for example in Zimbabwe (i.e. had antibodies in their blood which revealed the presence of the Human Immunodeficiency Virus); and that 25–40 per cent of babies born to these mothers would also be infected, and would die before they were five years old. By the end of the twentieth century the number of people living with HIV exceeded 33 million, and was increasing by about 10 per cent per year, up to the end of 1998. Over 13 million children had lost their mother, or both parents, to AIDS since the epidemic began. In Botswana life expectancy at birth had fallen from 70 to around 50 years. Although AIDS in the developing countries was seen initially to be largely an *African* problem, WHO estimated that by the turn of the twenty-first century one-quarter of people with AIDS were in Asia, especially India.

Recognition that AIDS was a *global* problem only slowly took force, but by 1987 the WHO, with financial assistance from many donors, established the *Global Programme on AIDS*, and began to fund AIDS programmes in low- and middle-income countries. Uganda was one of the first countries to launch a national programme, and by 1990 well over 125 countries had established national AIDS programmes, usually administered by ministries of health (Figure 8.15).

Because AIDS is a disease that transgresses the boundaries of ministries of health, others also became involved, from religious and non-governmental organisations, to other government sectors such as education or the military. In Uganda,

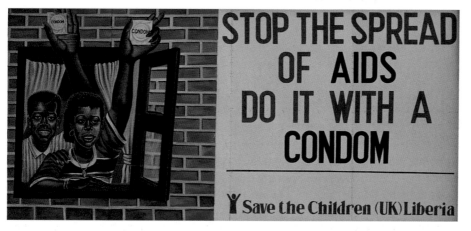

Figure 8.15 *Health education campaigns aimed at preventing the spread of AIDS began to appear in affected countries in the late 1980s and 1990s, as here in Monrovia, Liberia. (Source: Giacomo Pirozzi/ Panos Pictures)*

[10] The epidemiology of AIDS and HIV infection is discussed in *World Health and Disease* (Open University Press, 3rd edn 2001), Chapter 8; the biological aspects appear in *Human Biology and Health: An Evolutionary Approach* (Open University Press, 3rd edn 2001), Chapter 6; and the socio-political and personal dimensions are analysed in *Experiencing and Explaining Disease* (Open University Press, 3rd edn 2002), Chapter 4.

Noerine Kaleeba, whose husband had died of AIDS, joined with others to form the first indigenous AIDS support group:

> When we first began we were just a group of lunatic people, some of whom had AIDS. We met to talk, to cry, to pray, to share, to let off steam. Soon we realised we needed to do more than that, especially in relation to medicine and clinical care, professional support and welfare support. (Kaleeba *et al.*, 1991, p. 44)

The Ugandan AIDS Support Organisation (TASO) began in 1987 with 16 people, 12 of whom had AIDS. Within one year those 12 founders had died, but in the same year 850 other people used TASO's services. By the 1990s, TASO was providing counselling, information, medical and nursing care, and material assistance to over 6 000 families or people with HIV or AIDS. By then many African countries had also introduced such services, including health education programmes for the whole population, sometimes targeting special groups such as the army or sex workers.

For many developing countries, the burden of care was overwhelming. With falling GNP and smaller health budgets, the harsh reality was that the expensive antibiotic therapies for 'opportunistic' infections (which flourish only when immunity is deficient), or the anti-retroviral drugs brought on to the market in the late 1990s to help treat HIV-positive people, were simply not affordable for hard-pressed governments and their citizens in poor countries.

In 1999, for example, Olivia Verkade, working in Kenya for Médecins Sans Frontières (a non-governmental organisation), pointed out that the drug of choice for a lethal AIDS-related opportunistic infection called *cryptococcal meningitis* is fluconazole, produced and marketed by the American company Pfizer. The first two weeks of intensive treatment with fluconazole costs 60 000 Kenyan shillings (US$800), but patients have to continue taking the drug for much longer. An average monthly wage in Kenya is 10 000 Kenyan shillings (US$130), and most do not earn even that. Compared with Kenyans, Thais with AIDS-related meningitis are lucky — fluconazole costs only US$0.70 per dose because the drug is made in Thailand and is not patent protected.

By the early years of the twenty-first century, some concessions had been wrung from the pharmaceutical companies through the pressure from activists or NGOs, although battles continued on how far such concessions would be allowed. For example, in April 2000, Pfizer offered to donate fluconazole to AIDS patients in South Africa suffering from cryptococcal meningitis (affecting about 10 per cent of people with AIDS), but not to those who had thrush, a fungal infection which affects many more patients (around 40 per cent) and for which the drug is particularly effective. As AIDS manifests its devastating impact on Sub-Saharan Africa, and the inequitable access to drugs became more apparent, so discussion has grown among international and national policy makers, the private sector and non-governmental organisations on devising an ethical drugs policy to fight the disease.[11] We return to discuss the pharmaceutical industry and its influence on health care in Chapter 9, where we again highlight the affordability of drugs to treat AIDS in South Africa.

---

[11] An article by Thomas Garrett and David Finkel in *Health and Disease: A Reader* (Open University Press, 3rd edn 2001) contrasts the availability and affordability of combination drugs to treat AIDS in two businessmen — one a New Yorker, the other Malawian. It is set reading for Open University students during *Experiencing and Explaining Disease* (Open University Press, 3rd edn 2002), Chapter 4 — but if you have time it would be useful to read it now.

8.7 Emerging and re-emerging infectious diseases

AIDS was not the only new disease to create concern. At the end of the 1990s there were outbreaks of unfamiliar diseases such as a bird influenza, affecting humans for the first time, ebola haemorrhagic fever, variant Creutzfeldt–Jakob disease (vCJD), as well as unexpected outbreaks of 'old' diseases such as plague, cholera and typhoid. Further, some diseases, such as malaria and tuberculosis which had all but disappeared from industrialised countries, re-appeared, often with the added complication of drug resistance.

Malaria, for example, was endemic in more than 100 countries in the world, with 300 million cases reported in 1998, of whom 1 million died. More than 90 per cent of these deaths occurred in Sub-Saharan Africa. The parasite and its mosquito vector became increasingly resistant to the cheaper drugs available; the fact that new drugs were 10 to 100 times more expensive, meant that most did not have access to treatment.

Similarly, tuberculosis, a disease that was curable in 1945, was declared by WHO in 1993 to be a 'global emergency', with an annual rate of 8 million *new* cases of clinical tuberculosis diagnosed, and 2.9 million people dying of the disease. The complications of treating the disease (patients had to take drugs daily for up to six months) and growing drug resistance, meant people were dying, because even combining many different drugs to treat them (a very expensive proposition), sometimes did not work.

● Can you suggest why (a) malaria and (b) tuberculosis re-appeared in the industrialised world in the 1990s?

■ (a) Malaria was re-imported by international travel (which rose from two million airline passengers in 1950 to over 1.4 billion a year in the 1990s); passengers or crew members infected others and malaria-infected mosquitoes arrived in baggage holds.

(b) The HIV/AIDS epidemic unleashes latent TB infections when the virus destroys the immune system. In both diseases, multidrug resistance and adverse socio-economic factors such as poor nutrition are factors.

These were not problems that could be tackled by ministries of health alone. They were *public health* issues, which crossed the normal boundaries of the health sector. They affected people in low- and middle-income countries, but also those in the industrialised world, which had been free of many of these infectious diseases for years.

Partly because such diseases affected people in high-income countries, there was increased concern about the very limited scope of available treatments and alarm about drug-resistance. Public health professionals began calling attention to the lack of research on potential remedies and the high cost of new medicines, for diseases such as AIDS, malaria and TB among others. Such concern prompted greater discussion between private and public sectors, to find ways to work together. Thus, by the early twenty-first century the health landscape was dotted with many new partnerships of international organisations, governments and industry, working together to solve particular health problems. For example, the International AIDS Vaccine Initiative was established to find an AIDS vaccine; several pharmaceutical firms joined with governments or the WHO to address problems with treating

Figure 8.16 *The biggest mosquito net in the world was erected to house an international conference of African leaders and health agencies on the prevention of malaria, held in Abuja, Nigeria, in April 2000. (Source: Philip Ojisua/AFP)*

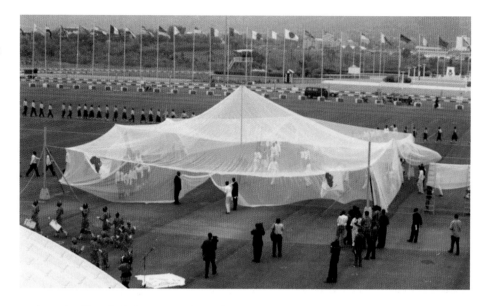

malaria (Roll Back Malaria campaign, Medicines for Malaria Venture, the Malarone Donation Programme; Figure 8.16). Some of these ventures were based on one particularly successful collaboration between a number of different organisations to tackle the problem of river blindness, as described in Box 8.6.

Box 8.6   Controlling river blindness: a win-win partnership?

Onchocerchiasis is a vector-borne disease, often called river blindness, because the blackflies that transmit the disease survive only within a certain distance of rivers, and so infect populations living in the vicinity. It is a serious public health problem, affecting over 17 million people in Africa, in 27 countries. Although only a minority of people become blind as a result of the disease, it causes a great deal of misery, including skin changes and itching. One of the ways of controlling the disease is by adding chemicals (larvacides) to rivers to prevent the fly larvae from hatching. Adding larvacides to rivers was used extensively in the Onchocerchiasis Control Programme (OCP) in West Africa, established in 1974 by a coalition of donors: the World Bank, UNDP, and WHO, with considerable success.

However, this method of control is not appropriate to all sites where the disease exists, and in 1987, the drug firm, Merck, seemed to provide a better answer. Its oral drug, Mectizan (ivermectin MSD) needed to be taken only once a year, in tablet form. In 1987 Merck held a press conference to announce that it would supply as much of the drug as was needed, for the treatment of river blindness to everyone who

needed it, at no charge, and for as long as necessary. It was able to do this because the drug had been originally developed for veterinary use, the company had made huge profits from its sale, and although testing its usefulness for humans had incurred development costs, the overall cost of production was low, and it would be needed for a geographically well-defined population.

The Mectizan Donation Programme was the largest donation programme ever made by a commercial company, and provided free Mectizan, not only for the West Africa OCP, but for many other programmes in other countries, often through NGOs, but also through governments. In 1997 about 16 million people received Mectizan for the prevention of river blindness. This example of private-public partnership has been described as a win-win situation: many people in Africa formerly vulnerable to the disease, are protected from it, and the programme has served to 'enhance Merck's corporate image and increase recognition of Merck's name and helped build relationships and alliances between its key constituents'. (Colatrella, 1998; Supplement p. S154)

● Do you see an echo of the selective PHC approach in these partnerships? Can you think of problems with such public-private programmes?

■ Some of the concerns voiced about public-private partnerships is that they focus on particular diseases, often create vertical programmes for their implementation, work only in a selected number of countries. It is not clear who they are accountable to, and there may be real problems of sustainability, if a pharmaceutical donation is withdrawn or reduced.

But infectious diseases were not the only environmental problem facing developing countries.

8.8 Ecological deterioration: polluting the land

In the 1970s, community health workers were taught the importance of environmental cleanliness at the domestic level. They tried to raise consciousness about clean water, the need to build latrines and to pen animals so that they did not wander inside the house. But the greater environmental problems were ones of deforestation, falling or insufficient water levels, creeping desertification, overgrazed land—all taxing the survival tactics of many rural populations — and threats for which community health workers had no tools or even answers. What else could women do than go further and further afield to find wood to burn, so they could cook?

By the 1990s more than 500 million acres of tropical rain forest had been felled and nearly 500 billion tonnes of topsoil lost (equivalent to the entire cropland of the USA). The combination of unfavourable winds and drought, coupled with forest fires in Indonesia led to blankets of fog all over South-East Asia in 1997, and an increase of respiratory disorders in those countries. More than I million hectares of Indonesian forest had been destroyed through logging for provision of paper and palm oil. The effects on health were probably short-lived in comparison with the long-term disturbances to the ecosystem from carbon dioxide released by slow-burning peatlands, species loss, and food chains broken by non-pollination (McMichael and Haines, 1997).

While these problems had implications for everyone, it was above all in the *cities* that environments were particularly at risk (see Figure 8.17 overleaf). At the turn of the century over 80 per cent of the world's people were urbanised, and many of them were living in conditions that gravely affected their health for the worse. Between 30 and 60 per cent of urban dwellers in poor countries lived in squatter or tenement areas in cities.

The rapid urban growth witnessed over the past three decades had not been accompanied by sufficient investment in services in urban areas. Even though many slum and squatter communities showed considerable ingenuity and capacity for organisation and planning, they could not address the problems of providing paved roads, drains, sewers, piped water, garbage collection or services. Many governments were unable to keep up with the need for such infrastructures; nor had they installed sufficient safety mechanisms to avoid the tragedies of industrial disasters:

> Industrial development may bring many bonuses, but it also opens up new possibilities of accidents involving transport accidents, chemical spills, fires and explosions, toxic wastes (including gases) and mass poisonings. A few dramatic events of recent years,

Figure 8.17 *Urban slum and squatter areas are often unhealthy environments, crowded precariously on steep inclines, without water and sewerage services or electricity, and prone to collapse or flooding during the rainy season. As in this district, Dona Marta favella, outside Rio de Janeiro, industrial pollution is also a common hazard. (Source: John Maier/Still Pictures)*

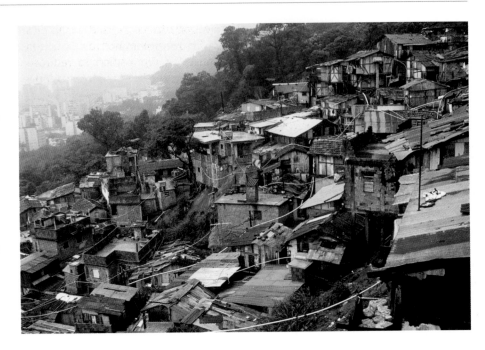

including the accidental release of chemicals at Bhopal (1984) and Seveso (1976), the gas explosions in Mexico City (1984) and the explosion of the nuclear power station at Chernobyl (1986) as well as many other close calls, have served to draw public, governmental and expert attention to the growing problem ... It is in the Third World regions with rapid urban population-growth that urban planners face the greatest problems in managing urban expansion and in so doing, limiting the risks arising from the close proximity of people, industrial production and pollution, risks accentuated by poverty. (Hardoy *et al.*, 1990, p. 220)

Environmental problems that affect health, go well beyond cities and countries. By the end of the century increasing attention was being drawn to environmental problems such as global warming, and its consequences for health (such as exposure to thermal extremes, with an increasing frequency and severity of extreme weather events; creating hospitable ecosystems for mosquitoes carrying diseases such as dengue and malaria), potential conflicts over water (for instance 97 per cent of Egypt's water originates from outside its borders), challenges to biodiversity (through the production of genetically-modified seeds for example), and damaging use of energy, leading to air and water pollution, acid precipitation, land degradation, emissions of carbon dioxide and other greenhouse gases, and the production of toxic and hazardous wastes.

On many of these issues the prospects for getting changes, at least in the short term, lie in direct action by consumers and non-governmental organisations against the multinational corporations. For instance, when faced by a high-profile campaign, the multinational biotechnology company Monsanto agreed it would not pursue its 'terminator' seed technology, which would have rendered genetically-modified crops sterile.

However, addressing the most important global environmental problems relies on inter-governmental co-operation. This is proving difficult to realise. Many environmental issues, and the solutions proposed to address them, have been strongly contested on scientific, economic and political grounds. For example, the

Global Climate Coalition (a group of oil companies and others) exerted continuous pressure throughout the 1990s to persuade the US government not to take action on reducing the production of 'greenhouse gases'.[12] Opposition to reduced emissions from fossil fuels was maintained despite evidence from the International Panel on Climate Change, which demonstrated the likely effects on global warming. In response to adverse publicity about its lobbying against American reductions in fuel consumption, in 2001, Exxon, the giant American oil company, announced a gift of US$1.3m for the treatment of malaria, out of profits which, in the first three months of 2001, amounted to US$5 billion.

Against such opposition, it is evident why the modest Kyoto Protocol on International Climate Change, concluded in Japan in 1997 after ten years of hard negotiation, remains unimplemented at the time of writing in Spring 2001. Progress towards ratification has been consistently obstructed by the USA, and this opposition has become sharper since the election of President George W Bush. Further rounds of diplomacy, aimed at rescuing the Kyoto Protocol are scheduled for Bonn in July 2001, but the USA, as the dominant producer of greenhouse gases, is not expected to make more than a token concession to reducing this major threat to the stability of the global environment.

8.9 PHC or health sector reform: rhetoric and reality

This chapter has described how ideas and policies about health and health care shifted considerably over the second half of the twentieth century, from PHC to health sector reforms. Nevertheless, even though the PHC approach was displaced by the emphasis on health sector reforms, many of the basic principles of PHC are still used to measure the effectiveness of reformed health systems. For example, commitment to immunisations, including new vaccines, remains high; oral rehydration solutions are still promoted; equity remains high on the agenda, and research and evaluation are being undertaken to find out how people's access to health services is being affected in the move towards more private care, or 'fee-for-service' provision. Where activities were undermined by economic factors (support for community health worker programmes for example), lessons have been noted and ways of involving community members in decentralised bodies (such as district hospital boards or district councils) have been sought.

While policies have shifted, so too have the international actors involved in health. WHO and UNICEF, once the two main agencies involved in health, have been joined by many others (as Box 8.1 showed). Where once there was considerable distance between the public and private sectors — the UN organisations and industry for example — that is no longer the case. Not only are public-private partnerships increasingly common, but NGOs are playing a much greater role in international health policy development and service delivery than ever before. This diversity is bringing new resources into the health arena — for example in 1999 the Bill and Melinda Gates Foundation announced a US$6 billion investment in developing new vaccines — making the Foundation the largest charitable donor of the twentieth

---

[12] The effects on the upper atmosphere and climate from the build-up of certain gases (popularly known as 'greenhouse gases' because they promote global warming), and the health consequences of pollution in the lower atmosphere, are discussed in *Human Biology and Health: An Evolutionary Approach* (Open University Press, 3rd edn 2001), Chapter 10.

century. While clearly welcomed, such sums dwarf WHO's annual budget of US$1 billion for diverse world-wide health activities, and places the Foundation, accountable only to its Board, in a highly influential position.

Finally, oscillations in policy remain rhetoric if they do not take into account the realities facing developing countries. While international agencies have acknowledged that poverty must be tackled — the mission of the World Bank for example, is to 'fight poverty with passion and professionalism', and many agencies have devised 'pro-poor' policies, it seems as if the policies emanating from such concerns are quite selective, and narrowly focused. For example, an essential PHC package has been devised (Bobadilla *et al.*, 1994)[13], recommending what basic services countries should provide for the very poor, with strong expectations that the market will solve the resource problems in health for the rest of the population.

Thus, while the rhetoric firmly addresses poverty, and the problems facing very poor and vulnerable populations, and policies are increasingly linked to the needs of these groups, the reality is that the health reform language still dominates most health policy discussion, and debates continue to be about health financing and organisational issues. What remains to be seen is whether these shifts in policy and thinking result in changing realities, and alleviate some of the existing inequalities, which remain stark both within and between countries.

[13] See *World Health and Disease* (Open University Press, 3rd edn 2001), Chapter 3, Table 3.8, for a detailed discussion of the components and costs of the minimum package of health services for low-income countries.

OBJECTIVES FOR CHAPTER 8

When you have studied this chapter, you should be able to:

8.1 Define and use, or recognise definitions and applications of, each of the terms printed in **bold** in the text.

8.2 Use appropriate examples to illustrate a discussion of the four main areas of influence on the shift towards primary health care in the 1960s and 1970s:

(a) experiments in different countries;

(b) changing ideas about poverty, health and development;

(c) population growth; and

(d) the role of international organisations.

8.3 Describe training programmes for community health workers and traditional midwives in general, and comment on their strengths and limitations in the 1970s and 1980s.

8.4 Distinguish between the goals of comprehensive and selective primary health care, using appropriate examples to illustrate problems in implementation.

8.5 Describe the key characteristics of health sector reform, and how these differed from the primary health care approach (PHC); trace the shifts in funding away from the public to the private sector.

8.6 Discuss the direct political and economic factors that undermined PHC, as well as the indirect pressures from AIDS, emerging and re-emerging infectious diseases and environmental damage, all of which led to health sector reform.

QUESTIONS FOR CHAPTER 8

1 (*Objective 8.2*)

Community participation was a basic principle of primary health care. Where did the idea come from?

2 (*Objective 8.3*)

What is the rationale for shifting the boundaries between lay and formal care by training community health workers or traditional midwives in elements of formal practice?

3 (*Objective 8.4*)

Compare the main weaknesses of selective PHC with the main limitations of comprehensive PHC.

4 (*Objective 8.5*)

What were the key components of health sector reform? Which reforms reflected lessons learned during the PHC era?

5 (*Objective 8.6*)

What factors led to the emphasis on health sector reform in the late 1980s?

CHAPTER 9

International patterns of health care, 1960 to 2001

9.1   Introduction   296

9.2   The cost of formal health care   296

9.2.1 Health expenditure per person   296

9.2.2 Trends over time   300

9.2.3 The distribution of health
       expenditure   303

9.3   Health expenditure: why does it vary
       between countries?   304

9.3.1 Definitions of health care   304

9.3.2 Variations in health activities   305

9.3.3 Variations in costs   306

9.3.4 Variations in ill-health   306

9.4   Why does health expenditure vary
       over time?   308

9.5   Funding and provision in developed
       countries   308

9.5.1 Public and private funding for
       health care   309

9.5.2 Health funding in the USA   310

9.5.3 Health funding in the UK   310

9.5.4 Funding from out-of-pocket
       expenses   311

9.5.5 Other private funding sources   312

9.5.6 Trends in public expenditure
       on health   312

9.6   Funding health care in developing
       countries   314

9.6.1 Sources of funding   314

9.6.2 Effects on use of services   315

9.7   Methods of health care provision and
       remuneration   316

9.7.1 Providers of health care   316

9.7.2 Paying the doctor   317

9.7.3 Paying for hospitals   318

9.8   Contemporary health care:
       an international trade   319

9.8.1 Migration of health workers   319

9.8.2 The world pharmaceutical
       industry   321

9.8.3 A world health-care system   325

Objectives for Chapter 9   325

Questions for Chapter 9   326

Study notes for OU students

This chapter builds on knowledge of patterns of health and disease in industrialised and developing countries as described in *World Health and Disease* (Open University Press, third edition 2001), in particular Chapters 7 and 8, which discuss the effects of economic development on these patterns. The television programme about health care in South Africa entitled 'Catching the good health train' and Video 1 entitled 'South Africa: health at the crossroads', are also relevant to this chapter.

9.1   Introduction

This chapter, like the previous two, is concerned mainly with the period from the early 1970s to 2001, but we also look back briefly to the 1960s. The first aim is to try to uncover some recurring patterns within the diversity of health care in different countries. The second aim is to place health care in the UK within the context of other industrialised countries. The third is to consider some of the main similarities and differences between the health systems of industrialised and the developing countries.

The chapter focuses on a set of questions that tend to dominate contemporary comparative research on health care world-wide, and on which at least some information is available:

1   How much do different countries *spend* on their health services, how has it changed over time, and why is there so much variation between them?

2   What are the main *ways of funding* health care, and what kinds of organisations are involved in *providing* health services?

3   Are such things as migration of health workers and multinational pharmaceutical companies reducing diversity and creating a *world health-care system*?

These questions have been studied most closely in the industrialised countries of the world, and especially among the member states of the Organisation for Economic Cooperation and Development (OECD): that is, the industrialised countries apart from some of the former socialist economies (FSEs) of Eastern Europe and the Soviet Union.[1] In addition, published data normally refer only to *formal* health care. However, we have tried where possible to extend the discussion to developing countries, and to include some references to lay, traditional and public-health provision, in keeping with the themes of this book as set out in Chapter 1.

9.2   The cost of formal health care

9.2.1   Health expenditure per person

We begin by trying to establish what resources are devoted to formal health care in different countries. One way of attempting to measure this is to try to express the total amount spent on formal health care as a *sum per head of population*, converted into a standard currency so that different countries can be compared. The most

---

[1] Trends in health profiles in the FSEs and the factors underlying changes since the 1990s are discussed in *World Health and Disease* (Open University Press, 3rd edn 2001), Chapter 7.

obvious way of putting everything onto a comparable basis is to calculate everything in terms of one currency — such as British pounds or US dollars — using the prevailing exchange rate. However, exchange rates between currencies can fluctuate sharply over short periods, perhaps because of an election, political problems or a whole variety of other reasons that have little to do with the actual price levels in a particular country. For example, between July 1999 and May 2000 the number of French francs one dollar could buy fell from 6.5 to 6.0 and then rose again to 6.8. So if French health expenditure had been expressed in terms of US dollars using prevailing exchange rates, the quite misleading impression would be created that it fluctuated sharply.

One way of avoiding such problems with exchange rates is to calculate a *stable conversion rate* between currencies which makes them comparable in terms of the prices for similar goods and services within different countries, and this rate is called the **purchasing power parity** (**PPP**). It can be calculated in any currency, but is most commonly calculated in US dollars and referred to as PPP$. Figure 9.1 shows the expenditure per person on health care in a range of countries in 1999, calculated on the basis of PPP$.

The countries in Figure 9.1 are arranged in ascending order of **Gross Domestic Product** (**GDP**) per person, which, like **Gross National Product** (**GNP**), is a measure of *national wealth*. GDP and GNP are both measures of national income: the money

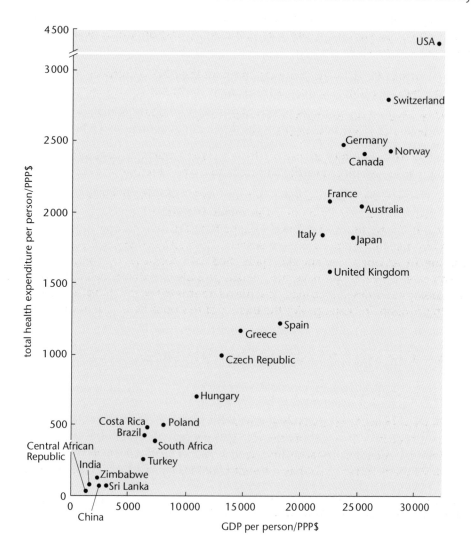

Figure 9.1 *Health expenditure per person, and GDP per person, for 16 OECD countries and eight developing countries, in US dollars using purchasing power parities (PPP$), in 1999 or nearest year. (Data from OECD, 2000, OECD Health Data 2000, CREDOC/OECD, Paris; United Nations Development Programme, 1999, Human Development Report 1999, Oxford University Press, Oxford, Table 1; World Health Organisation, 2000, World Health Report. Health Systems: Improving Performance, WHO, Geneva, Table 8)*

value of all the goods and services available to the nation. The main difference between them is that GDP includes only income from *domestic* economic activity, whereas GNP also includes income from abroad, for example from foreign investments.

Even within the group of mainly industrialised, mostly Western European, and relatively wealthy countries towards the top right of Figure 9.1, there are wide differences in the amount spent each year on formal health care per person: twice as much in Germany as in Spain, for example, or twice as much in the USA as in Norway. (Note the break in the vertical scale; the USA's expenditure per person on health is even greater than it appears at first glance.) The UK in 1999 was at the lower end of this group, spending less on health care than countries such as France, which has a similar level of GDP per person.

●   What does Figure 9.1 reveal about the differences in health expenditures between rich and poor countries?

■   Whereas the former commonly spent around 1 500 to 2 500 PPP$ per person on health care in 1999, the majority of the developing countries in the figure had health expenditures of less than one-tenth of this, and in some cases under 50 PPP$ per person per year.

This gulf becomes even more striking when the formidable health problems facing most developing countries are recalled.[2] Not surprisingly in these circumstances, large portions of the population in many developing countries are effectively not provided with any formal health care.

Using the United Nations Development Programme's definition of **health service access** — the percentage of the population that can reach appropriate local health services on foot, or by the local means of transport, in no more than one hour — over one-quarter of the population of the developing countries as a whole did not have access to health services in the early 1990s, rising to almost half the population in the countries of Sub-Saharan Africa. Such very limited resources for formal health care were, of course, the background for many features of health care in developing countries discussed in Chapter 8: notably the reliance of many people on lay carers, traditional practitioners and community health workers.

An obvious reason for variations between countries in the absolute amount spent on formal health care per person is that countries vary in their level of national income. The broad picture revealed by Figure 9.1 is that as national income per person increases, spending on formal health care rises, just as in richer countries people on average spend more on clothes or cars or food. However, what is interesting is that higher-income countries seem systematically to devote a larger and larger *proportion* of their income to formal health care. Figure 9.2 shows formal health-care expenditure as a proportion of GDP for the same countries listed in Figure 9.1; again, the countries are arranged in ascending order of GDP per person.

If the USA or Switzerland, for example, were each devoting the *same* proportion of their GDP to formal health care as the UK was in 1999, health-care spending per person would have been much higher in these countries than in the UK because their GDP per person is consistently substantially higher than in the UK. But the *proportion* of GDP these two countries devote to formal health care is also consistently much higher than that of the UK — in 1999 it was close to 14 per cent in the USA and 10 per cent in Switzerland, compared to 7 per cent in the UK.

[2] See *World Health and Disease* (Open University Press, 3rd edn 2001), Chapters 2–4, 7, 8 and 11.

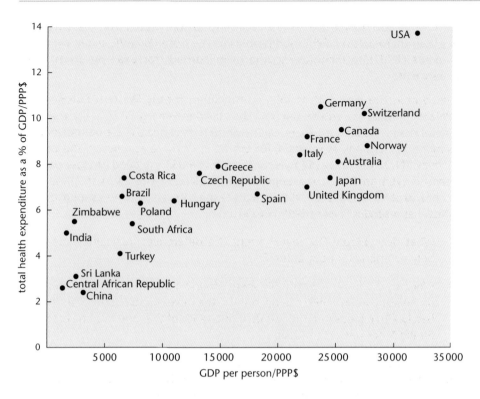

Figure 9.2 *GDP per person, and health expenditures as a percentage of GDP, for 16 OECD countries and 8 developing countries, in US dollars using purchasing power parities (PPP$), in 1999 or nearest year. (Data from OECD, 2000, OECD Health Data 2000, CREDOC/OECD, Paris; United Nations Development Programme, 1999, Human Development Report 1999, Oxford University Press, Oxford)*

Broadly, therefore, countries with a higher GDP per person also devote a larger share of their national income to health. Figure 9.2 shows that formal health services now consume on average between 8 per cent and 10 per cent of the total national income of the richest industrialised countries, and ranging as high as 14 per cent (one-seventh of total national income) in the USA.

● What proportion of national wealth is devoted to formal health services in low-income countries?

■ The average is under 5 per cent; for some countries shown in Figure 9.2 it is less than 3 per cent.

Findings such as these convey an important message: that there seems to be no ceiling or limit to how much can be spent on formal health care, and the richer a country becomes the more it will tend to spend. Indeed, it has sometimes been suggested that national income is by far the best predictor of formal health-care spending. A number of studies conducted at different times and using different samples of countries (mainly industrialised countries) have all found that approximately 90 per cent of the variation in formal health-care spending per person could be statistically 'explained' by variations in national income per person.

Superficially, this would seem to leave very little room for such things as national health policies, or methods of funding, provision and remuneration to exert any influence. However, this would be a quite misleading conclusion. It is clear that very few countries exactly fit the pattern, some spending much more and others much less than might be predicted on the basis of their national income.

● South Africa is a middle-income country with a GDP per person of just over 7 000 PPP$. How does its health expenditure per person (Figure 9.1) and as a per cent of GDP (Figure 9.2) compare with that of Costa Rica?

■ In 1999 South Africa spent less *per person* on health than Costa Rica, which has a lower national income (around 6 600 PPS$), and it devoted a lower *proportion* of its GDP to health (around 5.5 per cent) than did Costa Rica (around 7.5 per cent).

● Now compare the position of the UK in 1999 as shown in Figures 9.1 and 9.2 with that of our closest European neighbour, France.

■ The GDP per person in the two countries is identical, at 2 000 PPP$, but the UK spent much less per person on health than did France (around 1 500 PPP$ compared to over 2 000 PPP$), and devoted a lower share of national income to health (around 7 per cent in the UK, compared to over 9 per cent in France).

More fundamentally, when examining patterns of health expenditure it is important to remember that many other aspects of a health system may influence the type, amount, quality and distribution of services: there are important differences between the kind of system that developed in which patients' access to hospitals is controlled by GP referrals, and a system in which the public have direct access to specialists (for example, recall the comparison of methods of referral in the UK and the USA, as described in Rosemary Steven's article which you read with Chapter 4). And, as discussed in Chapter 6, spending was very little higher under the NHS than it had been under the arrangements existing prior to 1948, but the NHS nevertheless fundamentally changed many aspects of health provision. So national income is only one factor influencing health expenditure, which in turn is only one factor influencing a health system.

9.2.2 Trends over time

Chapters 6 and 7 traced the way in which a long period of unprecedented economic growth after 1948 was accompanied by a massive expansion of welfare provision; this was interrupted by the oil price rise in 1973, after which economic growth deteriorated and welfare policies were placed under increasing economic and political pressure. These patterns of spending on welfare are reflected in expenditure on health services. Figure 9.3 attempts to trace these changes by showing the percentage of GDP devoted to health care, averaged across the main OECD countries over the period from 1960 to 1997; it shows this as a 'weighted average', which

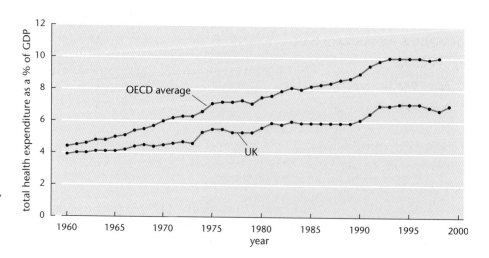

Figure 9.3 *Health expenditure as a percentage of GDP in all OECD countries and the United Kingdom, 1960–1999. (Data from OECD, 2000,* OECD Health Data 2000, *CREDOC/OECD, Paris)*

takes account of the absolute size of each country's economy. Figure 9.3 also shows the same information for the UK separately, to assess whether the British experience was in any way untypical.

Figure 9.3 reveals that across the OECD countries as a group, there has been a clear trend since 1960 towards formal health care taking a larger and larger slice of national income: in 1960 around 4 per cent of GDP was devoted to health, but by 1985 this had doubled to 8 per cent, and by 1998 it was 10 per cent. However, Figure 9.3 indicates that this trend has gradually become less pronounced, and indeed since 1993 the proportion of GDP devoted to health care in these countries has been fairly stable.

● What does Figure 9.3 reveal about the UK's health spending compared to that of the OECD as a whole?

■ In 1960, the UK was devoting almost an average amount of GDP to health, but from then until the later 1990s it fell steadily further behind.

Thus the bearing down on health and welfare provision described in Chapter 7, which has formed a constant backdrop to policy towards the NHS in the UK, is graphically illustrated by Figure 9.3. (It is also worth noting that health expenditure's share of the national 'cake' can change *either* because of a change in health expenditure *or* a change in the size of the national cake. For example, the severe recessions in Britain in 1973–74 and again in 1980–81 reduced the overall size of the national economy, with the result that health expenditure's *share* suddenly increased, even though the total amount spent on health care remained unchanged.)

In 2000, the Labour government announced that it planned to close the gap between the UK and other European countries, bringing the UK's health expenditure up to the average by a sustained increase in public expenditure. This announcement was sufficiently vague to spark a heated debate on which countries were included in the comparison, how the average should be measured, and so on. However, the Budget of April 2000 laid out more detailed spending plans for the period from 2000 to 2004, allowing comparisons with previous spending on the NHS to be made. Table 9.1 shows some of these comparisons.

Table 9.1   Real increases in NHS spending over various periods.

	Average annual real increase (%)
Planned April 2000 to March 2004	6.1
By parliament:	
April 1992 to March 1997	2.6
April 1979 to March 1997	3.1
Highest 5-year period of growth in history of NHS (April 1971 to March 1976)	6.4
Entire history of NHS (April 1950 to March 2000)	3.4
History of NHS excluding initial years (April 1954 to March 2000)	3.7

Data derived from Emmerson, C., Frayne, C. and Goodman, A. (2000) *Pressures in UK Health Care: Challenges for the NHS*, Institute for Fiscal Studies, London.

● According to Table 9.1, how did the increase in planned NHS expenditure announced in April 2000 compare with NHS spending in previous parliaments and over the history of the NHS?

■ The plan announced in 2000 was to increase average annual spending to 6.1 per cent for the next 4 years. This is more than twice the rate of growth in the previous parliament (1992 to 1997) and almost twice the rate of growth over the Conservative years in office, from 1979 to 1997. It compares favourably with an average growth rate over the history of the NHS (excluding the first few years, when there was a severe squeeze on spending as described in Chapter 6) of 3.7 per cent per annum.

● Was the increase in planned NHS expenditure announced in April 2000 'by far the largest sustained increase in NHS funding of any period in its 50-year history', as stated at the time by the Chancellor?

■ Not quite. During the five-year period 1971–1976, the annual growth rate in real spending on the NHS was 6.4 per cent.

Once again, comparable data for developing countries are very hard to obtain and should be treated with some caution, but Figure 9.4 shows total expenditure on health as a percentage of GDP in 10 developing countries in 1990 and 1997.

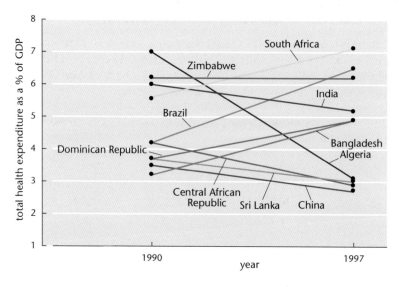

Figure 9.4 *Total health expenditure as a percentage of GDP in 10 developing countries, 1990 and 1997. (Data from World Bank, 1993,* World Development Report, *Oxford University Press, Oxford and New York, Table A.9; World Health Organisation, 2000,* World Health Report. Health Systems: Improving Performance, *WHO, Geneva, Table 8)*

It is not possible to draw firm conclusions from Figure 9.4, as the countries may not be representative. However, it does suggest that health spending did not rise uniformly during the 1990s (although it did increase in both South Africa and in Bangladesh, among others), and in fact in 5 of the 10 countries included in the figure the proportion of GDP devoted to health care *fell* during this period. Some of the possible reasons for this were discussed in Chapter 8, including structural adjustment policies, slow economic growth or even falling incomes, high levels of debt, and, in China, a combination of rapid economic growth and market-oriented reforms that disrupted many features of the health-care system.[3]

---

[3] See also the article 'Health sector reform: lessons from China' by Gerald Bloom and Gu Xingyuan, which was set reading for Chapter 8 of this book, and appears in *Health and Disease: A Reader* (Open University Press, 3rd edn 2001).

9.2.3 The distribution of health expenditure

So far, we have been comparing *average* levels of formal health-care spending per person in *different* countries, but at several points in this book we have also noted the existence of substantial variations in the way health spending is distributed *within* countries. For example, Chapter 5 discussed the unequal geographical distribution of voluntary hospitals and health services provided by local authorities in Britain between the two World Wars. Such variations are still commonplace. For example, in 1998/99, eight Health Authorities in England were each receiving at least £10 million more than the target indicated by a formula intended to distribute resources equitably across the country, while another nine Health Authorities were at least £10 million below their target level. Such differences have persisted despite the existence for many years of a variety of formulae intended to share out resources more equally.

Research in other European countries has found similar variations. So, for example, France may have spent more per person on health than did the UK in 1999 (as shown in Figure 9.1), but this was not distributed equally across different regions of France. Such regional differences in expenditure are only one form of inequality in health care within nations, but they do illustrate the shortcomings of relying on very simple aggregated measures when making international comparisons: as the data are disaggregated, so more and more diversity becomes exposed.

The same kinds of differences can be found between the different countries of Britain, with the result that, for example, Scotland receives at least 20 per cent more per person in total health expenditure than do England or Wales.

Such differences in health provision within countries are even more pronounced in developing countries. Table 9.2, for example, displays some data collected from a small number of countries in the 1980s on the distribution of population and of government health spending between the rural and urban areas.

Table 9.2 The distribution of government health expenditure and population in five developing countries, early 1980s.

	Share of government health spending (%)		Share of total population (%)	
	rural	urban	rural	urban
China	29	71	79	21
Colombia	19	81	38	62
Indonesia	77	23	83	17
Malaysia	57	43	60	40
Senegal	57	43	81	19

Data from Jiminez, E. (1986) The public subsidisation of education and health in developing countries: a review of equity and efficiency, *World Bank Research Observer*, **1**, p. 120, Table 9.

● What pattern is revealed by the data in Table 9.2?

■ The urban areas generally attracted a disproportionately large share of health expenditure. In some instances, the imbalance was fairly small, but in China, for example, four-fifths of the population lived in rural areas, but received less than 30 per cent of government health expenditure. (This may remind you of David Morley's 'three-quarters rule' described in Chapter 6.)

In summary

The main points to note are:

1 Higher-income countries tend to devote a higher *proportion* of their national income to health care than do lower-income countries.

2 Among the OECD countries, health care has been taking a growing share of national income for many years, but the share has been static since the early 1990s. In many developing countries, pressure on health spending was severe during the 1990s.

3 Health expenditures are often distributed very unevenly within countries — for example, between different regions or between rural and urban areas — and this should be recalled when comparing national averages.

9.3 Health expenditure: why does it vary between countries?

So far, we have been concerned mainly to establish *levels* of health expenditure in different countries and how they have *changed*. Amidst the diversity, and the many different policy influences and historical contingencies that have been richly documented in earlier chapters, can any more systematic reasons be discerned for these variations between countries?

9.3.1 Definitions of health care

One obvious reason for variations between countries in health spending is that they are likely to differ in what they define as 'formal health care'.

● In which areas would you particularly expect there to be international differences in what is referred to as formal health care?

■ One of the vaguest boundaries is between formal health care and informal or lay care. In some countries, for example, all nursing work in hospitals is performed by paid staff, whereas in others the relatives of patients may provide a good deal of nursing care, as well as supplying food, laundry and other services. Next, traditional healers, complementary medicine, or health-related activities such as attending health spas may be included in some countries but not in others. Community health workers — a sizeable part of the workforce in many countries, as Chapter 8 showed — may or may not be included. Another hazy boundary is between formal health care and the social welfare services; a wide range of social welfare services are included as formal health care in some countries but excluded in others. Similarly, there is often an overlap between formal health care and education services, which often provide some health services for children.

The groups that often straddle such boundaries include people with physical and/ or mental disabilities, elderly people in residential and private nursing homes, and others such as people who are addicted to drugs. However, although these differences do cast light on the way in which the boundaries of formal health care vary, they explain only a small proportion of the variation in spending discussed earlier in this chapter.

9.3.2 Variations in health activities

Another potential explanation for differences in health spending between countries relates to the activities actually undertaken by their health-care systems. In particular, evidence has gradually been amassed that **activity rates** — the rates at which many medical and surgical procedures are performed — vary widely between (as well as within) countries. Figure 9.5 illustrates this with data on the rate at which two common surgical operations — Caesarian section during delivery of a baby and cholecystectomy (removal of the gall bladder) — were performed in seven developed countries around 1997.

Figure 9.5 shows very wide variations between countries in the rates at which these two procedures were performed. For example, the rate at which Caesarian section was performed was nine times higher in the USA than in Ireland.

The reasons for surgical interventions are many and complex, and can be influenced by a range of factors, most obviously the *prevalence* and *incidence* of disease. However, it is not conceivable that this could explain all the variation shown in Figure 9.5. Other factors include clinical judgement, or prevailing customs, traditions and beliefs. It is also plausible to suggest that such variations are connected to different levels of *income*.

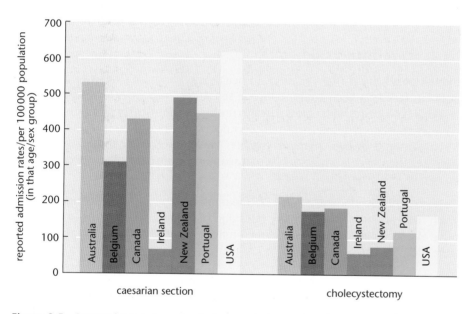

Figure 9.5 *Reported admission rates for two surgical procedures in seven industrialised countries, 1997 or nearest year. (Data from OECD, 1999,* OECD Health Data 99, *CREDOC/ OECD, Paris)*

In high-income countries such as the USA, it is more likely that operations will be sought by patients and performed by surgeons when they offer a small measure of reassurance to the patient, even when symptoms are slight or possibly absent. The spectre of 'preventive hysterectomy' is alarming, but equally, in a society concerned about the risks of cancer, it would be an economically 'rational' choice for someone afraid of the disease, having a great need for reassurance, and having a high enough income to pay for it. Finally, there is again some evidence that health-care activity rates may be influenced by the way in which health care is funded and provided, the way doctors and hospitals are remunerated, and so on. We will also return to this below.

9.3.3 Variations in costs

Although *purchasing power parities*, or PPPs, as described earlier in this chapter, are a much better basis on which to make international comparisons than are exchange rates, nevertheless they are normally calculated for an economy as a whole, and it remains a possibility that it may be relatively much more expensive in some countries than in others to buy the things needed to run a health system. For example, there can be very big differences from one country to another in the prices charged for pharmaceuticals. Similarly, doctors are much better paid in some countries than in others, even after differences in purchasing power are taken into account. In the UK a doctor, on average, earned around two and a half times the national average wage in 1998, but in the USA the figure was closer to four times their national average wage.

These differences are the result of many different factors, including the bargaining strength of doctors, the way they are remunerated, and their general social standing and status; (for example, Chapter 6 described how the status of GPs tended to decline in post-war Britain). Whatever the reasons for such variations, the consequence is that in some countries doctors are relatively much more expensive than in others, and this means that more money is devoted to health care. Once more, however, this only explains part of the variations in health spending that actually exist.

9.3.4 Variations in ill-health

Another possibility is that variations in health spending are related to the health problems faced by each country. In one sense this seems clearly untrue, in that developing countries with colossal health problems spend on health care a fraction of the amount spent by industrialised countries, whose health problems seem minor in comparison. However, many researchers have turned this question round, and asked whether there is any evidence that spending *more* on health care creates any discernible improvement in health.

There are indeed a number of well-documented examples of developing countries which have attained low mortality rates and high life expectancy by means of a range of policies including relatively well-funded health services: examples include Costa Rica, Sri Lanka and Cuba.[4]

More perplexing has been the poor correlation between the amount spent on health care by Western industrialised countries and commonly-used indirect measures of health such as the infant mortality rate (IMR). For example, Figure 9.6 is a scattergram showing the IMR per 1 000 live births and health expenditure per person for a range of OECD countries in 1999.

●   How would you describe the pattern revealed in Figure 9.6?

■   There is a slight inverse correlation (countries with a low level of health spending have higher infant mortality rates), but the association between the two variables is not very strong. Some countries such as the USA, Japan and Finland seem to have much higher (USA) or lower (Japan and Finland) IMRs than might be expected on the basis of their health expenditure.

[4] These countries are sometimes categorised as 'superior health achievers' and are discussed in *World Health and Disease* (Open University Press, 3rd edn 2001), Chapter 8.

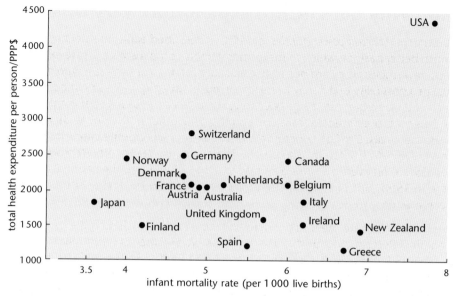

Figure 9.6 *Infant mortality rates per 1 000 live births and health expenditure per person (PPP$) in 23 OECD countries, 1999 or nearest year. (Data from OECD, 2000, OECD Health Data 2000, CREDOC/OECD, Paris)*

What does this apparently weak correspondence between the level of health-care spending in industrialised countries and mortality mean? There are many difficulties involved in trying to assess the relationship between health care and health. First, the measurement of health-care resources is difficult, as discussed earlier in this chapter. Second, just because a country spends heavily on health care and does not have comparably low mortality rates, it does not follow that the health care was ineffectual: mortality rates might have been even higher without large amounts of health care. And third, we are only assessing the effect of health care in terms of *mortality*, and at a very aggregate level of measurement, which might be quite unrealistic. It may be better to focus on specific *causes* of mortality where it is agreed that health care can have some impact, or to examine various measures other than mortality, for example, rates of morbidity or disability.

The problem with measures other than mortality is that it is so much more difficult to measure morbidity, or reductions in anxiety, or the level of comfort and reassurance. Despite such measurement problems, it is evident that it is necessary to consider much more than mortality rates when assessing the effect of formal health care. A significant number of activities are in no way intended to reduce mortality — hip replacement, for example, is an area of formal health-care provision that is intended primarily to improve the *quality* of life.

In addition, there is now virtually no limit to the amount of intensive care that can in theory be provided to a patient in the last stages of life: sometimes with a negligible effect on survival chances. Modern anaesthetics and surgical techniques make it possible to operate on very old people, when gains in life expectancy may be extremely small. Similarly, terminal care for people with cancers may have little impact on life expectancy, but may nevertheless transform the last stages of life from a painful deterioration into a relatively comfortable decline. Spending on formal health care in industrialised countries, on this account, may well have more influence on *health* than it does on *death*.[5]

[5] This point is addressed in an article 'Medicine matters after all' by John Bunker, which appears in *Health and Disease: A Reader* (Open University Press, 3rd edn 2001).

9.4 Why does health expenditure vary over time?

As we noted earlier, Chapters 6 and 7 showed how health and welfare provision expanded fairly rapidly during the long post-war phase of sustained economic growth, but came under increasing pressure after 1973. The reasons for the growth over time in health spending have been examined in some detail in the OECD countries, and the following factors have been identified:

- *Inflation* in the health sector has tended to be slightly higher than in the economy as a whole.

- *Demographic changes* have created extra demands on the health system, particularly from a growing proportion of older people who make more use of health care.

- *Intensity of use* of health services has been increasing constantly, with each individual on average making more use them: more consultations, more hospital admissions, more operations, and more prescriptions. In turn these are more expensive because of more advanced equipment, more and better-paid registered nursing and medical staff, higher standards and so on.

The effect of demographic changes on health care has been widely debated, with some commentators predicting the imminent collapse of health services under the pressure of an ageing population. However, the evidence is that this has not been a major factor either in explaining rising health expenditure in the past, or variations in health spending between countries. Even looking into the future, most predictions are that a maximum of less than 1 per cent per year growth in health expenditure will be necessary to keep pace with the increase in the proportion of old and very old people in the UK right into the middle decades of the twenty-first century. Indeed, some researchers have argued that even these estimates are too high, claiming that most of the association between old age and health-care costs is due to intense use of health services in the few months prior to death. On this account, increasing life expectancy increases the *number* of old people, but also *delays* the time when heavy health expenditure in the period preceding death is incurred.

Rising intensity of use of health services has been identified by most researchers as the most important factor behind increasing health expenditures, but the reasons why rates of use of health care should be rising so strongly are not clear. Among the possible explanations are, first, that patterns of disease may be changing towards more chronic illnesses that are not easily treated, and second, that new technologies, procedures and methods of diagnosis have expanded the range of treatments that health care can provide.[6]

9.5 Funding and provision in developed countries

Chapter 7 discussed the sequence of reforms to the NHS in the period after 1989, such as the creation of an internal market and a purchaser–provider split. This distinction between *health-care funding* and *health-care provision* is very important and sounds simple, but in practice is often complex. Health services may be funded in one way and provided in another: for example, hospice care may be funded by

---

[6] The impact of new medical technologies on health-care provision is discussed in *Dilemmas in UK Health Care* (Open University Press, 3rd edn 2001), Chapter 7, and in a television programme for OU students associated with that book, entitled 'Hospitals: who needs them?'.

charitable donations, but provided in a building owned by local government, with staff employed by the Department of Health through a Health Authority. To take another example, residential care for elderly people may be provided by private nursing or residential homes, but be paid for by the government via Social Security payments.

In the UK, awareness of the distinction between funding and provision was for many years obscured by the fact that, since 1948, the great majority of formal health care has been provided by the NHS — a publicly funded *and* publicly provided system of health care.

There are wide variations between countries in the ways in which health care is funded, and even within a country many different sources of finance may be used in combination. The basic distinction is whether these sources are *public* or *private*.

9.5.1 Public and private funding for health care

Public sources of funding include general taxation, taxes which are specifically earmarked for health care, and compulsory health-insurance schemes. It is possible to think of various sub-divisions to these categories: for example, taxation can be raised nationally or locally. However, the essential feature of all these public sources of finance is that they are *compulsory*: people cannot choose whether to contribute the funds or to withhold them, irrespective of the use they may make of health care.

The main private sources of funding include voluntary health insurance, and direct or 'out-of-pocket' payments by individuals, such as over-the-counter purchase of drugs, or charges for particular services or treatments. The common attribute of these private sources of health finance is that they are either *voluntary*, or are tied to the *use* an individual makes of a particular service.

Unfortunately most countries use different accounting conventions, or publish some pieces of information but not others, so it is extremely hard to obtain comparable data. However, Table 9.3 shows some estimates of the sources of health-care funding in five industrialised countries around 1999, and amply illustrates the variations *between* countries as well as the use of a variety of funding sources *within* countries.

General taxation by national or local government invariably plays some role in the finance of health care, but the UK has been unusually reliant on this source. At the beginning of the NHS, almost 90 per cent of all health spending came from general taxation, but in 1999 the proportion was around 74 per cent.

Table 9.3 Percentages of total health expenditure funded from different sources in 5 industrialised countries, 1999 or nearest date.

	Government: general taxation	Social insurance schemes	Private for-profit insurance	Private not-for-profit insurance	Out-of pocket payments	All other private funds	Total
Canada	70	1	2	10	17	–	100
France	4	73	4	8	10	1	100
Germany	7	70	7	–	12	4	100
United Kingdom	74	10	4	–	11	1	100
USA	30	15	33	–	18	4	100

Data from OECD (2000) *OECD Health Data 2000*, CREDOC/OECD, Paris.

Compulsory or **social insurance** has become the dominant form of health-care finance in many countries, especially in Europe. Table 9.3 shows that France and Germany draw the majority of their health-care funding from this source. In the UK, health funding from this source is that part of the National Insurance contribution which is earmarked for the NHS; as the table shows, it only covers around 10 per cent of all health spending in the UK.

9.5.2 Health funding in the USA

The only developed country in the world not reliant on general taxation or social insurance for the majority of health funding is the USA. The American health-care system is unusually reliant on *voluntary* or **private health insurance**, purchased mainly by people in employment, and often involving contributions from employers.

However, reliance on private insurance creates a major problem: not everyone can afford the insurance premiums needed to obtain coverage, and, in particular, people who are old or in poor health (and therefore especially in need of health care) may be the least likely to be able to afford the higher payments they normally face. As a result, the American government finances medical programmes for Native Americans, armed forces veterans, the poor and elderly people, as well as various other school and public health programmes, which have grown in size and now account for almost half of all health spending.

Nevertheless, in 2000 over 44 million Americans, or around 18 per cent of the population, were not covered by these programmes and yet had no health insurance or were inadequately insured. In 1989, the equivilent number was 34 million, and the total is projected to increase to 55 million by the year 2015. Some of the uninsured population in 2000 were young people who, to some extent, were choosing to go uninsured on the assumption that they were a low-risk group; but those mainly affected were children, poor and middle-income families, blacks, Hispanics and unemployed or disabled Americans who were not eligible for government support, but were unable to afford private insurance.

9.5.3 Health funding in the UK

In the UK, ever since the beginning of the NHS, Conservative governments have generally encouraged the better-off to use private health services, believing that a combination of tax incentives and increasing wealth would lead an increasing proportion of the population effectively to 'opt out' of the NHS. The number of people covered by private health insurance policies did increase steadily in the early decades of the NHS, from around 0.5 million in 1955 to over 2 million by the late 1970s. However, it is not necessary to be insured to use private health services — they can be paid for directly. During the same period, **private spending on health** actually declined significantly — from about 15 per cent of all health spending in the early 1960s, to less than 10 per cent by the late 1970s — partly in response to diminishing tax incentives.

But the advent of the Conservative administration in 1979 under Margaret Thatcher marked a sharp break in these trends. Private health insurance was encouraged by a significant tax concession for employer-paid medical insurance premiums introduced in 1980, and the 1989 White Paper, *Working for Patients*, led to a similar tax concession for over-65s. As a result, the numbers of people with private health insurance rose, from just over 2 million in 1980 to around 7 million by 1999, and private spending on health more than tripled in real terms. By 1999, private spending on health had again risen to about 16 per cent of all health expenditure in the UK (that is, the sum total of private for-profit insurance, out-of-pocket payments and all other private funds in Table 9.3), and over 12 per cent of the population had private medical insurance.

However, encouragement of private health care by the Conservative government cooled in the post-Thatcher era, in part to avoid undermining public confidence in ongoing NHS reforms, and further changes occurred following the election of the Labour government led by Tony Blair in 1997. Tax relief on health insurance premiums for individuals aged over 60 was abolished in 1997, and in 2000 the government committed itself to a substantial increase in NHS expenditure, as discussed earlier. It remains to be seen whether this will affect the level of private health spending.

9.5.4 Funding from out-of-pocket expenses

Out-of-pocket expenses account for a significant proportion of health-care finance in most countries, and again the UK is unusual in the relatively low share of total expenditure (7 per cent) raised from this source — although it is much more important in particular areas, such as dentistry or optician services.

These out-of-pocket expenses may cover a range of different items:

- **direct health charges** levied on users of health services, for example the prescription charges or charges for glasses provided by the NHS in the UK;
- *co-payments*, whereby people who are insured have to pay a proportion or a set amount of any claim made on the insurance policy;
- *fees* paid directly to privately-practising doctors or other health workers, or to private hospitals;
- *purchase costs* of other health-related products, such as non-prescription or over-the-counter drugs.

In total, it is not uncommon for such out-of-pocket expenses to provide up to one-fifth of all health-care finance in industrialised countries.

Since their first introduction into the NHS, *direct health charges* have been contentious. From the early years of the NHS their importance increased until by the early 1960s they were contributing almost 5 per cent of total NHS expenditure. However, Labour governments in the 1960s and 1970s held health charges down and by 1978–9 they constituted only 2 per cent of total NHS expenditure — the lowest percentage yield from such charges since 1952.

From 1979 onwards, the policy of successive Conservative governments was to raise the yield from direct charges: prescription charges were increased almost every year, from 20p in 1979 to reach £5.65 in 1997, when the Labour government was elected. Dental charges were similarly increased, while, in 1989, a charge for dental examinations was introduced. In 1984, the supply of spectacles under the NHS ended and a voucher scheme was substituted to help the needy. Also in 1989, a charge for sight tests was introduced, except for the needy.

Although the rises in direct charges were offset by exemptions and voucher schemes, the system has inevitably acted as a disincentive to poor and elderly people. For instance, the ending of the free sight-test was associated with an immediate 50 per cent reduction in the numbers offering themselves for sight tests. The charging system has also contributed to the steady withering away of NHS dentistry. As a result of these policies, the contribution of direct charges increased to almost 4 per cent of the total cost of the NHS by the early 1990s.

The Labour government elected in 1997 made one substantial change to the charging system that it inherited, reintroducing the free sight-test for those above the age of 60. The rate of increase in direct charges was also reduced, and by 1999–2000, these charges had once again fallen to contribute around 2 per cent of all NHS costs.

9.5.5 Other private funding sources

The final item listed in Table 9.3 is funding from *all other private funds*, which includes sources such as philanthropic and voluntary organisations. These often provide care without formal payment, and hence are often excluded from measures of health-care expenditure, so their contribution is normally underestimated. In fact, they continue to play a significant role in most countries, and in some countries their contribution may be of similar magnitude to funds from private health insurance. In the UK, one estimate in the 1980s suggested that voluntary help to hospitals was equivalent to around 300 000 full-time workers, spending around 50 per cent of their time on fund-raising and administration (CIPFA, 1984, p. 33). And this estimate still omits the activities of informal carers in the home, who remain the main source of health care, as Chapter 7 showed.

9.5.6 Trends in public expenditure on health

In 1960, public expenditure on health in most OECD countries was between 60 per cent and 70 per cent of total health spending, but in some countries such as the USA this share was as low as 25 per cent, with the remainder met privately. But during the 1960s, the public-sector share of health expenditure rose rapidly as many governments shouldered additional responsibilities for the health care of their citizens. This development was part of a wider 'mobilisation for total welfare', similar to that discussed for the UK in Chapter 6, and was also manifested in the USA with the creation and expansion of some government-funded health services directed at the poor, elderly people and armed-services veterans. As a consequence, the public-sector share of total health spending across the OECD rose steadily. Figure 9.7 shows these changes: one line on the chart shows the average public-sector share of health spending as a crude average, taking no account of differences in the size of countries; the other line shows the same information, but weighted according to the size of each country's economy.

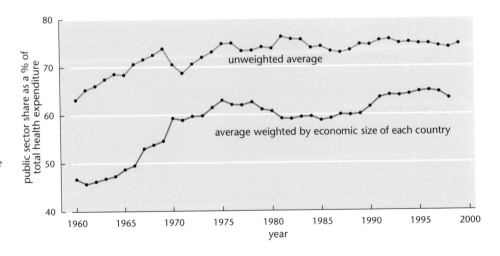

Figure 9.7 *The public-sector share of total health expenditure in the OECD countries, 1960–99. (Data from OECD, 2000, OECD Health Data 2000, CREDOC/ OECD, Paris)*

● Recalling Chapter 7, how would you explain the pattern shown in Figure 9.7 from the mid-1970s to about 1990?

■ After the oil price rise of 1973, many governments became concerned at the ever-expanding importance of public spending in their economies, and attempted to rein back public expenditure in areas such as health, while encouraging the private sector. As a consequence, in many countries the public share of total expenditure on health levelled off and even began to decline in the 1970s before stabilising at a lower level throughout the 1990s.

However, the weighted line, which takes account of the relative size of each economy, did rise slowly during the 1990s. The explanation lies in the greater influence of the USA on this weighted average (because of the size of its economy): there, the public share of health spending has continued to creep upwards, from 40 per cent in 1990 to around 45 per cent by 1999.

Finally, it is illuminating to compare public and private health expenditure as a percentage of GDP in a selection of industrialised countries, as shown in Figure 9.8.

● What strikes you about this comparison?

■ Public expenditure on health as a per cent of GDP is quite similar across these countries, and the UK is not significantly out of line. Most of the variation in total health expenditure as a share of GDP arises because of differences in *private* spending, and in this regard the UK stands out as having a very low level of private health expenditure.

On this account, the UK's low levels of expenditure on health care could be said to have arisen at least in part because of a failure to find an acceptable way of mobilising additional *private* spending on health care.

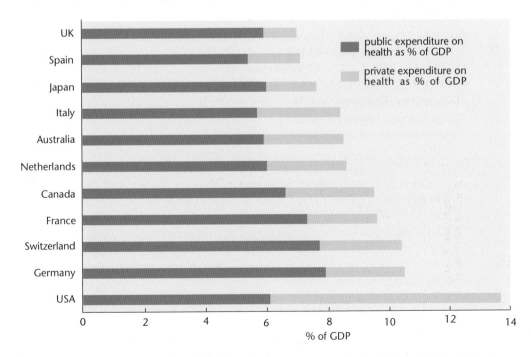

Figure 9.8 *Public, private and total health expenditure as a percentage of GDP in 10 industrialised countries, 1999 or nearest date. (Data from OECD, 2000, OECD Health Data 2000, CREDOC/OECD, Paris)*

9.6 Funding health care in developing countries

9.6.1 Sources of funding

The same broad categorisation of funding sources already discussed for industrialised countries can be applied to developing countries, but if anything there is even more variation between them. Table 9.4 shows some information from 11 developing countries in 1999.

Table 9.4   Sources of health expenditure in 11 developing countries, 1999.

	Public funding	Out-of-pocket payments	All other private funds
Bangladesh	46	54	0
Brazil	49	46	6
Central African Republic	69	31	0
China	25	75	0
Costa Rica	77	22	1
Dominican Republic	39	37	25
India	13	85	2
South Africa	47	46	7
Sri Lanka	45	52	3
Uganda	35	48	17
Zimbabwe	43	38	18

Data from World Health Organisation (2000) *World Health Report. Health Systems: Improving Performance*, WHO, Geneva, Table 8.

● How does the distribution of funding in Table 9.4 compare with the information in Table 9.3 for industrialised countries?

■ There is a lot of variation between countries, but broadly the public sector has a smaller role in developing countries — accounting for around 40–50 per cent of total health expenditure — while out-of-pocket payments (which include direct health charges) are much more important.

Direct health charges to users are also sometimes described as *cost recovery programmes*. The main arguments used in their favour are that they generate additional income which can be used to expand health care, they provide users and providers with information about the cost of different services, and they deter 'frivolous' use and therefore favour users with the greatest need. They have a long history of use in mission hospitals and clinics, which often provide high quality care to those most in need of it. However, it has also been argued that direct charges can deter the very patients who are at greatest risk and who would benefit most from health care, that they can be costly and difficult to collect, and that often they are not accompanied by any improvement in quality of service.

Ultimately, these arguments will only be resolved by recourse to evidence, which is still accumulating. One survey of the experience of a number of African countries in the 1980s concluded that on average 5 per cent of the total running costs of health services could be recouped in this way, with a range of between 2 per cent and 15 per cent (Vogel, 1990). Against this has to be set the cost of collection, which in some instances is considerable. Moreover, in many instances part or all of the income generated from direct charges is not retained for use in the health sector, but is returned to government finance ministries. Overall, therefore, direct charges are not a proven way of making a major contribution to health-service finance.

9.6.2 Effects on use of services

The most clearly documented effects of imposing direct charges are on the *use of services*. One study in Kenya found that the imposition of uniform charges for government hospital services in 1989 led to a fall in attendances at out-patient departments of between 29 per cent and 41 per cent, while attendances at dispensaries — which continued to provide services free of charge — increased sharply. When the charges were subsequently removed, the number of out-patient attendances surged, while visits to mission and private clinics declined. Finally, the study showed that demand for out-patient services following the introduction of charges fell *most* in the 'ultra-poor' households and to a lesser degree in the 'middle-poor' and 'least-poor' households (Mbugua *et al.*, 1995).

- What does this sequence of events suggest about the impact of charges on demand for health services?

■ First, patients do react to the cost of services, and demand for services falls when the cost increases. Second, patients tend to seek alternative sources of health care when the cost of a service increases: in other words, they are sensitive to the *relative* price of different health services. Third, uniform charges tend to have greatest impact on the poorest households and are therefore regressive in their impact.

These findings have been replicated in many different settings, and underline the need to consider all the costs and benefits of different options when formulating strategies to finance health care. In particular, it has been argued that policy makers who advocate charges too often focus on the 'targeting error' that results in people receiving free benefits which they could afford to pay for, while ignoring targeting errors that result in people who require services being excluded from them (Cornia and Stewart, 1995). A good example of this has been documented in Swaziland (Yoder, 1989), where those most deterred by charges were people with sexually transmitted diseases, respiratory diseases, and other infectious diseases — an outcome that severely hampered policies to control infectious diseases such as AIDS.[7]

9.7 Methods of health care provision and remuneration

The diversity in the ways that health systems are funded is matched by a tremendous amount of variation in the ways they are provided and the methods by which providers are paid. And these differences in turn can exert a major influence on the degree of access to health care, the cost of providing it, and the type and quality of services provided.

[7] The rapid spread of AIDS since the mid-1980s was discussed in Chapter 8 of this book, and is also addressed in *World Health and Disease* (Open University Press, 3rd edn 2001), Chapter 8, and in *Experiencing and Explaining Disease* (Open University Press, 3rd edn 2002), Chapter 4.

9.7.1 Providers of health care

Providers of health care fall into three basic categories. The first is *government institutions*, such as hospitals owned and managed by public bodies. In comparison with most other European countries, the UK has been unusually reliant on this method of provision, whose historical origins — culminating in the nationalisation of almost all hospitals in 1948 — has been traced in earlier chapters.

The second main category of providers, *non-government institutions*, can be subdivided into two sub-groups: *not-for-profit* and *profit-making*. Not-for-profit providers, including charitable hospitals and homes, seldom account for a large proportion of health expenditure in industrialised countries. The exception is the USA, where *Health Maintenance Organisations* (HMOs), mainly (but not exclusively) non-profit associations which provide health care to subscribers, had expanded to cover around 84 million Americans by 1998. *Profit-making institutions* include private hospital chains and insurance companies, and a minority of HMOs.

The third category of providers consists of *individual practitioners in private practice*. In the UK, a small proportion of doctors rely on private practice for most or all of their income. GPs in the UK are also nominally independent self-employed individuals, but their contracts to supply certain services to the NHS provide most of their income. Private practitioners also include the *self-employed indigenous and traditional practitioners,* such as the traditional midwives discussed in Chapter 8, who comprise the bulk of people involved in health care in many countries of the world (Figure 9.9). In India, for example, up to 40 per cent of health care is estimated to be provided by indigenous practitioners, compared with 20 per cent by Western medicine, and 40 per cent by lay care.

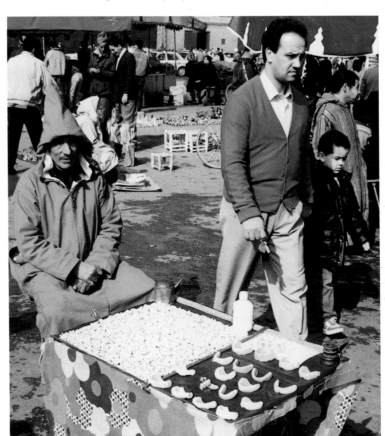

Figure 9.9 *Self-employed indigenous practitioners supply the majority of health services in many low- and middle-income countries. Here, dentures are sold and repaired from a market stall in Morroco. (Source: Michel Bergsma)*

9.7.2 Paying the doctor

The way in which *doctors* are remunerated has already been discussed at various points in this book: for example Chapter 6 described the way in which GPs held out against the salaried service to which hospital specialists agreed in 1948. In practice, there are three main ways of paying doctors (although they may be used in various combinations):

- a *salary* agreed in advance;
- *capitation*, in which payment is related to the number of people for whom a doctor is responsible, e.g. in a general practice;
- *fee-for-service*, where a doctor receives payment according to the services she or he performs.

The UK system of remunerating GPs has involved a mixture of capitation payments, fee-for-service payments for particular items, and a salary element. By the mid-1980s these three elements contributed roughly equal shares to an average GP's total remuneration, although the NHS reforms since then have tended to increase the importance of capitation payments and fee-for-service payments for meeting particular targets, such as pre-set levels of child immunisation. Most other OECD countries pay GPs on a fee-for-service basis or — if working from health centres — by means of a salary. And although the NHS system of salaries for hospital-based specialists is found in a number of other OECD countries, including France, Italy and Germany, fee-for-service is also widespread, as it is in UK private hospitals, although the details vary considerably.

The fact that the remuneration system clearly has some influence on a doctor's activity raises a more general issue concerning the doctor's ability to *influence the demand* for his or her own services. In most instances where goods or services are being exchanged, the roles of the person demanding and the person supplying are taken by two people assumed to be equally well informed about the item being exchanged. The patient 'demanding' formal health care, however, is frequently in a bad position to know what to demand.

● Why might this be so?

■ First, the patient may be unconscious or in need of emergency treatment. Second, the patient will frequently be at a disadvantage over information about what is wrong, or the range of options for dealing with the problem, their availability and their likely consequences. Even after treatment, the patient may find it difficult to assess the outcome, or the quality of the work performed.

In short, there is an *asymmetry* in the information available to doctor and patient, which places the doctor in the position of having to make the key decisions about what to supply to the patient.[7] This is sometimes referred to as an **agency relationship**, in which the doctor acts as the agent of the patient, making decisions on the patient's behalf. But once this situation exists, the possibility arises that the doctor will supply more health care than the patient would have chosen had the patient been fully informed. The doctor in such circumstances can be said to be inducing a demand for her or his own services, and hence this phenomenon has come to be called **supplier-induced demand**.

[7] Agency relationships and other aspects of 'supply and demand' for health services are discussed further in *Dilemmas in UK Health Care* (Open University Press, 3rd edn 2001), Chapter 2.

● Under what circumstances might doctors have particular incentives to create supplier-induced demand?

■ If they are paid according to the number of services that they provide, then they will have a financial incentive to induce as much demand for their services as possible.

It is fairly clear that the existence of a fee-for-service payment system, as for example in the USA, has a significant influence over the rates of *surgical intervention*, which are considerably higher than rates in the UK's National Health Service, where surgeons are paid by a salary that is independent of the volume of work done. This is one factor in the variations in surgical intervention rates discussed earlier. But the crucial question that the discussion of supplier-induced demand raises is not whether the rates of surgical intervention in, for example, the USA, are higher than in the UK, but whether they are higher than patients in the USA *would be willing to tolerate if they were fully informed*. So far research on this question has not provided any unambiguous findings.

9.7.3 Paying for hospitals

The other major category of health provider that can be paid for in various ways is the *hospital*. In countries such as the UK, Sweden and the Netherlands, most hospital costs are paid for on the basis of an *annual global budget* which is set *prospectively*. This system makes it easier to control health spending, although it may achieve this by reducing access or quality, or by passing costs on to patients — for example in the form of long waiting times for admission.

In a number of other European countries, hospitals are not controlled by any global budget, but instead are refunded their running costs *retrospectively*, for example by insurance companies on the basis of a set rate per patient per day: this is known as *per diem* payment (from the Latin word *dies*, day). Retrospective payment systems avoid some of the problems associated with global budgets, but they also remove incentives for hospitals to keep costs down. For example in Germany, where the *per diem* system is widespread, average lengths of stay are comparatively long, and by the 1990s there were more hospital beds relative to the population than in most other European countries, in turn making the health system expensive to operate.

In response to this type of problem, a number of countries, such as France and the Netherlands, dropped the *per diem* system during the 1980s in favour of setting annual global budgets for hospitals. In the USA prior to 1984, the Medicare programme for elderly people involved the government in picking up the bill retrospectively for any treatment that hospitals saw fit to provide. In 1984, concern over rapidly rising costs led to a system in which American hospitals were paid *prospectively* the amount deemed reasonable to treat particular problems, classified by *Diagnosis Related Groups*. A variant of this system, which is intended to give providers more incentive to keep costs down, is also playing an increasing role in the service agreements in the UK within the NHS. It is still too early to say with any confidence what effect this form of hospital reimbursement will have on the quality or volume of care, on access, or indeed on costs in the UK.

In summary

Looking back over Sections 9.4 to 9.7, you should note the following points:

1   There are many possible reasons for variations in health spending between countries. Factors such as different definitions of health care or rates of activity

explain only a small part of the variation. Level of national income is a very important influence, but by no means the only one.

2   The correlation between levels of health spending and levels of mortality are fairly weak, especially among the industrialised countries. This may be because mortality is not the best or only way of measuring the effect of health care.

3   Health expenditure has grown mainly because of rising utilisation of services, measured by higher admission rates, operation rates, and so on.

4   The basic distinction in methods of funding health care is between public and private sources of funds. The public share of health expenditure in industrialised countries rose rapidly during the 1970s to around three-quarters of the total, but has been fairly stable since the 1980s. The public sector share of health spending is lower in developing countries.

5   The way in which health care is provided, in particular the way in which providers such as doctors and hospitals are remunerated, can have a powerful effect on the quality and quantity of health care.

9.8   Contemporary health care: an international trade

So far, the main concern of this chapter has been to explore the *diversity* of health systems around the world, particularly in terms of their funding and type of provision, and to assess the extent to which the UK is typical of, or different from, systems elsewhere. But you have repeatedly seen how health systems have been subject to influences from other countries, ranging from the colonial interventions described in Chapters 3–6, to the policies of international organisations such as the WHO discussed in Chapter 8.

●   Drawing on earlier chapters, can you suggest some ways in which such international influences on health care occur?

■   There are many, but four of the main ones are:
1   The migration of health workers, in particular doctors and nurses.
2   The movement of ideas and knowledge via journals, books, conferences and, increasingly, broadcasting and the Internet.
3   The trade in drugs and medical equipment.
4   The provision of health services by international agencies such as the WHO.

This final section considers such *international exchanges,* and whether they might have the effect of *reducing* health-care diversity. We will look in more detail at two aspects — the migration of health workers and the pharmaceutical trade.

9.8.1   Migration of health workers

The migration of doctors and nurses from certain developing countries was discussed in Chapter 6, and one feature of this was that it often represented a huge donation from poorer to richer countries. These flows from poorer to richer countries are also found within the European Union (EU), whose doctors have in theory been free to work in any other member country since 1977; an increasing proportion of the EU's 800 000 doctors have taken the opportunity to do so. By 2000, of the 65 000 medical staff working in hospitals in England, around 3 400 had qualified in other EU countries. However, no fewer than 16 700 had qualified in countries outside the EU.

Among nurses, there has also been an increasing amount of movement between countries. In 2000 for example, around 7 400 overseas-trained nurses and midwives came to the UK to start work, the highest number ever recorded (UKCC, 2000). Within this total, only around 1 400 came from EU countries (mainly Finland, Germany, Ireland and Spain). The biggest suppliers were South Africa, with 1 460, followed by Australia (1 166), the Philippines (1 052, see Figure 9.10), New Zealand (461), the West Indies (425) and Zimbabwe (221).

The reasons for migration can be divided into two broad categories: factors that tend to *push* health workers out of donor countries, and factors tending to *pull* health workers into recipient countries. Among the push-factors, the fundamental one is that some countries train more doctors and nurses than they can afford to employ. This lack of connection between the number of doctors or nurses a country trains and the number it can afford to employ is compounded by the fact, mentioned in Chapters 6 and 8, that the type of training is often based on teaching curricula that have been transferred from much richer countries.

On the other side of this equation, the main pull-factor is that some of the richer countries train an insufficient number of doctors for their needs, and can therefore offer employment opportunities to immigrants. In the 1960s, the lowering of immigration barriers and the granting of employment permits by richer recipient countries brought forth a large increase in the number of doctors and nurses who migrated. However, in the late 1970s and early 1980s, immigration barriers were raised again and qualification criteria tightened to reduce the flow. This was because the rich industrialised countries of Western Europe and North America were then producing enough, or even too many, of their own doctors.

The movement of a health worker between countries is likely to involve various losses or gains to the countries involved, but these may be hard to assess. If we were to assume for a moment that all workers who in fact migrated had stayed in their country of origin, then broadly the industrialised countries would be slightly

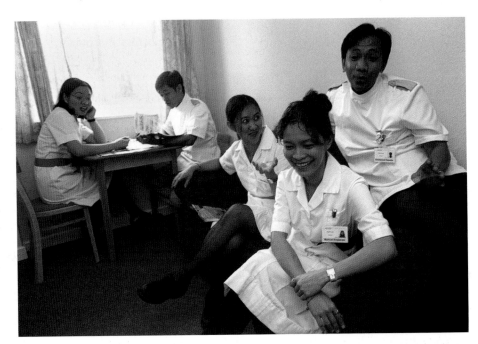

Figure 9.10 *These five nurses from the Philippines working at a hospital in Leeds, were among the 1 052 nurses from that country to start work in the UK in 2000. (Source: Joan Russell/Guzelian)*

worse off and developing countries better off than they are in reality. But these differences are insignificant in comparison with the gulf in the overall level of provision between the industrialised and developing countries. With or without migration, the former have between five and ten times as many doctors and nurses per head of population as the latter. And, as you saw earlier, one important reason for migration is the lack of employment in donor countries, or the low incomes in posts that are available. If every migrant doctor or nurse were to go back to the country they trained in, it could not be assumed that they would be employed. So the loss to donor countries is partly the loss of a doctor or nurse; it also represents a transfer from poor to rich countries of the scarce resources invested in their training.

9.8.2 The world pharmaceutical industry

The world pharmaceutical industry merits attention not least because its products have had a significant impact on mortality and morbidity patterns in most parts of the world. The industry performs in a very political and highly regulated environment, where the safety, effectiveness, prices and marketing of its products may all be subject to public scrutiny and legislation. This has contributed to an atmosphere of secrecy around most large drug companies, and as a consequence detailed information on the industry is limited.

The pharmaceutical industry has a very unusual structure, with the actual production of drugs sandwiched between a powerful scientific research effort and a vigorous and sophisticated marketing system. The marketing end of the industry is genuinely global, in that the largest companies increasingly operate around the world and sell products in almost all national markets. However, research and production remain concentrated in a few countries, and the pattern of consumption is also highly uneven.

Research and development

The most striking area of concentration is in research and development (R&D); spending on these activities can reach as much as 18 per cent of annual sales, compared to 5 per cent or less on R&D in most other industries. One standard measure of research effort and success is the number of new products or *new molecular entities* that are developed by a company and then marketed on a worldwide basis (that is, on at least six of the world's major national markets). In 1987, a total of 60 such products were launched, but by 1997 this had fallen to 37, despite a rapid rise in spending on R&D by the pharmaceutical industry — from $5.4 billion in 1981 to more than $40 billion by 1998 (measured in US$ here, and in the following discussion).

● What might explain this pattern of rising R&D expenditure and fewer new drugs being marketed?

■ The cost of developing new pharmaceutical products and bringing them to the market has been rising, mainly due to tighter regulations and controls.

The research and development costs for each new product brought to the market rose from around $110 million in 1976 to between $500 million and $600 million by 1997. In addition, although fewer new products were launched in 1997, a higher proportion of them were genuinely 'new', rather than 'me-too' or follow-up products to others already on the market. Around 75 per cent of these new products came from companies based in just four countries: the USA, Switzerland, Germany and the UK, with the USA by far the dominant country.

The core producers

Most of the manufacture of pharmaceuticals also remains concentrated in a core group of countries in which the modern industry emerged — these are in North America, Western Europe and latterly Japan. In 1999 over 80 per cent of the world's drugs (measured by value) were made in these regions. However, although world manufacture has remained heavily concentrated in these regions, the 1990s saw an increasing dominance by American companies. In 1990, 13 of the 25 top-selling drugs were manufactured in Europe, but by 2002 this will have fallen to just 3 — while 20 of the top 25 will be American.

Although many thousands of small and medium-sized companies are involved in the pharmaceutical industry, the top 25 pharmaceutical companies accounted for approximately half of total production in 1999. Despite the enormous size of the largest pharmaceutical companies (which account for eight of the world's top 25 companies by market value), none in 2000 had a market share of more than 6.5 per cent. But the 1990s and early 2000s saw a hectic pace of amalgamation in the industry: for example, Glaxo merged with Wellcome, SmithKlein merged with Beecham, and the two merged companies joined forces in 2001 as GlaxoSmithKlein — creating one of the world's largest companies. By comparison, leading car manufacturers typically have 15–20 per cent of a country's market in new cars.

However, unlike the market for cars or television sets, the market for pharmaceuticals is very fragmented, with almost as many sub-markets as there are diseases and treatments. If we define the market for drugs in terms of products that are genuine substitutes for each other, a different picture emerges. For example, the two leading anti-ulcer drugs — one of the most profitable drug categories of the 1980s and 1990s — together had a two-thirds share of the market in 2000. And the more precisely the market is defined, the higher the market shares tend to be.

●   Why might a lack of vigorous competition in sub-markets for drugs be of concern to policy makers or to consumers?

■   The main concern is that the prices charged for drugs may be higher than would be the case if markets were more competitive.

Unequal access

Patterns of world consumption of pharmaceuticals closely parallel the pattern of production. In 1999, 80 per cent of total world sales of pharmaceutical products were accounted for by just 15 industrial countries. In contrast, only 9 per cent of sales were in Asia (excluding Japan), containing almost 60 per cent of the world's population; many other developing countries import an even lower share of the global market in medical drugs (Figure 9.11).

Although the absolute amount spent on pharmaceuticals in developing countries is low, they spend proportionately far more of their health budget on pharmaceuticals — up to half of all health-care expenditure, compared to an average of 10 per cent or less in industrialised countries. Partly this is because of less regulated access to drugs: whereas in industrial countries medicines are mainly sold on a prescription basis or via chemists' shops, medicines in developing countries are often dispensed by hospital pharmacies or sold from relatively uncontrolled sources. For example, in China in 1999 about 85 per cent of all drugs were dispensed by hospital pharmacies, and drugs accounted for almost 60 per cent of all health expenditure. As hospitals can effectively charge what they want, there are strong

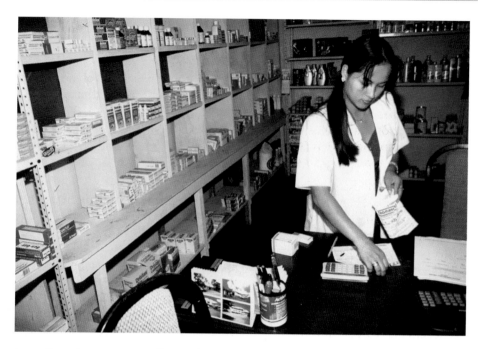

Figure 9.11 *Sales of pharmaceutical products to developing countries account for a tiny proportion of the global market; this cooperatively-run pharmacy in Versalles, Colombia, provides essential drugs at low cost for community members, but frequently runs short of basic supplies. (Source: WHO/HPR/TDR/ Crump)*

incentives to over-prescribe and over-charge. Similar problems exist in many developing countries, and policies designed to improve matters are frequently not enforced through lack of money or because of corruption.

One policy that has gained ground in many developing countries is to obtain better value for money by cutting back on the purchase of non-essential drugs and concentrating on a limited number of drugs that are of proven efficacy and cost-effectiveness. In 1991, for example, the United Nations Development Programme estimated that drug consumption per person in developing countries was $5.40 in 1985, but that basic and essential drugs could be provided for around $1.00 per person. This approach has been encouraged by the WHO, which has produced listings of interventions — including drugs — that are judged to be the most efficacious and cost-effective in relation to the therapeutic needs of developing countries.

However, despite the gradual adoption of such policies in many countries, many people worldwide have little or no access to essential drugs, and some researchers have argued that this is because the R&D efforts of the pharmaceutical industry effectively ignore the health concerns of the developing countries. Of a total of 1 233 drugs licensed worldwide between 1975 and 1997, only 13 were specifically related to tropical diseases, and of these, two were developed primarily for the American armed forces and five resulted from veterinary research.

In 1998, the Wellcome Trust (a leading medical charity) estimated that worldwide research on malaria totalled $84 million annually, for a disease that kills around 860 000 people every year. So R&D expenditure was equivalent to around $100 for each malaria fatality, or about 4 US cents for each person vulnerable to malaria. In contrast, research funding for asthma was around $800 million annually; asthma was the cause of around 140 000 deaths per year, so the R&D expenditure on this disease was approximately $5 700 per fatality.

In response, the pharmaceutical industry has argued that the health problems of the developing countries are not confined to the tropical diseases, and that research on cardiovascular therapies, antibiotics, anti-cancer therapies and indeed asthma drugs will eventually benefit everyone. In addition, some specific collaborations between the pharmaceutical industry and governmental and international agencies were agreed in the late 1990s, which aimed to improve the supply of existing and new vaccines and other drugs for diseases such as malaria, bilharzia and elephantiasis.

Another major source of friction between the pharmaceutical industry and developing countries has been the desire of the industry to protect its patented drugs against cheaper generic substitutes. This issue came to a head in the late 1990s when the South African government, which claimed that it was entitled under World Trade Organisation rules to import cheaper generic copies of patented drugs to treat people with AIDS, had to defend a legal action brought against it by 39 leading pharmaceutical companies. These companies argued that the powers claimed by the South African government gave it the freedom to override any patent protection, to the ultimate detriment of research and innovation.

Faced with increasingly hostile public opinion (Figure 9.12) and the risk of long-term damage to their image, the companies eventually abandoned their action against the South African government in 2001. But, at the time of writing (Spring 2001), other countries such as India and Brazil continue to be involved in legal disputes with the pharmaceutical industry, and it remains to be seen whether international trade rules will protect or disadvantage developing countries seeking to lower the cost of effective drugs.

More generally, it is clear that the global configuration of the modern pharmaceutical industry to a large extent mirrors the distribution of world income, with drug research, production and consumption concentrated in the countries with the largest markets. In 2001, the leading developed countries agreed to establish a drugs fund worth approximately £2 billion, to help provide new drugs and vaccines against HIV/AIDS, tuberculosis and malaria in some of the poorest countries. Nevertheless, it remains an uncomfortable fact that far more is spent on helping an obese Westerner to lose a few pounds, or an elderly male in a rich country to maintain an erection, than is devoted to saving people in developing countries from tuberculosis, malaria or AIDS.

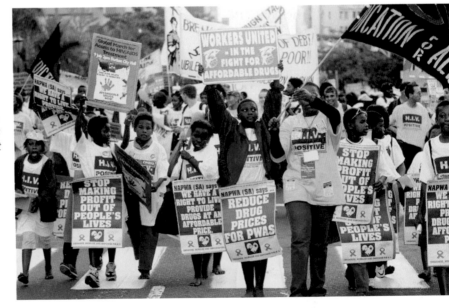

Figure 9.12 *Protesters at a rally in Durban, South Africa, 9 July 2000, demand affordable access to drugs for the treatment of HIV and AIDS; at the time, pharmaceutical companies had brought a court action against the government for attempting to import cheaper generic versions of these drugs. (Source: Obed Zilwa/ Associated Press)*

9.8.3 A world health-care system

These briefly considered aspects of international health care suggest that, although some common patterns and trends can be detected in the health-care systems of different countries, the degree of diversity remains almost overwhelming. Moreover, as noted at several points, apparent similarities seem to dissolve or slide out of focus on closer inspection. Nevertheless, there does exist something that might be called a **world health-care system**. Western models of health care and medicine tend to dominate in this system, and this is reflected in pharmaceutical production, consumption and research priorities, medical education and technology, the migration of health workers, and the organisation of health care.

This dominance is partly related to the comparative effectiveness of Western medicine in dealing with specific diseases, but it also reflects patterns of economic strength and weakness, custom and culture. Not least, it is an example of how the modern world reflects the past, for many aspects of international health care can be traced to developments discussed earlier in this book, particularly to the gap that opened up between Europe and the rest of the world from around the late fifteenth century. When studying the diversity of health care in the contemporary world, the consequences of this gap form a constant companion.

OBJECTIVES FOR CHAPTER 9

When you have studied this chapter, you should be able to:

9.1 Define and use, or recognise definitions and applications of, each of the terms printed in **bold** in the text.

9.2 Discuss variations between different countries and over time in the resources committed to formal health care, and the difficulties involved in making comparisons.

9.3 Summarise the main ways in which formal health care may be financed and provided, using examples to illustrate variations between and within countries.

9.4 Describe ways in which methods of funding and providing health care may influence the volume or quality of services.

9.5 Use the examples of migration of health workers and the international pharmaceutical industry to illustrate international influences on health care.

QUESTIONS FOR CHAPTER 9

1 (*Objective 9.2*)

'Spending on formal health care increases in direct line with national income.' Is this statement true?

2 (*Objective 9.3*)

On the evidence of this chapter, to what extent is the way in which health services are funded in the UK typical of other industrialised countries?

3 (*Objective 9.4*)

Under what circumstances might a 'shortage' of doctors *not* be overcome by increasing the number of doctors at work?

4 (*Objective 9.5*)

'Pharmaceutical companies will develop products if markets for them exist. Therefore they will not neglect common diseases.' Evaluate the strength of this claim.

CHAPTER 10

Conclusions

10.1   Introduction   328

10.2   Health care: a universal phenomenon   329
    10.2.1   The classical tradition   329
    10.2.2   Religion and healing   329
    10.2.3   Pluralism of health-care practices   330
    10.2.4   Ethical concerns   330

10.3   Characterising health care in Britain   331
    10.3.1   Secularisation and the expansion of local government   331
    10.3.2   The rise of state intervention   331
    10.3.3   Resource inadequacies   332
    10.3.4   Inequalities in health care   332
    10.3.5   The diversity of health care   333

10.4   Health care: in whose service?   333
    10.4.1   Mutations of the hospital system   333
    10.4.2   Reshaping the health-care system   334

10.5   Limits to a world health-care system   335
    10.5.1   Convergence   335
    10.5.2   Global medicine   336
    10.5.3   Global retrenchment   336
    10.5.4   Global exploitation   337

10.6   Poverty and health   337

Study notes for OU students

This short chapter concludes the book by summarising the main themes developed over the course of Chapters 1–9. Its aim is to assist you in drawing together your thoughts about the material you have been studying and to consolidate your understanding of the content of this book, before moving on to *Dilemmas in UK Health Care* (Open University Press, third edition, 2001). There are no new terms or concepts and no Objectives or self-assessment questions at the end of the chapter.

10.1 Introduction

The preceding chapters contain many reminders of the long shadow cast by past events. The first chapter of this book was concerned with basic questions of orientation. It argued for a broad-ranging social–historical approach and pointed out the limitations inherent in conventional triumphalist representations of the past. Subsequent chapters make it clear that historical constructions in terms of 'the conquest of disease' or the 'triumph of modern medicine' provide impoverished and misleading impressions of events on the ground. It is of course tempting to focus on the heroic successes of biomedical scientists, such as 'microbe hunters'; indeed a book of this title by Paul de Kruif is a famous history-of-medicine classic from the 1920s.

In the course of time, realism has necessitated a more guarded approach to assessing the impact of medical discoveries. Nevertheless, echoes of triumphalism are not difficult to locate. For instance, in the Reith Lectures in 2001, Professor Tom Kirkwood, the influential gerontologist, elaborated upon scientific developments that had facilitated a 'longevity revolution'. He described the 'taming of the age-old scourge of premature and preventable death' as the 'greatest triumph that our species has achieved' (Kirkwood, 'Brave Old World', Reith Lecture 1, BBC Radio 4, 4 April 2001).

● On what grounds could Kirkwood's conclusion be considered triumphalist?

■ Triumphalist constructions tend to gloss over the scale of the problem of translating scientific findings into tangible health benefits; living longer does not inevitably mean gaining more years in good health. And the grim conditions of existence experienced by much of the world's poor are not reflected in the state of affairs he portrays. In Sub-Saharan Africa, life expectancy at birth is falling, not rising, in all classes and income-groups as a result of the AIDS epidemic and other infections that follow in its wake (e.g. TB).

On the basis of the wider frame of reference adopted in this book, we have observed a striking paradox. As Kirkwood has observed, especially in the course of the twentieth century, the capacities of curative medicine have been transformed. Yet health care in the UK has drifted inexorably into a state of crisis. The perception of malaise also applies in some other advanced Western economies and throughout the developing world. This situation has forced health care to the head of the political agenda. Everywhere there is a frantic search for policies capable of preventing the escalation of public health catastrophes, reducing glaring health inequalities, and providing the basics of health care for all those in need.

The power of the past to overshadow the present therefore emerges as more than a theme for idle antiquarian curiosity. You have noticed that modern health-care systems have not evolved into perfect functional constructions. Rather they are imperfect hybrids, bearing the marks of a wide range of political, economic and social determinants. Many of these influences represent forces acting over long duration. This element of historical determination becomes all the more evident and compelling with fuller investigation. Such factors can then be granted their proper weight in explaining the sources of our current turmoils. On the same grounds, this historical perspective needs to be taken into account in deliberations on policy options for the future. Consequently, despite modern society's zest for novelty, and the continuing revolutionary progress of medicine, the historical frame of reference retains a remarkable degree of relevance in our discourse about the major policy predicaments of health care. This final chapter summarises some of our main points of emphasis under five headings.

10.2 Health care: a universal phenomenon

Maintenance of health and elaboration of appropriate health-care systems represent a universal phenomenon, applying as much in the past as in the present, and not limited to the developed world.

10.2.1 The classical tradition

Although we have concentrated on events since 1500, it is clear that the expanding empire of Western Europe was drawing on a cultural tradition of long ancestry. Europe, as the seat of the Renaissance, took over a system of medical ideas that was formed before the time of Aristotle and Plato. This classical reference-point of modern medicine has lost none of its resonance. For example, Charles Winslow, the respected American medical thinker, from whom we derive the modern definition of public health, described classical Greek thinking as the greatest single event in the history of Western civilisation and 'the rock upon which the science' of modern medicine was founded (Winslow, 1952, pp. 8–10).

More recently, in the context of the perceived crisis of confidence afflicting general practice in the UK, the leaders in this field insisted that the profession's 'ancient values distilled over time remain a vital asset' as a buttress against 'the demands of business management, bureaucratic accountability and information overload' being imposed by modern government (Morrell, 1998, pp. 18–19). On careful reflection, it is evident that the message of Greek medicine is not interpreted with consistency. Whereas Winslow admired the Greeks for their rejection of animism and their pursuit of rationalism, Professor Morrell appealed to the more intangible, charismatic values of the doctor, which he believed were ranged against the forces of modernisation associated with bureaucracy.

10.2.2 Religion and healing

European Christianity traditionally placed primacy on obligation to the poor and treatment of the sick, and believed — on the basis of New Testament authority — that the miracle of healing was freely available to believers. As evident from the early chapters of this book, the Reformation and fragmentation of the church did nothing to obscure its healing and charitable mission. The commitment of the medieval church to healing, and the dedication to the sick of spiritual leaders such as Julian is evident from the example of Norwich given in Chapter 1 (see Figure 1.3). Church organisations have remained prominent even as providers of hospital services in the Western industrial economies. Also they are particularly dominant in NGOs and in primary health-care work in the developing world.

Magical healing associated with the Christian church provides a striking analogy with traditional societies. These also evolved parallel and elaborate systems for coping with distress and disease, involving modes of treatment that were integrated into their frameworks of religious belief and magical practice.

In all societies the health-care system reflects the delicate web of values devised for maintaining social equilibrium. Accordingly, health-care systems are not a modern creation dependent on the existence of operating theatres, intensive care units, or doctors with scientific training. Early Christianity and Islam made use of hospitals for the sick, and highly trained corps of doctors were common in remote antiquity. But neither doctors nor hospitals are essential to health care, the greater part of which has always been provided by the family or local community. Consequently this book has attempted to avoid equating health care with formally constituted health services and professions, although it naturally draws attention to the growth of health services and health-care professions as an important element in modern Western society.

10.2.3 Pluralism of health-care practices

The continuing involvement of family, community and many facets of the social infrastructure in health maintenance, have determined that health services reflect all the diversity of our cultural and political atlas. This variety accounts for the difficulty pointed out in Chapter 9 in adopting simple typologies of health care for the purpose of international comparison. Migration of peoples and the more cosmopolitan approach to culture in the modern world have served to strengthen links between East and West.

Consequently, although this book has attached importance to the process of *modernisation*, and to such associated phenomena of secularisation, bureaucratisation and professionalisation, we are constantly reminded of the *pluralism* of health care, even extending to the persistence of beliefs and practices which are rooted in the pre-modern era. Paradoxically, while Western medicine has been advancing in developing countries, a plethora of alternative medicines of ancient and largely religious origin, from China, India and Japan, have been making notable headway in the West. Although, as indicated in Chapter 9, it is difficult to quantify such changes in the pattern of health care in any country, it is obviously unrealistic to confine attention to developments connected with Western biomedical science, as if all other dimensions of health care are an irrelevant and obsolete legacy from a discredited pre-scientific past.

10.2.4 Ethical concerns

Even in cases where Western high-technology medicine is supreme, a purely technical approach to health care has proved impracticable. Ethical problems impinge on health care at so many points that the practice of medicine and conduct of health-service personnel are everywhere regulated on the basis of codes evolved with respect to legal, philosophical and religious criteria.

- ● Select some notable examples in health care where the application of technical innovations has been influenced by the above criteria.

- ■ Birth control and abortion provide the most obvious examples. Numerous other examples mentioned in this book or others in the series include: enforced confinement and treatment of people who are mentally ill or have learning disabilities; questions of consent raised, for instance, in transplantation; *in vitro* fertilisation and experiments on embryos; gene therapy and the creation of genetically-modified organisms for therapeutic uses; or compulsory blood-testing for HIV infection. Immunisation, blood transfusion, and water fluoridation have all met with opposition on ethical grounds.

These examples demonstrate that, even in its most secularised phase, health care and medical practice all over the world have become exposed to controls stemming from religious or quasi-religious sources.

10.3   Characterising health care in Britain

Our account of developments in Britain (latterly the United Kingdom) has provided a specific and detailed insight into the manner in which the informal and formal aspects of the health-care system have been moulded by the values, cultural norms and institutions prevailing in a modern nation-state.

10.3.1   Secularisation and the expansion of local government

In the course of our account of modernisation in Chapter 1 we drew attention to the importance of secularisation. Of all countries in Europe, Britain led the way in this trend; secularisation in health care was evident early in the Reformation and it proceeded quickly thereafter. Over a long period, as described in Chapter 2, Britain's medical charities, voluntary hospitals, university medical schools, nursing organisations and philanthropic bodies were characterised by religious inspiration and they retained generalised religious links. However, they were predominantly non-denominational in character and administered in a largely secular manner, partly because Britain was unusual in Europe in possessing no religious denomination sufficiently dominant to control medical philanthropy. Religious organisations have of course continued to be active in charities relating to health and social care, and indeed in some cases such as the Salvation Army, they are still involved as providers for groups liable to fall through the net of services provided by public agencies.

With the collapse of church ascendancy in medical philanthropy during the Reformation, the pathway was clear for the dominance of *lay organisations* in the administration of poor relief and medical care. From the Elizabethan period onwards, the parish became the major provider. Then, in the later nineteenth century, parishes were superseded by newer forms of local government, which were granted greater powers to levy local taxation. This arrangement provided a sufficient basis for the funding of health services until the inception of the NHS.

10.3.2   The rise of state intervention

In the course of the nineteenth century a mounting body of national statutes were enacted to ensure the uniformity of local government provision. In the twentieth century, central state involvement expanded rapidly and increasingly entailed direct subsidy from general taxation. Health and welfare services thereby offered opportunities for redistribution of wealth and reduction of inequality. This trend culminated in 1948 with the establishment of the NHS, which, as pointed out in Chapters 6 and 9, was the first major health service in the Western world to be supported almost entirely by general taxation. Establishment of the NHS marked the end of a long period of local government ascendancy in the field of health care, and the beginning of a phase of dominance of the central state, which continues into the new millennium.

As indicated by Chapters 6 and 7, the character of lay accountability within the health services was transformed during the second half of the twentieth century. On the eve of the NHS, public-health services were controlled by elected local government councils; under the NHS these were replaced by bodies nominated by central government; then since the 1980s these nominated bodies have declined in importance owing to the rising management authority of central government-appointed bureaucrats. This trend has led to the complaint that health care is alone among personal welfare services in lacking any significant element of local democratic accountability.

10.3.3 Resource inadequacies

You have discovered from Chapter 9 that the UK demonstrates the perhaps unexpected combination of high state-involvement in health care together with low expenditure, relative to countries with comparable incomes as measured by a number of separate criteria. This parsimony is deep-rooted historically and it is arguably explained by the traditionally strong links between health care and the poor law. This conclusion was reached in consideration of each of the periods discussed in Chapters 2, 3 and 4. The state assumed responsibility for the care of the sick, but the close ties between sickness, poverty and social deviance entailed, as noted in Chapter 3, intrusion of the principle of *less eligibility* into health care. Because the treatment of the poor was financed by taxes levied on the rich, the secular authorities were always vulnerable to political pressures to minimise this imposition, even if this acted to the detriment of the health of the poor.

In the second half of the twentieth century, appeals to altruism with implications of higher taxation to support health care notionally gained general assent, but for most of its history, the NHS remained a low spending-priority of governments and the temptation of low taxation has prevailed at the ballot box. As indicated in Chapters 7 and 9, it was not until the profound crisis affecting the NHS at the turn of the millennium that the UK government conceded a pledge to raise health-service spending to the European average.

10.3.4 Inequalities in health care

Throughout the twentieth century, the adverse effects of low spending have been compounded by entrenched irrationalities in the distribution of human and material resources within the publicly-funded health services. As indicated by Chapters 7 and 9, this has resulted in the perverse consequence that the NHS itself has reinforced inequalities in health.

● Can you suggest examples of this?

■ Significant geographical variations were identified in the 1990s in the availability of services provided under the NHS (treatment for infertility is one example), and in the length of time patients wait to see a consultant or to receive specialist treatment for certain conditions. These variations became known as the 'postcode lottery' in health care, since inequalities in provision were based on where patients lived.

The fact that the problem of inequalities was not granted anything like its proper recognition until the late 1990s arguably points to the tenacious hold of prejudices rooted in the idea of 'less eligibility'.

As a recent report sponsored by the mental-health charity Mind (formerly, MIND) has confirmed, vulnerable groups continue to suffer from a great sense of injustice and social exclusion. One witness to the Mind report said that 'people need to be educated about the past of psychiatry' in order to appreciate the wide range of persons (he listed 'single mothers, lesbians and gay men, slaves who tried to escape') who have been arbitrarily labelled as mentally ill and thereby consigned to the ranks of the less eligible (quoted in Dunn, 1999, p. 29). It is notable that the UK has evolved a health service which is notionally generous, supportive in principle of universal access and designed to combat inequality, but in practice is no more kind to the poor or other vulnerable groups than systems founded on less-enlightened principles. Also, the Cinderella status of services available to vulnerable groups, such as people with mental-health problems, exacerbates their sense of exclusion in the marginalised under-classes.

10.3.5   The diversity of health care

It is evident that the evolution of health care and social support, including the health and personal social services, is determined by a wide range of economic, political and social factors that are specific to any national and local situation. The detailed consideration of Britain in the previous chapters confirms that although there was a broadly similar pattern of change throughout the Western economies, the British model possesses a characteristic imprint and is not replicated elsewhere, even among neighbours displaying the closest similarity in development of their welfare states.

The British case-study therefore underlines the phenomenon of diversity. Although not described in detail, it is also evident that there has existed considerable room for separate development in England, Wales, Scotland and Northern Ireland. Indeed, the stepping up of devolution at the beginning of the new millennium will increase the scope for further divergence. Diversity within the UK has also been increased by the devolved pattern of health-service administration, which follows the precedent set under the voluntary hospitals and local government. As noted in Chapter 7, in recent years this devolved system has been subject to critical comment owing to variations in management efficiency, lack of professional accountability, and irrationalities in levels of service provision. When the informal sector is taken into account, the diversity of health care is even greater.

10.4   Health care: in whose service?

The growing volume of resources devoted to health and social support has undoubtedly yielded real and measurable benefits. On the other hand our case-study of Britain has cited many instances where these resources have not been utilised to the maximum beneficial effect. Of course, many erroneous policy decisions were made in good faith; they seemed fair and appropriate at the time. Nevertheless, it is important to appreciate the extent to which major choices about the distribution and use of human and material resources in health care were dictated by the social objectives of the ruling elite, or self-interest of the medical profession, rather than by the real needs of the people.

10.4.1   Mutations of the hospital system

It is difficult to argue that the huge system of workhouses, asylums, mental deficiency institutions, sanatoria, or infectious-diseases hospitals built up in the nineteenth and first part of the twentieth century represented a necessary response to real need. More appropriate, humane and cheaper alternatives were available, for instance by more determined commitment to the sanitarian programme, providing relief within the community, or more prompt use of vaccination and immunisation. Such alternatives were justified at the time by experts in the respective field using cogent arguments. In the event, these non-institutional alternatives were rejected. Instead, partly on grounds of less eligibility, the strategies of incarceration and building of vast hospital networks were adopted. It so happened that these policies also extended the career options and advanced the status of certain sections of the medical profession. Developments within the hospital system were therefore very much tied up with the balance of power within medicine.

Several chapters in this book outline the manner in which the acute medical specialisms and their general hospitals assumed ascendancy in the twentieth century. The vast institutional system inherited from the previous century then became an embarrassment and those medical specialists concerned with long-stay patients were relegated to second-class status. The later chapters of this book describe the rise and slow collapse of this system. In line with the above trend, under the NHS the limited resources available for development were largely swallowed up by intrinsically expensive Teaching Hospitals and District General Hospitals. Although public health, primary care and community care represented integral elements of the NHS and supplied many essential services, for a long period they occupied low status, with the result that these relatively economical and effective services remained underdeveloped.

This process was in effect a re-enactment of developments in the previous century. In both cases, expensive institutional services were provided when much cheaper non-institutional alternatives could have been implemented. In both cases the bias towards concentrating resources in expensive institutional services coincided with the preferences of the most powerful elements within the hierarchy of the medical profession.

● What parallels can you find for this trend in developing countries?

■ As we observe in Chapters 6, 8 and 9, the acute-hospital system was exported to the former colonies of Western powers, where its huge expense proved unsustainable and subversive to the campaign to establish a viable system of primary care in rural areas. The central position accorded to large hospitals in the health systems of poor countries until the 1990s was largely in pursuit of the prestige attached to 'disease palaces' modelled on European lines and ruled by a medical elite.

Dismantling of the long-stay hospitals in the UK only occurred with the demotion in status of the professional groups possessing a vested interest in these institutions. Equally, as shown in Chapter 7, the more recent decline of beds within the acute-hospital sector (a trend accelerated by the transfer of hospital building to the Private Finance Initiative), and tentative moves towards reducing dependence on expensive hospital services, has coincided with distinct loss of authority and decline of public confidence in the current hospital-medical elite.

10.4.2 Reshaping the health-care system

Dominance of the hospital system in its various forms tended to delay the introduction and implementation of care alternatives that were often less expensive and more appropriate. In Chapters 6 and 7 it has been observed that community care was first adopted as policy in the 1960s, primary health care in the 1970s, the new public health in the 1980s, and health promotion in the 1990s. However, it was not until the 1990s that all of these alternatives to acute-hospital care moved to the forefront of policy. By the turn of the millennium the NHS had become at least notionally 'primary-led', while preventive and promotive health care were regaining the prominence that they had assumed in the policies of the Victorian sanitarians.

The attempt to achieve a more satisfactory balance between primary and secondary health care, discussed in detail in Chapter 7, in many respects represented a revival of the philosophy of the Dawson Report (Chapter 5), or the health-centre programme in vogue at the end of World War II (Chapter 6). Both of these earlier initiatives foundered on account of opposition from the medical profession.

As noted in Chapter 7, it took determined effort by governments with strong electoral mandates to generate momentum for change. The new public management reforms instituted by the Conservatives in the early 1990s were reinforced by the modernisation plans introduced by Labour after 1997. You have attained some insight into the massive effect of these policies, which have already brought about a total reshaping of the NHS, and are likely to generate further radical changes.

Although the UK and the countries of the developing world represent very different health-care environments, Chapters 7 and 8 reveal striking parallels in the general direction of policy in the 1990s.

● Briefly summarise this common ground.

■ A change in economic philosophy, in line with the thinking of the World Bank, the International Monetary Fund, and the OECD, dictated moves towards market-oriented, competitive and privatised arrangements for health care, under the general banner of health sector reform.

Despite superficial differences in political rhetoric, this change of direction was broadly embraced by governments of both right and left political persuasion. As a consequence of the above policies, the absolute power hitherto exercised by the medical profession is gradually being eroded. This represents an epoch-making change. If carried to its logical conclusion, this will result in health care becoming the responsibility of a truly multi-disciplinary partnership of health-care professions.

Changes of this kind would bring about convergence in character between primary care teams in the UK and their developing-world equivalents. Primary care in a Western economy would thereby achieve some of the accessibility that has long characterised primary health-care initiatives in developing countries.

10.5   Limits to a world health-care system

10.5.1   Convergence

This book has underlined the historical basis for the *persisting* diversity (and by implication substantial inequalities) of health care. This argument needed to be developed to combat the once-dominant opinion in Western social science that differences between one place and another were confined to inessentials. Having established the importance of diversity and the local socio-political environment, it is necessary to acknowledge that economic development and modernisation have irrevocably produced a large measure of social and economic uniformity. The examples of medicine and health care illustrate this conclusion. The tried successes of biomedical science have given Western medicine an assured standing throughout the world. Numerous conditions are treated everywhere in the same manner, by medical personnel trained similarly, and all linked by a universal system of professional organisations and a body of advanced knowledge enshrined in academic journals. The evidence of migration of all types of medical personnel given in Chapter 9 draws attention to the uniformity of medical and nursing training.

10.5.2   Global medicine

'Western' medicine has become something of a misnomer: 'Western' relates to remote historical origins. Since the beginning of the twentieth century biomedical science has provided the universal language of medicine, used and understood throughout the world, and applied with dramatic effect. The advancement of medicine is the work of scientists of every nationality. Uniformity of standards and practices has permitted the mobilisation of medical expertise on a massive scale, as witnessed by the remarkably impressive campaigns of immunisation and vaccination described in Chapter 8.

● What major infectious diseases have been brought at least substantially under control in both developed and developing regions by immunisation and vaccination?

■ Diphtheria, polio, smallpox, whooping cough, measles, and, until recently, TB.

As noted in Chapter 3, vaccination for smallpox dates from 1798. This simple intervention was destined to become the single most effective medical discovery made before 1900, and perhaps the only one to have had significant worldwide demographic effect. The definitive triumph for preventive medicine was announced in 1980 when WHO declared that its global campaign to eliminate smallpox had been successfully concluded. In the course of the nineteenth century, the main demographic impact of medicine came through the various avenues of 'public health'; however, many of these interventions were only 'medical' in the most limited sense.

● List some public-health interventions in which the 'medical model' of health care was extremely limited or absent.

■ You may have thought of the provision of services such as sanitation, sewage disposal and a clean water supply; action on town planning, housing standards and overcrowding; environmental controls governing pollution and food safety; education access programmes, particularly to increase participation in primary schooling by children and to raise literacy rates among women; and legislation to protect workers from occupational injury, among other examples.

Most of the advances in immunology, chemotherapy and surgery which have transformed the capacity of medicine to save lives and improve the quality of life belong to the twentieth century, although of course they were the fruit of researches begun in previous centuries.

10.5.3   Global retrenchment

For much of the twentieth century medical advance proceeded at an almost exponential rate. There was always a time-lag in the wholesale application of these advances, explicable in various ways, but often involving the ingredient of resource limitation. As explained in Chapters 7 and 9, since the oil crisis of 1973, even the most wealthy economies have experienced profound difficulties in guaranteeing access to the latest benefits of modern medicine to their entire populations. The 'taming of the age-old scourge of premature and preventable death' (Kirkwood, Reith Lecture 1, 2001) was therefore a benefit that was indefinitely postponed as far as most of the world's population was concerned. This economic downturn converted health care into one of the most intractable policy problems facing Western governments. As a consequence, the 1990s were characterised by a wave of efforts at major reform. Chapters 7 and 8 considered these changes in some detail with respect to the Western and developing-world contexts. As in the past the results of these reforms are characterised by some generic similarities, but they have also contributed to the continuing diversity of health-care systems.

10.5.4   Global exploitation

When stark economic realities forced Western industrialised nations to reassess their spending on health care, through vehicles such as the International Monetary Fund, they made sure that the developing world responded to the same pressures. Even minor cutbacks in already hard-pressed health-care systems had a crippling effect. In many respects globalisation has worsened the plight of developing countries. For instance, some low-income countries have experienced erosion of all classes of their trained health personnel. Since its creation, the NHS has relied heavily on immigrant professionals such as doctors from the Indian subcontinent and nurses from the West Indies — a dependence that sharply increased in the 1990s, as indicated in the later chapters of this book.

Many other advanced Western economies also turned to the developing world for their supply of doctors, nurses and auxiliary staff. For the West this represented a cheap source of labour that was in short supply at home, producing an unfortunate domino effect. The UK has recruited staff from South Africa, which in turn has poached from its northern neighbours; these countries have been forced into desperate measures such as contracting medical and nursing staff from China. This unsavoury trade has exercised a destabilising effect, with the poorest countries being the worst sufferers.

The above examples show that expectations that such factors as liberalisation of trade, the growth of information technology, the improvement of training, and greater availability of new therapies would unify and equalise health care systems have proved to be wildly overoptimistic. The idea that the world economic system would generate even an effective 'trickle down' effect is not borne out by experience. Indeed the world economic system might well exacerbate the handicaps of low and middle-income economies. The failure of the malaria eradication campaigns mentioned in Chapters 6 and 8 indicate that relatively simple interventions have failed owing to the absence of stable, elementary welfare infrastructures.

10.6   Poverty and health

Finally, this book has demonstrated that although medical services have contributed to controlling certain diseases, they have played only a limited part in the optimisation of health. The latter depends for the most part on effective measures to combat poverty and economic exploitation. As we are reminded by many illustrations included in this book, low family income, unemployment and adverse working conditions have always been passports to malnutrition and diseases associated with bad housing conditions and unhealthy occupations. Of course, entirely different diseases stem from affluence, but the burden is nothing like that carried by the poor. Indeed, the poor in all parts of the world are also afflicted by impediments to health connected with affluent lifestyle and imported or even imposed on them from the richer economies.

● What examples of such imports to developing countries spring to mind?

■ Feeding babies with formula milk, the fashion for canned soft drinks, or Western food habits. Even more pernicious: alcohol, organised prostitution, changes in nutrition consequent on enforced transition to cash crops including tobacco, or inducement to become engaged in the production and distribution of other addictive drugs.

Of course, alcohol, addictive drugs and prostitution are not creations of the advanced economies, but the scale of their impact has been exacerbated by Western influence.

For the above reasons, it is clear that any realistic programme of health maintenance must be based on the attainment of higher living standards and achievement of social justice for the entire population. Consequently our historical review has paid attention to environmental regulation, sanitation and water supply, and also education and the wider economic and political sources of inequality. As indicated in Chapter 2, the traditional 'best practices' of the religious institutions of poor relief embodied the assumption that social support and maintenance of independent subsistence were the main guarantee of sound health. Chapter 4 reminds us of the benefits stemming from the Victorian sanitarian programme which gave priority to environmental regulation. After this heroic inception, the momentum of public health was gradually lost. In the course of the twentieth century, Western health planners became increasingly preoccupied with facilitating the expanding capacities of curative medicine. For the people, this switch of priorities had disastrous consequences, since it enabled governments to evade their preventive responsibilities and avoid confronting the many powerful corporate interests whose wealth depended on the neglect of public health.

Appreciation of the unity of factors relevant to health prompted the famous dictum by Rudolph Virchow, the German pioneer of health reform: 'Medicine is social science, and politics is nothing more than medicine on a grand scale' (quoted in Rather, 1985, p. xiii). In the 1940s the conception 'social medicine' encapsulated this idea. In Britain, the Black Report (1980) and the World Health Organisation's primary health-care, health-promotion and new public-health initiatives, discussed in Chapters 7, 8 and 9, have represented recent statements of the inseparability of social justice and health care. This principle is easier to enunciate than to follow. Mass experience of extreme social adversity ceased in Europe only after World War II. Thereafter destitution and poverty were reduced, but never became things of the past, even in North America or Western Europe.

Nevertheless, the problems of the poor in Europe and other Western economies are on nothing like the scale experienced in the developing world. Long ago the influential Swiss medical thinker Henry Sigerist warned that 'to immunise coloured people against disease with the one hand and to exploit them into starvation with the other is a grim joke' (Sigerist, 1943, p. 236). As our book demonstrates, despite all the urgent efforts of relief agencies, large tracts of the developing world are facing starvation under the relentless pressures of exploitation, political instability, environmental degradation and uncontrolled population increase. Such phenomena as global warming will undoubtedly worsen this disastrous situation.

Although immunisation programmes are one of the most successful elements in the primary health-care initiative, they will constitute no more than a minor palliative unless basic problems of poverty are addressed. Accordingly, without substantial measures of social justice there is no likelihood of enduring relief from the unremitting succession of health crises that are endemic to large parts of the developing world.

Although inequalities in health stemming from poverty in the Western economies are of a lower order, they nevertheless represent a severe problem. Since the UK has done much less than its Western neighbours to bridge the gap between rich and poor, its problem of health inequality is proportionately greater. The poorer parts of cities like Glasgow rate among the most unhealthy in Europe. Glasgow today is the counterpart of Manchester and Liverpool in 1850. As was appreciated in a long series of classic reports ranging from Engels' *The Condition of the Working Class in England* to the Black Report and its subsequent updates, a broad programme of measures to enhance social justice represents the only effective means to close the health gap between rich and poor.

In recognition of the essential global similarities of the problem of inequalities in health, the World Health Organisation has, since 1970, evolved initiatives in primary health care, public health and health promotion intended to apply in all countries regardless of their wealth. All the reform programmes of the 1990s respond in some way to these initiatives. For the first time in history the achievement of 'health for all' has become adopted worldwide as a practicable objective. For the attainment of this almost utopian goal and the creation of appropriate systems of health care, the WHO rightly appreciates the need for a much greater exercise of 'national will' for health, which — in the more graphic language of earlier decades — was called by Sigerist the 'peoples' war' for health (Sigerist, 1952, p. 362). It is the task of the historians to monitor the ability of governments to turn this ideal into reality.

References and further sources

References

Abbott, P. and Meerabeau, L. (eds) (1998) *The Sociology of the Caring Professions,* UCL Press, London.

Abel-Smith, B. (1964) *The Hospitals, 1800–1948*, Heinemann, London.

Abrams, P. (1980) Social change, social networks and neighbourhood care, *Social Work Service*, No. 22, pp. 12–23.

Acheson Report (1988) *see* Department of Health and Social Security (1988).

Acheson Report (1998) *Independent Inquiry into Inequalities in Health,* The Stationery Office, London.

Allan, J. (1992) *Berthold Lubetkin: Architecture and the Condition of Progress*, RIBA, London.

Armstrong, D. (1983) *Political Anatomy of the Body: Medical Knowledge in Britain in the Twentieth Century*, Cambridge University Press, Cambridge.

Arnold, D. (1993) *Colonising the Body: State Medicine and Epidemic Disease in Nineteenth-Century India*, University of California Press, Berkeley.

Ashton, J. and Seymour, H. (1988) *The New Public Health*, Open University Press, Milton Keynes.

Austoker, J. (1988) *The History of the Imperial Cancer Research Fund 1902–1986*, Oxford University Press, Oxford.

Baker, N. and Urquhart, J. (1987) *The Balance of Care for Adults with a Mental Handicap in Scotland*, Scottish Health Service Information Services Division, Edinburgh.

Balfour, A. and Scott, H. H. (1924) *Health Problems of the Empire*, Collins, Glasgow.

Balint, M. (1956) *The Doctor, His Patient and The Illness*, Pitman, London.

Bannington, B. G. (1929) *English Public Health Administration*, 2nd edn, P. S. King & Son Ltd., London.

Bayly, C. A. (1988) *Indian Society and the Making of the British Empire,* Cambridge University Press, Cambridge.

Berridge, V. (1979) Opium and oral history, *Oral History*, **7**, pp. 48–58.

Berridge, V. (1990) 'Health and medicine, 1750–1950', in Thompson, F. M. L. (ed.) *The Cambridge Social History of Britain, 1750–1950*, Vol. 3, Cambridge University Press, Cambridge.

Berridge, V. (1996) *AIDS in the UK. The Making of Policy, 1981–1994*, Oxford University Press, Oxford.

Berridge, V. and Edwards, G. (1987) *Opium and the People: Opiate Use in Nineteenth-Century England*, Yale University Press, New Haven.

Beveridge, W. (1942) *Report on Social Insurance and Allied Services*, Cmd. 6404, HMSO, London (the 'Beveridge Report').

Bloom, G. and Xingyuan, G. (1997) Health sector reform: lessons from China, *Social Science and Medicine*, **45**, pp. 351–60. An edited extract from this article appears under the same title in Davey, B., Gray, A. and Seale, C. (eds) (2001) *Health and Disease: A Reader*, 3rd edn, Open University Press, Buckingham.

Blyth, M. (1986) A century of health education, *Health and Hygiene*, **7**, pp. 105–15.

Bobadilla, J. L., Cowley, P., Musgrove, P. and Saxienien, H. (1994) 'Design, content and financing of an essential national package of health services', in Murray, C. J. L. and Lopez, A. D. (eds) *Global Comparative Assessments in the Health Sector: Disease Burden, Expenditure and Intervention Packages*, WHO, Geneva.

Bosanquet, N. and Salisbury, C. (1998) 'The practice', in Loudon, I., Horder, J. and Webster, C. (eds) *General Practice under the National Health Service 1948–1997*, Clarendon Press, Oxford.

British Medical Association (1938) *A General Medical Service for the Nation*, BMA, London.

British Medical Association (1986) *Alternative Therapy*, BMA, London.

British Medical Association (1993) *Complementary Medicine: New Approaches to Good Practice*, Oxford University Press, Oxford.

Brockington, C. F. (1965) *Public Health in the Nineteenth Century*, Livingstone, Edinburgh.

Brook, C. (1945) *Battling Surgeon*, The Strickland Press, Glasgow.

Brookes, B. (1988) *Abortion in England, 1900–1967*, Croom Helm, Beckenham.

Bulmer, M. (1987) *The Social Basis of Community Care*, Allen and Unwin, London.

Burgess, M. (1990) Milk shake-up, *The Guardian*, 20 November.

Buse, K. (1994) Spotlight on international organisations … The World Bank, *Health and Policy Planning*, **9**, pp. 95–9.

Caldwell, J. C. (1986) Routes to low mortality in poor countries, *Population and Development Review*, **12**, pp. 171–220.

Cassels, A. (1995) Health sector reform: key issues in less developed countries, *Journal of International Development*, Special Issue, **7**, pp. 329–48.

Chowdhury, M. and Vaughan, J. P. (1988) Perception of diarrhoea and the use of a homemade oral rehydration solution in rural Bangladesh, *Journal of Diarrhoeal Diseases Research*, **6**, pp. 6–14.

CIPFA (Chartered Institute of Public Finance and Accountancy) (1984) *Health Care UK 1984: An Economic, Social and Policy Audit*, CIPFA, London.

Cipolla, C. M. (1976) *Public Health and the Medical Profession in the Renaissance*, Cambridge University Press, Cambridge.

Colatrella, B. D. (1998) Corporate donations, *Annals of Tropical Medicine and Parasitology*, **92**, Supplement, p. S154.

Comptroller and Auditor General (2000) *Inpatient Admissions and Bed Management in NHS Acute Hospitals*, The Stationery Office, London.

Constantine, S. (1983) *Social Conditions in Britain, 1918–1939*, Methuen, London.

Consultative Council on Medical and Allied Services (1920) *Interim Report on the Future Provision of Medical and Allied Services*, Cmd. 693, HMSO, London (the 'Dawson Report').

Corfield, P. J. (1982, reprinted 1989) *The Impact of English Towns 1700–1800*, Oxford University Press, Oxford.

Cornia, G. A. and Stewart, F. (1995) 'Two errors of targeting', in van de Walle, D. and Nead, K. (eds) *Public Spending and the Poor: Theory and Evidence*, Johns Hopkins University Press, for the World Bank, Baltimore and London.

Crosby, A. W. (1974) *The Columbian Exchange: The Biological and Cultural Consequences of 1492*, Greenwood, Westport, Connecticut.

Crosby, A. W. (1986) *Ecological Imperialism: The Biological Expansion of Europe, 900–1900*, Cambridge University Press, Cambridge.

Davies, C. (1988) The health visitor as mother's friend: a woman's place in public health, 1900–14, *Social History of Medicine*, **1**, pp. 39–59.

Davies, C. (1995) *Gender and the Professional Predicament in Nursing*, Open University Press, Buckingham. An edited extract from Chapter 7 of this book appears under the title 'Professionalism and the conundrum of care', in Davey, B., Gray, A. and Seale, C. (eds) (2001) *Health and Disease: A Reader*, 3rd edn, Open University Press, Buckingham.

de Morgan, S. E. and Smith, D. E. (eds) (1915) *A Budget of Paradoxes*, Vol 1, 2nd edn, The Open Court Publishing Co., Chicago and London.

Denoon, D. (1989) *Public Health in Papua New Guinea: Medical Possibility and Social Constraints, 1884–1984*, Cambridge University Press, Cambridge.

Department of Health (1992) *The Health of the Nation*, Cm. 1986, HMSO, London.

Department of Health (1997) *The New NHS Modern Dependable*, Cm. 3807, The Stationery Office, London.

Department of Health (1998) *Informal Carers: Results of an independent study carried out on behalf of the Department of Health as part of the1995 General Household Survey*, The Stationery Office, London.

Department of Health (1999) *Our Healthier Nation*, Cm. 3852, The Stationery Office, London.

Department of Health (1999a) *Smoking, Drinking and Drug Use among Teenagers, 1998, Volume 1: England*, The Stationery Office, London.

Department of Health (2000) *Shaping the Future NHS: Long Term Planning for Hospitals and Related Services; Consultation document on the findings of the National Beds Inquiry*, The Stationery Office, London.

Department of Health (2000a) *The NHS Plan*, Cm. 4818, The Stationery Office, London.

Department of Health and Social Security (1971) *Better Services for the Mentally Handicapped*, Cmnd. 4683, HMSO, London.

Department of Health and Social Security (1976) *Prevention and Health: Everybody's Business*, DHSS, London.

Department of Health and Social Security (1980) *Inequalities in Health, Report of a Working Group*, DHSS, London (the 'Black Report').

Department of Health and Social Security (1981) *Drinking Sensibly*, DHSS, London.

Department of Health and Social Security (1988) *Public Health in England*, HMSO, London (the 'first Acheson Report').

Diesfeld, H. J. and Hecklau, H. K. (1978) *Kenya: A Geomedical Monograph*, Springer-Verlag, Berlin.

Digby, A. (1989) *British Welfare Policy: Workhouse to Workfare*, Faber and Faber, London.

Digby, A. (1994) *Making a Medical Living. Doctors and Patients in the English Market for Medicine, 1720–1911*, Cambridge University Press, Cambridge.

Digby, A. and Bosanquet, N. (1988) Doctors and patients in an era of national health insurance and private practice, 1913–38, *Economic History Review*, **41**, pp. 74–94.

Dingwall, R., Rafferty, A. M. and Webster, C. (1988) *An Introduction to the Social History of Nursing*, Routledge, London.

Djukanovic, V. and Mach, E. P. (1975) *Alternative Approaches to Meeting Basic Health Needs*, UNICEF/WHO, Geneva.

Doyal, L. and Pennell, I. (1979) *The Political Economy of Health*, Pluto Press, London.

Draper, P. (ed.) (1991) *Health Through Public Policy: The Greening of Public Health*, Greenprint, London.

Dunn, C. L. (1952) *Emergency Medical Services*, Volume 1 from the series *Medical History of the Second World War*, HMSO, London.

Dunn, S. (1999) *Creating Accepting Communities. Report of the Mind inquiry into social exclusion and mental health problems*, Mind Publications, London.

Dunnell, K. and Cartwright, A. (1972) *Medicine Takers, Prescribers and Hoarders*, Routledge, London.

Dupree, M. W. (1995) *Family Structure in the Staffordshire Potteries, 1840–1880*, Clarendon Press, Oxford.

Dutt, R. P. (1940) *India Today*, Victor Gollancz, London.

Eckstein, H. (1958) *The English Health Service*, Harvard University Press, Cambridge, Massachusetts.

Edelstein, L. (1967) *Ancient Medicine*, Temkin, O. and Temkin, C. L. (eds) The Johns Hopkins University Press, Baltimore.

Elias, N. (1978) *The Civilising Process. I: The History of Manners*, translated by Jephcott, E., Basil Blackwell, Oxford.

Elliott-Binns, C. P. (1973) An analysis of lay medicine, *Journal of the Royal College of General Practitioners*, **23**, pp. 255–64.

Elliott-Binns, C. P. (1986) An analysis of lay medicine: 15 years later, *Journal of the Royal College of General Practitioners*, **36**, pp. 542–4.

Emmerson, C., Frayne, C. and Goodman, A. (2000) *Pressures in UK Health Care: Challenges for the NHS*, Institute for Fiscal Studies, London.

Engels, F. (1845) *The Condition of the Working Class in England*, reprinted in 1969 with introduction by E. Hobsbawm, Panther, London. An edited extract appears under the title 'Health: 1844' in Davey, B., Gray, A. and Seale, C. (eds) (2001) *Health and Disease: A Reader*, 3rd edn, Open University Press, Buckingham.

Eyler, J. M. (1979) *Victorian Social Medicine: The Ideas and Methods of William Farr*, The Johns Hopkins University Press, Baltimore.

Finch, J. and Groves, D. (eds) (1983) *A Labour of Love: Women, Work and Caring*, Routledge, London.

Fisher, P. and Ward, A. (1994) Medicine in Europe: complementary medicine in Europe, *British Medical Journal*, **309**, pp. 107–11.

Flinn, M. W. (ed.) (1965) *Report on the Sanitary Condition of the Labouring Population of Great Britain, by Edwin Chadwick, 1842*, Edinburgh University Press, Edinburgh.

Flora, P. and Heidenheimer, A. J. (eds) (1981) *The Development of Welfare States in Europe and North America*, Transaction Publishers, Piscataway, New Jersey.

Flynn, R. and Williams, G. (1997) *Contracting for Health*, Oxford University Press, Oxford.

Forsyth, G. (1963) *Doctors and State Medicine*, Pitman, London.

Foster, W. D. (1978) *Sir Albert Cook: A Missionary Doctor in Uganda*, Newhaven Press, Newhaven, Sussex.

Foundation for Integrated Medicine (1997) *Integrated Healthcare: A Way Forward for the next Five Years*, FIM, London.

Fraser, D. (1973) *The Evolution of the British Welfare State*, Macmillan, London.

French, R. D. (1975) *Antivivisection and Victorian Society*, Princeton University Press, Princeton and London.

Gilbert, B. B. (1966) *The Evolution of National Insurance in Great Britain*, Michael Joseph, London.

Gillam, S. (1999) Linkworkers in primary care (Editorial), *British Medical Journal*, **319**, p. 1215.

Godber, G. (1975) *The Health Service: Past, Present and Future*, Athlone, London.

Godber, G. (1983) The Doomsday Book of British Hospitals, *Bulletin of the Society for the Social History of Medicine*, **42**, pp. 4–13.

Graham, H. (1979) 'Prevention and health: every mother's business; a comment on child health policies in the 1970s', in Harris, C. (ed.) *The Sociology of the Family*, New Directions for Britain, Keele.

Graves, C. (1947) *The Story of St Thomas's 1106–1947*, Faber and Faber Ltd., London.

Gray, N. (1986) *The Worst of Times: An Oral History of the Great Depression in Britain*, Wildwood House, London.

Griffiths, R. (1983) *NHS Management Inquiry*, DHSS, London. [The first 'Griffiths Report' was in the form of a 24-page letter from Roy Griffiths (later, Sir Roy Griffiths) to the Secretary of State for Health, Norman Fowler, which was never formally published. The full text appears as an Appendix, pp. 157–77, in Harrison, S. (1994) *National Health Service Management in the 1980s*, Avebury, Aldershot.]

Griffiths, R. (1988) *Community Care: Agenda for Action*, HMSO, London (the second 'Griffiths Report').

Griffiths, S. and Hunter, D. (eds) (1999) *Perspectives in Public Health*, Radcliffe Medical Press, Abingdon.

Guillebaud Report (1956) *see* Ministry of Health (1956).

Gunning, O. (2000) Overseas nurse recruitment soars, *Nursing Times*, 15 June.

Hardoy, J., Cairncross, S. and Satterthwaite, D. (1990) *The Poor Die Young*, Earthscan Publications Ltd., London.

Haynes, B. (1991) *Working-class Life in Victorian Leicester: The Joseph Dare Reports*, Leicestershire County Council, Leicester.

Headrick, D. R. (1988) *The Tentacles of Progress: Technology Transfer in the Age of Imperialism, 1850–1940*, Oxford University Press, Oxford.

Heggenhoughen, K., Vaughan, P., Muhondwa, E. and Rutabanzibwa-Ngaiza, J. (1987) *Community Health Workers: The Tanzanian Experience*, Oxford University Press, Oxford.

Helman, C. (1984, re-published 1995 and 2001) 'Feed a cold, starve a fever', in Davey, B., Gray, A. and Seale, C. (eds) *Health and Disease: A Reader*, 3rd edn, Open University Press, Buckingham.

Helman, C. (1990) *Culture, Health and Illness*, 2nd edn, Butterworth–Heinemann, Oxford.

Holland, H. (1958) *Frontier Doctor*, Hodder & Stoughton, London.

Horder, J. (1998) 'Developments in other countries', in Loudon, I., Horder, J. and Webster, C. (eds) *General Practice Under the National Health Service 1948–1997*, Clarendon Press, Oxford.

Hurst, J. (1985) *Financing Health Services in the United States, Canada and Britain*, King Edward's Hospital Fund for London, London.

Jeffery, P. *et al.* (1989) *Labour Pains and Labour Power: Women and Childbearing in India*, Zed Press, London.

Jeffery, R. (1988) *The Politics of Health in India*, University of California Press, Berkeley.

Jefferys, M. and Sachs, H. (1983) *Rethinking General Practice. Dilemmas in Primary Medical Care*, Tavistock, London.

Jenner, M. (1991) *Early Modern English Conceptions of 'Cleanliness' and 'Dirt' as Reflected in the Environmental Regulation of London c. 1530–c. 1700*, D. Phil. dissertation, University of Oxford.

Jewell, T. (1999) 'Public health practice in health authorities', in Griffiths, S. and Hunter, D. (eds) *Perspectives in Public Health*, Radcliffe Press, Oxford.

Jiminez, E. (1986) The public subsidisation of education and health in developing countries: a review of equity and efficiency, *World Bank Research Observer*, **1**, pp. 111–29.

Johnson, J. (1812) *The Influence of Tropical Climates, More Especially the Climate of India on European Constitutions; the Principal Effects and Diseases thereby Induced; and the Means of Preserving Health in Hot Climates*, J. Callow, London.

Jordan, B. (1989) Cosmopolitical obstetrics: some insights from the training of traditional midwives, *Social Science and Medicine*, **28**, pp. 925–37.

Kaleeba, N., Ray, S. and Willmore, B. (1991) *We Miss You All*, Women and AIDS Support Network (WASN), Zimbabwe.

Katz, A. and Bender, E. (1976) *The Strength in Us*, New Viewpoints, New York.

Kee, H. C. (1986) *Medicine, Miracle & Magic in New Testament Times*, Cambridge University Press, Cambridge.

Kelleher, D. (1994) 'Self-help groups and their relationship to medicine', in Gabe, J., Kelleher, D. and Williams, G. (eds) *Challenging Medicine*, Routledge, London.

King, M. (1966) *Medical Care in Developing Countries*, Oxford University Press, Oxford.

Kyd, J. G. (ed.) (1952) *Scottish Population Statistics*, Scottish Historical Society, Edinburgh.

Land, H. (1978) Who cares for the family? *Journal of Social Policy*, **7**, pp. 357–84.

Larkin, G. (1987) The licensing of health professions: medical or ministry control? *Bulletin of the Society for the Social History of Medicine*, **40**, pp. 51–3.

Lawrence, C. J. (1975) William Buchan: medicine laid open, *Medical History*, **19**, pp. 20–35.

Laybourne, K. (1990) *Britain on the Breadline*, Alan Sutton Publishing, Gloucester.

Lewis, J. (1980) *The Politics of Motherhood*, Croom Helm, Beckenham.

Lewis, J. (1986) *What Price Community Medicine? The Philosophy and Practice of Public Health 1918–1980*, Wheatsheaf, Brighton.

Llewellyn Davies, M. (ed.) (1915) *Maternity: Letters from Working Women collected by the Women's Co-operative Guild*, G. Bell & Sons, London; reprinted in 1978 by Virago, London.

Loudon, I. (1986) *Medical Care and the General Practitioner 1750–1850*, Clarendon Press, Oxford.

Loudon, I. (1991) On maternal and infant mortality, 1900–1960, *Social History of Medicine*, **4**, pp. 29–73.

Loudon, I., Horder, J. and Webster, C. (eds) *General Practice Under the National Health Service 1948–1997*, Clarendon Press, Oxford.

Lyons, M. (1988) 'Sleeping sickness, colonial medicine and imperialism: some connections in the Belgian Congo', in MacLeod, R. and Lewis, M. (eds) *Disease, Medicine and Empire: Perspectives on Western Medicine and the Experience of European Expansion*, Routledge, London.

M'Gonigle, G. C. M. and Kirby, J. (1936) *Poverty and Public Health*, Victor Gollancz, London.

MacFarlane, A. and Mugford, M. (1984) *Birth Counts: Statistics of Pregnancy and Childbirth*, HMSO, London; 2nd edn (2000), with Henderson, J., TSO, London.

Maggs, C. J. (1983) *The Origins of General Nursing*, Croom Helm, Beckenham.

Mahler, H. (1975) Health for all by the year 2000, *WHO Chronicle*, **29**, pp. 457–61.

Marks, S. (1988) The historical origins of National Health Services, in *Towards a National Health Service: Proceedings of the 1987 Namda Annual Conference*, Cape Town, South Africa.

Marland, H. (1987) *Medicine and Society in Wakefield and Huddersfield 1780–1870*, Cambridge University Press, Cambridge.

Martin, J. R. (1837) *The Medical Topography of Calcutta*, G. H. Huttman, Calcutta.

Maxwell, R. (1981) *Health and Wealth: An International Study of Health-care Spending*, Lexington Books, Massachusetts, USA.

Mbugua, J. K., Bloom, G.H. and Segall, M. M. (1995) Impact of user charges on vulnerable groups: the case of Kibwezi in rural Kenya, *Social Science and Medicine*, **41**, pp. 829–35.

McKeown, T. (1976) *The Modern Rise of Population*, Edward Arnold London. An edited extract from Chapter 5 of that book appears under the title 'The medical contribution', in Davey, B., Gray, A. and Seale, C. (eds) (2001) *Health and Disease: A Reader*, 3rd edn, Open University Press, Buckingham.

McMichael, A. and Haines, A. (1997) Global climate change: the potential effects on health, *British Medical Journal*, **315**, pp. 805–9.

McPake, B., Hanson, K. and Mills, A. (1993) Community financing in health care in Africa: an evaluation of the Bamako Initiative, *Social Science and Medicine*, **36**, pp. 1383–95.

McVie, G. (1999) quoted in 'Cancer cure explosion to plunge NHS into crisis', *The Guardian*, 21 October.

Milburn, A. (2000) quoted in 'Milburn says NHS too slow to change', *The Independent*, 19 May.

Ministry of Health (1944) *A National Health Service*, Cmd. 6502, HMSO, London.

Ministry of Health (1956) *Report of the Committee of Enquiry into the Cost of the National Health Service*, Cmd. 9663, HMSO, London (the 'Guillebaud Report').

Ministry of Health (1962) *A Hospital Plan for England*, Cmnd. 1604, HMSO, London.

Ministry of Health (1963) *Health and Welfare: The Development of Community Care*, Cmnd. 1973, HMSO, London.

Ministry of National Service (1919) *Report upon the Physical Examination of Men of Military Age by National Service Medical Boards from 1st November 1917 to 31st October 1918*, Cmd. 504, HMSO, London.

Mitchell, B. R. (1988) *British Historical Statistics*, Cambridge University Press, Cambridge.

Mitchell, B. R. and Deane, P. (1971) *Abstract of British Historical Statistics*, **316**, Cambridge University Press, Cambridge.

Morley, D., Rohde, J. and Williams, G. (1983, reprinted 1989) *Practising Health for All*, Oxford University Press, Oxford.

Morrell, D. (1998) 'Introduction and overview', in Loudon, I., Horder, J. and Webster, C. (eds) *General Practice Under the National Health Service 1948–1997*, Clarendon Press, Oxford.

Muraleedharan, V. R. (1987) Rural health care in the Madras Presidency: 1919–39, *Indian Economic and Social History Review*, **24**, pp. 323–34.

Newdick, C. (1995) *Who should we treat? Law, Patients and Resources in the NHS*, Oxford University Press, Oxford.

Newell, K. (1975) *Health by the People*, WHO, Geneva.

Newell, K. (1988) Selective primary health care: the counter revolution, *Social Science and Medicine*, **26**, pp. 903–6.

Newsholme, Sir A. (1925) *The Ministry of Health*, Putnams, London.

NHS Executive (1999) *Clinical Governance: Quality in the New NHS*, Health Service Circular 1999/065, Department of Health, Leeds.

OECD (1999) *OECD Health Data 1999*, CREDOC/OECD, Paris.

OECD (2000) *OECD Health Data 2000*, CREDOC/OECD, Paris.

Office of Health Economics (1999) *Compendium of Health Statistics*, 11th edition, OHE, London.

Office for National Statistics (1998) *Informal Carers, Supplement A, General Household Survey*, ONS, The Stationery Office, London.

Paediatric Intensive Care Taskforce (1997) *Nursing Standards, Education and Workforce Planning in Paediatric Intensive Care*, NHS Executive, Leeds.

Patterson, T. (1983) 'Science and medicine in India', in Corsi, P. and Weindling, P. (eds) *Information Sources in the History of Science and Medicine*, Butterworth, London.

PEP (1937) *The British Health Services*, Political and Economic Planning, London.

PEP (1939) *Britain's Health*, Pelican Special, London.

Pickstone, J. V. (1985) *Medicine and Industrial Society: A History of Hospital Development in Manchester and its Region, 1752–1946*, Manchester University Press, Manchester.

Porter, R. (1997) *The Greatest Benefit to Mankind*, HarperCollins Publishers, London. An edited extract from Chapter III appears under the title 'Hippocrates', in Davey, B., Gray, A. and Seale, C. (eds) (2001) *Health and Disease: A Reader*, 3rd edn, Open University Press, Buckingham.

Potter, A. R. (1991) Dealing with two Africas, *British Medical Journal*, **303**, p. 1558.

Pound, J. F. (1971) *The Norwich Census of the Poor 1570*, Norfolk Record Society, Volume XL, Norwich.

Power, M. (1997) *The Audit Society. Rituals of Verification*, Oxford University Press, Oxford.

Pringle, M. (2000) Participating in clinical governance, *British Medical Journal*, **321**, pp. 737–40.

Prochaska, F. K. (1980) *Women and Philanthropy in 19th-Century England*, Oxford University Press, Oxford.

Prochaska, F. K. (1992) *Philanthropy and the Hospitals of London*, The King's Fund, Clarendon Press, Oxford.

Rather, L. J. (ed.) (1985) *Collected Essays on Public Health and Epidemiology of Rudolph Virchow*, Science-History Publications, New York.

Reidy, A. and Kitching, G. (1986) Primary health care: our sacred cow, their white elephant? *Public Administration and Development*, **6**, pp. 425–33.

Rivett, G. (1998) *From Cradle to Grave: Fifty Years of the NHS*, King's Fund, London.

Roberts, E. (1980) 'Oral history investigations of disease and its management by the Lancashire working class, 1890–1939', in Pickstone, J. (ed.) *Health, Disease and Medicine in Lancashire, 1750–1950*, UMIST Occasional Publications, No. 2, Manchester.

Roberts, E. (1984) The working class extended family: functions and attitudes, 1890–1940, *Oral History*, **12**, pp. 48–55.

Roberts, F. (1952) *The Cost of Health*, Turnstile, London.

Roberts, R. (1971) *The Classic Slum*, Penguin, Harmondsworth.

Robinson, J. and Strong, P. M. (1987) *Professional Nursing Advice after Griffiths: An Interim Report*, Nursing Policy Studies Centre, University of Warwick, Coventry.

Rogers, A. and Pilgrim, D. (1998) *Mental Health Policy in Britain*, Macmillan, London.

Ross, J. S. (1952) *The National Health Service in Great Britain*, Oxford University Press, London.

Ross, R. (1923) *Memoirs*, John Murray, London.

Rowse, A. L. (1974) *The Casebooks of Simon Forman*, Picador, London.

Royal College of Physicians (1962) *Smoking and Health*, RCP, London.

Royal Colleges of Physicians, Psychiatrists and General Practitioners (1996) *Chronic Fatigue Syndrome. Joint Report of the Royal Colleges of Physicians, Psychiatrists and General Practitioners*, RCP, London.

Royal Commission on Long Term Care (1999) *With Respect to Old Age. Long Term Care – Rights and Responsibilities*, Cm. 4192, The Stationery Office, London.

Royal Commission on Medical Education (1968) *Royal Commission on Medical Education Report 1965–68*, Cmnd. 3569, HMSO, London (the 'Todd Report').

Royal Commission on the NHS (1979) *Report of the Royal Commission on the NHS*, Cmnd. 7615, HMSO, London.

Salvage, J. (1985) *The Politics of Nursing*, William Heinemann Medical Books, London.

Scally, G. and Donaldson, L. J. (1998) Clinical governance and the drive for quality improvement in the new NHS in England, *British Medical Journal*, **317**, pp. 61–5.

Scharlieb, M. (1907–8) Alcohol and the children of the nation, *British Journal of Inebriety*, **5**, pp. 59–82.

Schweitzer, P. (ed.) (1985) *Can We Afford the Doctor?* Age Exchange Publications, London.

Scull, A. (1979) *Museums of Madness: The Social Organisation of Insanity in 19th Century England*, Allen Lane, London.

Scull, A. (1993) *The Most Solitary of Afflictions: Madness and Society in Britain 1700–1900*, Yale University Press, New Haven, Connecticut.

Secretary of State for Health (1989) *Working for Patients*, Cm. 555, HMSO, London.

Shaw, M. *et al.* (1999) *The Widening Gap: Health Inequalities and Policy in Britain*, Policy Press, London.

Shellard, P. (1970) *Factory Life 1774–1885*, Evans Bros., subsequently HarperCollins Publishers Ltd., London.

Sheridan, R. B. (1985) *Doctors and Slaves: A Medical and Demographic History of Slavery in the British West Indies 1680–1834*, Cambridge University Press, Cambridge.

Sigerist, H. (1943) *Civilization and Disease*, Chicago University Press, Chicago.

Sigerist, H. (1952) 'Remarks on social medicine in medical education', in Roemer, M. L. (ed.) *On the Sociology of Medicine*, MD Publications, New York.

Simon, J. (1897) *English Sanitary Institutions*, 2nd edn, Smith, Elder & Co., London.

Slack, P. (1988) *Poverty and Policy in Tudor and Stuart England*, Longman, London.

Snell, K. D. M. (1987) *Annals of the Labouring Poor: Social Change and Agrarian England 1660–1900*, Cambridge University Press, Cambridge.

Sorsby, A. (1944) *Medicine and Mankind*, Watts and Co., London.

Stacey, M. (1988) *The Sociology of Health and Healing*, Unwin Hyman, London.

Starr, P. (1982) *The Social Transformation of American Medicine*, Basic Books, New York.

Stevens, R. (1966) *Medical Practice in Modern England: The Impact of Specialization and State Medicine*, Yale University Press, New Haven and London.

Stevens, R. (1976) The evolution of the health-care systems in the United States and the United Kingdom: similarities and differences, *Priorities in the Use of Resources in Medicine*, No. 40, Fogerty International Center Proceedings, US Department of Health, Education and Welfare. An edited extract from this article appears under the same title in Davey, B., Gray, A. and Seale, C. (eds) (2001) *Health and Disease: A Reader*, 3rd edn, Open University Press, Buckingham.

Summers, A. (1988) *Angels and Citizens*, 1st edn, Routledge, London; 2nd edn, (2000) Threshold Press, Newbury, Berks.

Summers, A. (1989) The mysterious demise of Sarah Gamp: the domiciliary nurse and her detractors, *c*. 1830–1860, *Victorian Studies*, **32**, pp. 365–86.

Swaan, A. de (1988) *In Care of the State: Health Care, Education and Welfare in Europe and the USA in the Modern Era*, Polity Press, Cambridge.

Szreter, S. (1988) The importance of social intervention in Britain's mortality decline *c*. 1850–1914, *Social History of Medicine*, **1**, pp. 1–37. An edited extract from this article appears under the same title in Davey, B., Gray, A. and Seale, C. (eds) (2001) *Health and Disease: A Reader*, 3rd edn, Open University Press, Buckingham.

Taylor, D. (1986) *A Tale of Two Villages*, New Internationalist Publications, Oxford.

Taylor, P. (1984) *Smoke Ring. The Politics of Tobacco*, The Bodley Head, London.

Thomas, K., Fall, M., Parry, G. and Nicholl, J. (1995) *National Survey of Access to Complementary Health Care via General Practice*. Report to the Department of Health, SCHARR, Sheffield.

Thompson, E. P. (1975) *The Making of the English Working Class*, Penguin, Harmondsworth.

Thompson, P. (1975) *The Edwardians: The Remaking of British Society*, Weidenfeld & Nicolson, London.

Titmuss, R. M. (1938) *Poverty and Population*, Macmillan, London.

Townsend, P. (1962) *The Last Refuge*, Routledge, London.

Townsend, P. and Bosanquet, N. (1972) *Labour and Inequality*, Fabian Society, London.

Tudor Hart, J. (1988) *A New Kind of Doctor. The General Practitioner's Part in the Health of the Community*, Merlin Press, London.

Turner, B. (1987) *Medical Power and Social Knowledge*, Sage Publications, London.

Turshen, M. (1989) *The Politics of Public Health*, Zed Press, London.

UKCC (1986) *Project 2000: A New Preparation for Practice*, United Kingdom Central Council for Nursing, Midwifery and Health Visiting, London.

UKCC (2000) Overseas trained nurses and midwives coming to the UK at record levels (press release), United Kingdom Central Council for Nursing, Midwifery and Health Visiting, London.

Ungerson, C. (1983) 'Why do women care?' in Finch, J. and Groves, D. (eds) *A Labour of Love: Women, Work and Caring*, Routledge, London.

UNICEF (1990) *The State of the World's Children*, Oxford University Press, Oxford.

United Nations Development Programme (1999) *Human Development Report 1999*, Oxford University Press, Oxford.

Vaughan, M. (1991) *Curing Their Ills: Colonial Power and African Illness*, Polity Press, Cambridge.

Vincent, D. (1991) *Poor Citizens. The State and the Poor in Twentieth Century Britain*, Longman, London.

Vincent-Priya, J. (1991) *Birth Without Doctors*, Earthscan, London.

Vogel, R. (1990) Trends in health expenditures and revenue sources in sub-Saharan Africa. Background paper prepared for *African Health Policy*, World Bank, Washington, DC.

Walker, A. (ed.) (1982) *Community Care: The Family, the State and Social Policy*, Basil Blackwell and Martin Robertson, Oxford.

Walsh, J. and Warren, K. (1979) Selective primary health care, *New England Journal of Medicine*, **301**, pp. 967–74.

Walt, G. (ed.) (1990) *Community Health Workers in National Programmes: Just Another Pair of Hands?* The Open University Press, Milton Keynes.

Webster, C. (ed.) (1979) *Health, Medicine and Mortality in the Sixteenth Century*, Cambridge University Press, Cambridge.

Webster, C. (1982) Healthy or hungry thirties? *History Workshop*, No. 13, pp. 110–29.

Webster, C. (1991) *Aneurin Bevan on the National Health Service*, Wellcome Unit for the History of Medicine, Oxford.

Weindling, P. (1989) 'Population policies under fascism: Germany, Italy and Spain compared', in Teitelbaum, M. S. and Winter, J. (eds) *Population and Resources in Western Intellectual Traditions*, Cambridge University Press, Cambridge.

Wellard's NHS Handbook 2000/01 (2000) JMH Publishing, Wadhurst, East Sussex.

Werner, D. (1978) 'The village health-worker: lackey or liberator?', in Skeet, M. and Elliott, K. (eds) *Health Auxiliaries and the Health Team*, Croom Helm, London. This article is reproduced in Davey, B., Gray, A. and Seale, C. (eds) (2001) *Health and Disease: A Reader*, 3rd edn, Open University Press, Buckingham.

Whitehead, M. (1987) *The Health Divide: Inequalities in Health in the 1980s*, Health Education Authority, London.

WHO (1973) *Organizational Study on Methods of Promoting the Development of Basic Health Services*, Annex II, Official Records of the WHO, No. 206, World Health Organisation, Geneva.

WHO (1984) *The supervision of traditional birth attendants*, Unpublished paper HMD/NUR/84.1, Division of Health Manpower Development, World Health Organisation, Geneva.

WHO (1999) *Removing Obstacles to Healthy Development*, World Health Organisation, Geneva.

WHO (2000) *World Health Report. Health Systems: Improving Performance*, World Health Organisation, Geneva.

WHO–UNICEF (1978) *Alma Ata 1978*, Primary Health Care 'Health for All' Series, No. 1, World Health Organisation, Geneva.

WHO–UNICEF (2000) *Global Water Supply and Sanitation Assessment 2000 Report*, World Health Organisation, Geneva.

Winslow, C-E. A. (1952) *Man and Epidemics*, Princeton University Press, Princeton, New York.

Winter, J. (1986) *The Great War and the British People*, Macmillan, London.

Woelk, H. (2000) Comparison of St John's Wort and imipramine for treating depression: randomised controlled trial, *British Medical Journal*, **321**, pp. 536–9.

Wohl, A. S. (1983) *Endangered Lives: Public Health in Victorian Britain*, Harvard University Press, Cambridge, Massachusetts.

Woodward, J. (1974) *To Do the Sick no Harm: A Study of the British Voluntary Hospital System to 1875*, Routledge, London.

Worboys, M. (1988a) 'The discovery of colonial malnutrition between the wars', in Arnold, D. (ed.) *Imperial Medicine and Indigenous Societies*, Manchester University Press, Manchester.

Worboys, M. (1988b) 'Manson, Ross and colonial medical policy: tropical medicine in London and Liverpool, 1899–1914', in MacLeod, R. and Lewis, M. (eds) *Disease, Medicine, and Empire: Perspectives on Western Medicine and the Experience of European Expansion*, Routledge, London.

World Bank (various years) *World Development Report*, Oxford University Press, Oxford and New York.

World Bank (1987) *Financing Health Services in Developing Countries: An Agenda for Reform*, a World Bank policy study, World Bank, Washington, DC.

World Bank (1993) *Investing in Health*, World Bank, Washington, DC.

Wyman, A. L. (1984) The surgeoness: the female practitioner of surgery 1400–1800, *Medical History*, **28**, pp. 22–41.

Yoder, R. A. (1989) Are people willing and able to pay for health services? *Social Science and Medicine*, **29**, pp. 35–42.

Young, M. and Cullen, L. (1996) *A Good Death: Conversations with East Londoners*, Routledge, London. An edited extract from Chapter 4 of this book, under the title 'The carer at home', appears in Davey, B., Gray, A. and Seale, C. (eds) (2001) *Health and Disease: A Reader*, 3rd edn, Open University Press, Buckingham.

Young, M. and Willmott, P. (1962) *Family and Kinship in East London*, Pelican, London.

Zollman, C. and Vickers, A. (1999) Users and practitioners of complementary medicine, *British Medical Journal*, **319**, pp. 836–8.

Zwi, A. and Mills, A. (1995) Health policy in less developed countries: past trends and future directions, *Journal of International Development*, Special Issue, **7**, pp. 299–328.

Zwi, A. and Ugalde, A. (1991) Political violence in the Third World: a public health issue, *Health Policy and Planning*, **6**, pp. 203–17.

Further sources

The following lists are designed to supplement the information contained in the References. We have confined this additional guidance largely to books, most of which are recent and reasonably accessible. The further sources is organised under the five recurrent themes specified in Chapter 1, preceded by items of a more general nature. This additional guidance on reading has been limited to sources that constitute a next step in complexity. These books will provide guidance on the more specialised literature.

As you will notice from the References, we have utilised an extremely wide range of sources. Consequently it is not possible to refer you to any book conveniently covering the entire, or even a major, part of our subject matter.

General

For introductory purposes you might like to read the relevant chapters from I. Loudon (ed.) (1997) *Western Medicine: An Illustrated History*, Oxford University Press, Oxford; also Chapters 4, 7 and 12 of R. Lowe's *The Welfare State in Britain since 1945*, and Chapters 1, 4, 13 and 14 of F. D. Powell and A. F. Wessen (eds) (1999), *Health Care Systems in Transition: An International Perspective* — both cited below in the section on health-care systems.

Armstrong, D. (1983) *Political Anatomy of the Body: Medical Knowledge in Britain in the Twentieth Century*, Cambridge University Press, Cambridge.

Berridge, V. (1999) *Health and Society in Britain since 1939*, Cambridge University Press, Cambridge.

Digby, A. and Stewart, J. (eds) *Gender, Health and Welfare*, Routledge, London.

Pierson, C. (1999) *Beyond the Welfare State? A New Political Economy of Welfare*, Polity Press, Cambridge.

Porter, R. (1997) *The Greatest Benefit to Mankind. A Medical History of Humanity from Antiquity to the Present*, HarperCollins Publishers, London.

Shryock, R. H. (1979) *The Development of Modern Medicine*, University of Wisconsin Press, Bloomington, Indiana.

Swaan, A. de (1988) *In Care of the State: Health Care, Education and Welfare in Europe and the USA in the Modern Era*, Polity Press, Cambridge.

Wear, A. (ed.) (1992) *Medicine in Society*, Cambridge University Press, Cambridge.

Lay care and formal care

Bartlet, P. and Wright, D. (eds) (1999) *Outside the Walls of the Asylum. The History of Care in the Community 1750–2000*, Athlone Press, London.

Bashford, A. (1998) *Purity and Pollution: Gender, Embodiment and Victorian Medicine*, Macmillan/ St. Martins Press, Basingstoke.

Drummond, J. C. and Wilbraham, A. (1991) *The Englishman's Food: Five Centuries of English Diet*, Pimlico, London.

Lindemann, M. (1999) *Medicine and Society in Early Modern Europe*, Cambridge University Press, Cambridge.

MacDonald, M. (1981) *Mystical Bedlam: Madness, Anxiety and Healing in Seventeenth-Century England*, Cambridge University Press, Cambridge.

Nagy, D. E. (1988) *Popular Medicine in Seventeenth-Century England*, Bowling Green State University Popular Press, Bowling Green, Ohio.

Pelling, M. (1998) *The Common Lot. Sickness, Medical Occupations and the Urban Poor in Early Modern England*, Longman, London.

Smith, F. B. (1979) *The People's Health 1830–1910*, Croom Helm, London.

Webster, C. (ed.) (1979) *Health, Medicine and Mortality in the Sixteenth Century*, Cambridge University Press, Cambridge.

Environmental and public health

Baldwin, P. (1999) *Contagion and the State in Europe 1830–1930*, Cambridge University Press, Cambridge.

Hamlin, C. (1998) *Public Health and Social Justice in the Age of Chadwick: Britain, 1800–1854*, Cambridge University Press, Cambridge.

Lewis, J. (1983) *What Price Community Medicine? The Philosophy, Practice and Politics of Public Health since 1919*, Harvester, Brighton.

Pelling, M. (1978) *Cholera, Fever and English Medicine 1825–1865*, Oxford University Press, Oxford.

Petersen, A. and Lupton, D. (1996) *The New Public Health. Health and Self in the Age of Risk*, Sage, London.

Porter, D. (1999) *Health, Civilization and the State. A History of Public Health from Ancient to Modern Times*, Routledge, London.

Rosen, G. (1993) *A History of Public Health*, The Johns Hopkins University Press, Baltimore, USA.

Rosenberg, C. (1992) *Explaining Epidemics and other Studies in the History of Medicine*, Cambridge University Press, Cambridge.

Rosner, D. and Markowitz, G. (eds) (1987) *Dying for Work: Workers' Safety and Health in Twentieth-Century America*, Indiana University Press, Bloomington, Indiana, USA.

Slack, P. (1985) *The Impact of Plague in Tudor and Stuart England*, Routledge, London.

Weindling, P. J. (ed.) (1985) *The Social History of Occupational Health*, Croom Helm, Beckenham.

Professionalisation

Cook, H. J. (1986) *The Decline of the Old Medical Regime in Stuart London*, Cornell University Press, Ithaca and London.

Digby, A. (1994) *Making a Medical Living. Doctors and Patients in the English Market for Medicine, 1720–1911*, Cambridge University Press, Cambridge.

Digby, A. (1999) *The Evolution of British General Practice, 1850–1948*, Cambridge University Press, Cambridge.

Freidson, E. (1988) *Profession of Medicine: A Study of the Sociology of Applied Knowledge*, Dodd, Mead & Co., New York.

Johnson, T., Larkin, G. and Saks, M. (eds) (1995) *Health Professions and the State in Europe*, Routledge, London.

Larkin, G. V. (1983) *Occupational Monopoly and Modern Medicine*, Tavistock, London.

Rafferty, A. M. (1996) *The Politics of Nursing Knowledge*, Routledge, London.

Health-care systems

Ham, C. (1999) *Health Policy in Britain*, Macmillan, London.

Lowe, R. (1999) *The Welfare State in Britain since 1945*, Macmillan, London.

Melling, J. and Forsythe, B. (eds) (1999) *Insanity, Institutions and Society, 1800–1914*, Routledge, London.

Powell, F. D. and Wessen, A. F. (eds) (1999) *Health Care Systems in Transition: An International Perspective*, Sage, Thousand Oaks.

Ranade, W. (ed.) (1998) *Markets and Health Care: A Comparative Analysis*, Longman, London.

Wall, A. (ed.) (1996) *Health Care Systems in Liberal Democracies*, Routledge, London.

Europe and the rest of the world

Harrison, M. (1994) *Public Health in British India. Anglo-Indian Preventive Medicine 1859–1914*, Cambridge University Press, Cambridge.

Harrison, G. (1978) *Mosquitoes, Malaria and Man: A History of the Hostilities since 1880*, John Murray, London.

Koivusalo, M. and Olliva, E. (1997*) Making a Healthy World: Agencies, Actors and Policies in International Health*, Stakes/Zed, Helsinki/London.

McNeill, W. H. (1976) *Plagues and Peoples*, Basil Blackwell, Oxford.

Walt, G. (1994) *Health Policy. An Introduction to Process and Power*, Zed Books, London.

Weindling, P. (1995) *International Health Organisations and Movements 1918–1939*, Cambridge University Press, Cambridge.

Internet database (ROUTES)

A large amount of valuable information is available via the Internet. To help OU students and other readers of books in the *Health and Disease* series to access good quality sites without having to search for hours, the OU has developed a collection of Internet resources on a searchable database called ROUTES. All websites included in the database are selected by academic staff or subject-specialist librarians. The content of each website is evaluated to ensure that it is accurate, well presented and regularly updated. A description is included for each of the resources.

The URL for ROUTES is: http://routes.open.ac.uk/

Entering the OU course code U205 in the search box will retrieve all the resources that have been recommended for *Health and Disease*. Alternatively if you want to search for any resources on a particular subject, type in the words that best describe the subject you are interested in.

Other useful websites include the Royal Historical Society (http://www.rhs.ac.uk), the Department of Health (http://www.doh.gov.uk/) and the electronic British Medical Journal (http://www.bmj.com/). The Office of Health Economics (OHE) commissions research and publishes reviews of UK health data, with an emphasis on economic aspects (http://www.ohe.org/). Scottish Health Information online (http://www.show.scot.nhs.uk/isd/index.htm) publishes a huge range of statistics and reports on topics including child health, coronary heart disease and mental health. The equivalent website for Northern Ireland is maintained by the Department of Health, Social Services and Public Safety (DHSSPS) at (http://www.dhsspsni.gov.uk). For Welsh health data and reports on births and deaths, lifestyle, prevalence of disease, access Statistics Wales (http://www.wales.gov.uk/statisticswales/walesinfigures/health/health.htm).

Answers to questions

Chapter 1

1   The imposing scale of the Great Hospital founded by a Bishop of Norwich, the building of the original Norfolk and Norwich Hospital with funding from voluntary subscriptions, and the unusual example of the Bethel Hospital (endowed by a woman for patients with mental illness), indicate the high status of philanthropy directed at caring for the sick. The Great Hospital (a monastic institution) also emphasises the capacity and willingness of the medieval church to engage in medical philanthropy, and the importance it attached to this work; notice also that the Lazar House was endowed by another Bishop of Norwich.

The remote situations of the Lazar House, the Workhouse Infirmary, the Norwich Isolation Hospital, the Norfolk County Lunatic Asylum, and (outside the boundaries of the map) the Hellesdon Mental Hospital, indicate the extent of fear of infection and the stigmatisation of people considered to be insane. Interestingly, the new purpose-built Norfolk and Norwich Hospital (due for completion in 2001) is also located 3 miles from the town centre, which could not have accommodated the large site now required for a modern hospital with a full range of specialist services (a photograph appears in Chapter 7; see Figure 7.7). However, at this distance, people who cannot afford a car may experience a similar disadvantage in access to hospital care as did the poor in former times.

The dismal appearance of publicly-funded institutions of the nineteenth century, such as the Workhouse Infirmary (later the West Norwich Hospital) and the Norwich Isolation Hospital (later the Julian Hospital) also reveals the prevailing view that the poor were deviant rather than unfortunate. These buildings, and their equivalents all over the country, often survived as geriatric or mental hospitals in the twentieth century, which perhaps indicates that discrimination against vulnerable groups persists to a greater degree than we generally appreciate.

2   Industrialisation and urbanisation generated ill-health through a combination of factors: overcrowding, damp, contagion and infestation in the tenements and shacks occupied by an impoverished workforce; disease outbreaks exacerbated by poor nutrition, pollution of the air and water, contact with hazardous chemicals and industrial waste, injury or strain from long hours of physically-arduous labour for those in work, and homelessness and destitution for the unemployed. Industrial pollution knows no political boundaries and environmental degradation has followed the rise of the industrial society. But as de Swaan comments, although the poor were hit hardest, the urban middle-classes were also at risk from epidemics and contamination of the air and the common water supply. Just as subscription to voluntary hospitals had been a philanthropic expression of their prosperity in the eighteenth century, so the 'established citizens' funded the provision of public-health reforms such as urban sanitation and sewerage systems in the nineteenth-century, as later chapters in this book will further exemplify. Urbanisation also facilitated other public health advances, including collectivisation of welfare provision and the organisational structures required to run a complex health system.

3   First among these interventions must come an increase in the general standard of education, particularly among women. Wherever developing countries have increased the literacy rate, there has been a significant fall in infant and child mortality and also in the birth rate. In the developed countries, education rates are positively associated with a reduction in potentially health-damaging behaviours (e.g. tobacco consumption), and an increase in health-promoting behaviours (e.g. exercise). Another important intervention outside the field of formal health care is the maintenance of food security and equity of access to the food supply; famines are generally the consequence of lack of entitlement of the poorest sections of society to the available food (e.g. through loss of land rights or wages), rather than to overall shortages of food within the country. Underpinning equity of access is both the political will to achieve it and the infrastructure necessary to deliver it. Income protection schemes and provision of social security or other welfare services for those in need of support can also be expected to reduce inequalities in health, as can improvements in the quality of housing and the urban environment in deprived areas. The other main area of intervention is what might be called 'health protection', for example in health and safety legislation in the workplace, since it is generally the lower-income occupations that expose their workforce to the greatest hazards to health.

4   Turner describes the advance of medicine in terms that are more usually associated with the control of criminality by policing agencies. Thus, in his account, doctors classify illness as 'deviance'; the professionals involved in dealing with the sick are said to be engaged in 'surveillance and control'. He refers to health and social care agencies as 'panoptic', a term borrowed from Jeremy Bentham's plan for a model prison, implying that doctors are a form of 'medical police' who incarcerate the sick in institutions. He describes new specialisms such as preventive medicine and community medicine invading more and more aspects of our social lives, until the 'doctor replaces the priest as the custodian of social values'. Critics of medicalisation such as Turner (and Ivan Illich, whose article 'The epidemics of modern medicine' appears in *Health and Disease: A Reader*, Open University Press, 2nd edn 1995; 3rd edn 2001), suggest that this trend has had a profound negative influence on Western cultures. Illich in particular claims that it has created dependency on doctors and other health professionals, which is itself detrimental to well-being.

Chapter 2

1   Women were involved in medical practice at many levels (though they were excluded from most formal systems of education). The example of Lady Margaret Hoby shows how a local gentlewoman could build up a reputation involving even serious surgical intervention, at least in desperate cases and in more remote areas. Figure 2.3 illustrates the importance of women in the routine care of children's health in the household. Figure 2.4 shows the role of more humble women, and in particular the midwife. Although men are shown in the background, casting the horoscope of the child about to be born, childbirth, even in a textbook, is still being shown as managed by women. We can also infer that Lady Margaret Hoby's patient was an infant, although it would be wrong to infer that she would never be asked to treat adults. Her case also shows the role of community sanction in the activities of lay practitioners. This can also be said of English midwives, because we know that the ecclesiastical system of regulation of midwives was very imperfect. (Formal training for midwives did exist in towns elsewhere in northern Europe.)

2   The quotation shows: lay people taking responsibility for potential threats to the public health; that conditions could be imposed on the use of buildings; that some control was exerted in cities on noxious trades; and that lay administrators were afraid of the concentration of infection from plague and venereal disease in particular. In addition, the quotation illustrates how many sick people could be accommodated outside hospitals; and how attempts were made during epidemics to restrict this common practice.

3   The poem implies (and other evidence confirms) that during epidemics the formally qualified physicians followed the example of their elite patrons by fleeing for safety into the country, leaving the less well-off to fend for themselves. (This was defended at the time in terms of the need for the elite to be able to call on medical advice, and the public value of physicians — and, by implication, their scarcity value.) Forman expresses the contemporary loss of faith in physicians and their search for status, as compared with the usefulness of the lower levels of practitioner, who were more prepared to treat the poor.

4   The quotation gives examples of the gradual discovery by the authorities of pre-industrial towns of the extent and causes of poverty among the 'respectable', resident poor. The reference to the 'storm of … sickness' shows an appreciation of how easily ill-health could lead to poverty, with the implication that timely assistance during sickness could prevent beggary and long-term dependence. The Cambridge authorities, like those of Sheffield, were driven to 'number the poor' in their community, but in their case the administrative response was caused by a crisis of epidemic disease. Few societies would think it appropriate or possible to provide institutional support for 36 per cent of their populations. Cambridge's experience suggests that epidemics underlined the need for flexible systems of out-door relief.

5   Like the epidemiological exchange described by Crosby and others, the exchange of medical knowledge was a very unequal one. Europeans in the tropics were confronted with diseases like yellow fever which they had never encountered before, and which took a heavy toll among them. Lacking knowledge of how to treat these diseases effectively, European practitioners initially became dependent on local medicinal plants (many of which were very effective) and, in many cases, on local medical practitioners. Medical knowledge and medicinal substances from Asia and the New World also found their way back to Europe, where they transformed the treatment and prevention of certain diseases. By contrast, Europeans were able to offer indigenous peoples little in return, and, in the case of slaves, only the most rudimentary health care was provided, in order to increase the profitability of the trade and of plantations.

Chapter 3

1   Both quotations illustrate the growth of class divisions during industrialisation, with the burden of the effects of industrialisation falling on the working class. You may feel that Johnson was not entirely serious, and you may suspect that some of the older towns, like Lichfield, were in some senses being 'left behind' by the industrial boom towns like Birmingham, 15 miles away. Nonetheless, Johnson betrays the gap already existing between the middle classes and the labouring poor. The second quotation shows how the situation had worsened in the intervening decades — and how necessary was the process of 'revelation' of which the Commission was itself a part. The physical proximity is greater —

Brook and Holroyd 'live within a few miles' — and they belong to professions which might be expected to be well informed about social conditions, yet they have to confess to not knowing what conditions in the mines were like. Their ignorance is also a measure of the lack of supervision or regulation of conditions at work, which of course affected men and women as well as children. (It may also strike you that poor working conditions made it possible for industrialists to produce coal and iron at the low cost essential for rapid economic growth.)

2   One aspect of urbanisation was the attempt by the middle classes in smaller centres to imitate the sophisticated amenities of larger towns — or even of the resorts of continental Europe. The search for health was a sufficiently strong motive for a health-related amenity to be a good commercial speculation, likely to improve local prosperity. At the same time, such resorts provided opportunities for social display and social contacts, which required agreeable surroundings. (For the middle classes, industrialisation may have sharpened enjoyment of such pastoral features as the rustic bridge — to which the 'rustics' themselves would not have had access.) It is possible, too, that the Lockwood entrepreneurs were hoping to capitalise on the sulphur well's local reputation for curative qualities.

3   The 'General Practitioner' label was relatively new in 1827, which was also a time of increased competition among practitioners for 'respectable' practice. General Practitioner would have hoped to improve his clientele by acquiring 'College and Hall' qualifications — the MRCS of the Royal College of Surgeons and the LSA of the Society of Apothecaries. However, this was well before the Medical Act of 1858 which, though limited, did offer some advantage to the formally qualified. In 1827, the MRCS and LSA would have improved General Practitioner's status, but would have had little effect on his unqualified competitors — who were very much in the majority. (Provisions in the Apothecaries' Act of 1815 against unqualified practice had had no effect.) General Practitioner's grievance is clearly also directed against the elites of the London medical organisations who put up barriers for rank-and-file practitioners to climb, without controlling unqualified practice or helping to guarantee an adequate return for the time and money involved in pursuing qualifications.

4   In political terms, environmental conditions were at this time 'no one's responsibility'. In better-off areas, the inhabitants could raise the funds and promote the legislation necessary for improving their surroundings. These were essentially local (or commercial) initiatives. By contrast, it was not possible for the poor to help themselves, and it was not yet perceived as in anyone else's interests to improve slum housing. The role of central government in health matters was extremely limited. Southwood Smith also makes the important point that the poor were obliged to live near their work — and were therefore most exposed to the effects of industrial pollution. You may also note, however, that Smith's account places the blame not on the workplaces of the poor, but on their living conditions — illustrating the Benthamites' limited willingness to interfere directly with the economy.

5   The quotation shows that the attitude of the poor to hospitals was not necessarily positive; that attendance as outpatients was often better suited to their circumstances; that it could be assumed that the living conditions of the poor did not include 'free air, wholesome ... diet, and clean ... attendance'; and that the medical and surgical procedures conducted in the voluntary hospitals could be relatively limited (partly to avoid deterring prospective

patients). You may also have noticed that, at this time, the hospitals were still functioning more like the pre-Reformation monastic foundations, rather than as acute hospitals in the modern sense (i.e. short-stay and emergency admissions); it was realised that good nutrition could do as much as medical intervention to improve the state of health among the poor. You might also have speculated that the poor's fear of hospitals could in part be based on experience of compulsory removal to pesthouses and mass burial during the plague epidemics of the previous century — and perhaps also on an increasing sense of social isolation.

6   These extracts signify two important developments which took place in colonial medicine in India in the 1820s and 1830s, both of which were associated with the growing influence of Benthamite principles. Indian medicine, along with Indian culture, morals and political institutions, were compared unfavourably with their Western counterparts, the latter supposedly being more rational, efficient, and enlightened. Whereas Europeans had once learned from indigenous medicine and hygienic practices, the Indian people and their customs were now identified as part of the sanitary problem confronting the British in India. But, like many of his contemporaries, Martin reserved a certain amount of admiration for the 'martial races' of northern India, whose physical appearance and culture were closer to those of the British.

Chapter 4

1   The quotation signals the change from thinking in terms of environmental causes, which were largely out of the poor's control, to a view focusing upon personal responsibility. In particular, we see the start of concern about the effects of the employment of mothers on the health of infants and children — 'maternal inefficiency' was stressed to explain why, at the end of the century (and in spite of sanitary reform), infant mortality had failed to fall as had adult mortality.

2   Although traditions of lay care remained strong, this quotation shows how homes were increasingly being invaded by outside help and advice. This advice also shows clearly the dual function of outside intervention: to help and advise, but also to provide moral leadership and to inculcate habits of thrift, cleanliness, and morality which were norms in middle-class society. The health visitor was also expected to emphasise the individual aspects of health. There is no appreciation in this advice that 'bad smells' and 'feeding and clothing' might also be dependent upon influences (such as drainage, and employment) outside the family's control.

3   Miss Phipps was, as a middle- to upper-class amateur nurse, in the *minority* at this time. Her practice among her 'farm people' links her with the gentlewoman practitioners you have met in earlier chapters. Her background experience shows her connections with philanthropic outlets for women. She may later have joined those pressing for professional status for nurses.

4   The British scheme had a number of advantages for insured people, compared with its German predecessor:

   (a) Contributions were not graduated, but paid at a flat rate.

   (b) Worker and employer contributed equal amounts, whereas German workers contributed twice as much as their employer.

   (c) Maternity benefits were paid to all working women in the British scheme, whereas in Germany they were discretionary.

(d) The scheme was open to all workers from the outset, whereas in Germany the scheme at first covered only certain categories of urban worker (but was extended to all later).

(e) Sexually transmitted diseases were not excluded in Britain, as they were in Germany before 1911.

However, the British scheme had certain significant limitations, which it shared with the German scheme:

(i) Dependants of the insured worker were excluded (although both schemes were modified at a later date to include them in limited ways).

(ii) Treatment options were limited; for example in Britain, hospital treatment was covered only for people with tuberculosis.

(iii) Cash benefits were a fixed amount regardless of the severity of an illness, accident or disability.

5   Colonial medical practitioners often claimed that it was the duty of Europeans to 'civilise' indigenous peoples by inducing them, through the provision of health care, to accept Christianity and other 'Western' values. The rhetoric of colonial medicine cast European civilisation in a superior light and portrayed indigenous peoples as morally as well as physically diseased. But, by 1918, colonial medicine had bestowed few medical benefits upon indigenous peoples, since, with the exception of medical missions, it continued to concentrate on the health of Europeans and on improving economic efficiency. Colonial medicine also expressed European fears of the indigenous population, with medicine providing a justification for racial segregation, which left indigenous Africans in settlements with inferior housing and poor sanitation.

Chapter 5

1   Health-care provision remained geographically patchy and uncoordinated. The location of voluntary hospitals was often unrelated to need (for example, see Figure 5.3), and their work was totally separate from that of the workhouse infirmaries and local authority hospitals. Local authorities provided an increasing range of services, from ante-natal clinics to 'VD' clinics. But there was no coordination with GP 'panel' services provided under the NHI scheme. There was no universal right of access to health services (women and children were particularly poorly served) and access to specialist hospital services was inequitable. Attempts to reform and rationalise the funding of services were prevented by economy measures taken by inter-war governments and by the attitude of the approved societies, which administered the NHI scheme.

2   This quotation indicates the continuing vitality of lay care and advice and the access to non-commercial means of self-medication. It also underlines the importance of the pharmacist in working-class health care. But the boundaries were beginning to shift towards a greater reliance on formal health-care provision. This tendency was most apparent in the area of childbirth and child care; hospital-based childbirth and the advice and assistance of outside 'experts' such as trained midwives and health visitors (including advice on birth control) became more common.

3   Nineteenth-century public health had seen its remit as covering environmental questions — housing, sanitation, and their effect on disease as well as matters of individual hygiene. In the twentieth century this focus narrowed to questions

of individual ill-health and the prevention of disease. In addition, in the inter-war years, MOHs in the local authorities took on a considerable range of administrative responsibilities, running local hospitals and a battery of local-authority services. Historians have argued that MOHs were simply taking on whatever activities offered themselves without thinking of what was distinctive about the public-health approach. There has also been criticism of the narrower focus on individual rather than environmental causes of ill-health.

4   In theory, the nurses achieved partial professional status in 1919. But many practising nurses did not meet the registration requirements and still wanted to continue nursing. The state and the voluntary hospital sector also had an interest in diluting professionalisation, since this kept nursing numbers up and costs therefore down. Trades-union activism spread among the unregistered nurses. A new and lower grade of nurse, the enrolled nurse, was recommended just before the outbreak of World War II. The move towards professionalisation was thus beset by internal and external difficulties — internally by different conceptions of nursing's role, and externally by the intervention of the Ministry of Health and the demands of government economic policy.

5   Dutt was undoubtedly correct in stating that the needs of the working population of India, as in other colonies, had not been adequately addressed by systems of health care which privileged white interests above those of the indigenous population. The colonial powers did practically nothing in this period to alleviate the widespread poverty and malnutrition which were the underlying causes of ill-health among indigenous peoples. Equally, the problem of chronic disease, as opposed to epidemic and infectious disease, was largely ignored. Yet Dutt fails to take account of the many genuine attempts that were made to improve the health of Indians and other colonial peoples in the inter-war period: attempts that constituted a significant shift from the limited interventionism of the nineteenth century.

Chapter 6

1   The acute hospital services were given priority when resources were scarce for a number of reasons:

   (a) The under-resourced hospitals inherited from the pre-NHS system were in urgent need of bringing up to the standard elsewhere in Europe and the USA.

   (b) The revolution in high-technology medicine created a demand for surgery, X-rays, pathology laboratories and blood transfusion services, all of which could only be supplied by hospitals. There was also increasing demand for childbirth in hospitals.

   (c) It was politically easier to focus resources on hospitals because they were under state control.

However, prioritising the acute hospitals meant that the bias in health care shifted towards the curative services. The preventive and primary health-care services, and in particular the services for people with mental-health problems and the frail elderly population, became 'Cinderellas', starved of resources and attention. Only after a long delay, with rising demand for community care and avoidance of unnecessary institutionalisation, was the concept of a first-class service altered to involve better balance between primary, secondary and tertiary care.

2   As indicated in Chapter 5, Bevan inherited the wartime faith in rational and integrated planning with a view to securing the most economical and effective use of scarce human and material resources. This ideally involved administration of all local health services by local government, which was also responsible for other personal social services such as housing and education.

However, the national government was forced into making concessions to medical vested interests. Unification of health services under local government was unacceptable to the medical profession. Because of opposition to integration by the BMA, primary care was administered by Executive Councils, which were merely updated National Insurance Committees. Also, to meet the demands of the powerful organisations representing consultants, each Teaching Hospital was given complete independence, while individual hospitals were granted a high degree of autonomy, under committees upon which consultants and former trustees of voluntary hospitals were dominant. Finally, the pattern of expenditure of the new health services replicated most of the inequalities of the pre-war system.

3   Community care in the immediate post-war period meant care at home, supported by a wide range of local-authority, voluntary and health-authority-provided services. In the 1950s and 1960s, it also came to mean residential care in the community in residential homes, for elderly people in particular (see Figure 6.7), and domiciliary care was downgraded. In practice, because of the poor coordination between different services providing domiciliary care and the patchy provision of residential accommodation, the role of lay care, i.e. care by family and friends, remained considerable.

4   The status of the GP in the immediate post-war period was low. The GP's rise in status between 1948 and 1974 involved: the establishment of a new image and function for GPs as 'family doctors' living among their patients and knowing them throughout their lives (see Figure 6.11); a new professional body, the College of General Practitioners; government support for general practice and primary health care, and GP management of other health-care occupations, e.g. health visitors.

5   Public-health doctors lost their hospital 'empires' and also lost control of social workers and sanitary inspectors in this period. Despite the new emphasis on 'community medicine', they failed to grasp the potential to become campaigners for improvements in public health on a wide range of issues. Instead, many health campaigns were run by single-issue pressure groups rather than involving public-health professionals; examples you could cite are campaigns on air pollution, birth control, abortion and housing.

6   Your answer should include some of the following points:
   (a) Strong confidence in, and the prestige associated with, Western medical and pharmaceutical technology led to the importation of expensive drugs and therapeutic and diagnostic equipment for the major urban hospitals. This skewed the health budget towards hospitals in capital cities.
   (b) Indigenous systems of medicine were undermined and devalued by the emphasis on the perceived scientific superiority of Western medicine.
   (c) The establishment of research bodies and medical schools run on European lines, with comparability of standards, led to the teaching of irrelevant curricula, and the perception that the best training could only be obtained

'abroad' (i.e. in the West). Health professionals often left their own countries to specialise in industrialised countries, and were not encouraged to return because they could not practise medicine under the same conditions, or earn as much.

(d) Social reform of the type that occurred in some European countries (e.g. West Germany and France) after World War II was discussed but not, on the whole, implemented in developing countries for a number of complex reasons, e.g. opposition from within the political and administrative structures, resistance of the medical profession to change, and 'cold war' ideology.

Chapter 7

1   The quotation represents an idealised statement about longer-term trends and the current state of affairs. In explaining why it does not reflect actual trends, you should include some of the following points:

(a) Under-investment and shortages of trained personnel in hospitals (e.g. specialist nurses to staff intensive therapy beds, see Figure 7.5), has restricted access to the latest forms of treatment; access may also vary between geographical locations (the 'postcode lottery').

(b) The long-term and massively expensive District General Hospital policy is still being pursued (as evidenced by the new Norfolk and Norwich Hospital, Figure 7.7). Change to an entirely different policy of secondary care provision can only be a distant possibility.

(c) The absence of adequate community-care support means that it is often not possible to discharge patients (especially frail elderly people) from hospital, and, if discharged prematurely, they are likely to need readmission. Local authorities experience severe difficulties in expanding their commitment to community care on account of lack of resources.

(d) The capacity to expand primary care depends on the ability to recruit larger numbers of GPs and other primary care staff, all of whom are in short supply and take many years to train.

(e) The status of GPs as independent contractors makes it difficult to negotiate contracts that facilitate adoption of new and expanded roles in primary care. The BMA has been highly effective in defending GPs against new responsibilities that could limit their traditional freedoms.

2   Power draws attention to the centrality of the consumer or taxpayer as a reference point in justifying the new public management (NPM). This carries the major implication that, in the context of the NHS, the patient as consumer would experience tangible benefits from NPM. A wide range of measures in the secondary acute-hospital sector have undermined what Power calls 'cosy self-regulation', directly to the benefit of patients. Starting in the 1980s, these measures have culminated in regulation by such bodies as NICE and CHI, and provide evidence of pressure on professionals to deliver the more up-to-date and uniform standard of care wanted by patients. Various initiatives were undertaken to increase direct responsiveness to the patient, e.g. facilitating the rights of patients to change their GP, aspirations enshrined in *The Patient's Charter*, improved access to information about services, waiting times pledges, more patient-friendly environments in hospitals, and introduction of standardised complaints machinery.

Within primary care more generally, consistent with NPM, the purchaser–provider split led to commissioning of secondary care by GPs. Commissioning was designed to help GPs to act more effectively as the surrogates of their patients in purchasing the most appropriate secondary care. However, consumer responsiveness is more difficult to achieve when almost all choices about treatment are not made directly by the patient as consumer, but by professionals on the patient's behalf. A succession of NHS scandals around the turn of the millennium provided many instances of system failures with respect to protection of the interests of patients.

3   Administrative fragmentation represents a problem of long duration in the field of community care. The problems highlighted by Martin Bulmer are rooted in the very structures adopted in 1948, central to which is the continuing fault-line between local government and the NHS. Since 1974, for all community care recipients, their social care has been provided by local government services, and their medical care by the NHS. In the conditions of severe resource constraint applying since 1974, each partner has inclined to shift the burden to the other, with the result that the relevant services are inadequately administered and the already difficult logistical exercise of inter-sectoral cooperation has been further undermined.

In some respects the problem has worsened since 1987, for instance owing to growth in numbers of elderly people needing long-term care, closure of long-stay hospitals, bed-reductions in acute hospitals, staff shortages in the hospital sector, and continuing retrenchment in local government services. A variety of policy initatives have aimed at improving harmonisation of effort in community care, for example the second Griffiths Report (1988), the development of multidisciplinary teamwork in general practice, and new public management innovations such as Health Improvement Plans.

4   Continuing professionalisation is assumed to benefit patients through increasing protection against inadequately-trained practitioners and ensuring that authorised practitioners deliver the best standard of care. Chapter 7 highlights continuing professionalisation in nursing, but the same process was occurring more widely, from NHS managers to local government environmental-health officers, and among the many groups involved in complementary and alternative medicine. State supervision of changes to professional practice is meant to ensure that each group uses its new status to benefit its patients/clients.

However, the quotation cites the qualms of Jane Salvage about trends within nursing, which she claims have transformed the profession in the interests of a dominant elite. Recent developments such as the introduction of Nurse Consultants and nurse practitioners prove that nurses have become more highly trained and more technically competent, and are taking on tasks that were formerly the province of doctors. It is less clear the extent to which the proposed reintroduction of the matron role represents part of the same trend. The available evidence suggests that there is a risk of creating a gulf between the graduate elite and the much larger number of less-qualified nursing personnel, who are likely to carry the main burden of the traditional nursing tasks; these lower grades work under worse conditions and without the superior remuneration that is associated with professionalisation. Critics such as Salvage believe this class distinction within nursing is unlikely to benefit patients.

5   In support of David Hunter's assessment, one could note that from the 1990s onwards, in response to pressures from outside agencies such as the European Union and the WHO's 'Healthy Cities' programme, successive UK governments introduced targets for improving health (e.g. in the White Papers *Our Healthier Nation* and *The Health of the Nation*). The Health Development Agency was formed to give greater effect to health promotion, and an effort was made to reinvigorate public health through official adoption of the 'new public health' initiative. In response to the BSE crisis a whole series of changes were set in motion, beginning with establishment of the Food Standards Agency.

However, in contradition of his optimism, you might suggest that the decline of public health as a specialised function has accelerated since 1974. From then onwards public health doctors became predominantly concerned with service planning and operational management within the hospital sector. The specialism was afflicted by low status and poor recruitment. The ineffectiveness of the public health system was evident in such diverse areas as fluoridation of water, policy over tobacco advertising and alcohol, environmental pollution, and inequalities in health. The extreme dangers of this situation were demonstrated by the BSE crisis and by the massive foot-and-mouth disease outbreak in 2001, which — although not a direct threat to human health — provided additional proof of the weakness of the public health system.

Chapter 8

1   Your answer should include some of the following points:
   (a) The Chinese barefoot doctor was a stimulus for thinking about the mutually beneficial relationship between community and health worker.
   (b) Social research encouraged ideas that lay people were already, and could be more, involved in health care, providing a link between formal health services and communities.
   (c) Concern about consumer dissatisfaction within international organisations such as the WHO led to active searching for ways in which communities could be involved in health and health care.

2   Your answer should include some of the following points:
   (a) Low-income countries cannot afford to train doctors and nurses in the necessary numbers to ensure that the whole population has access to a health professional. Many community health workers (or traditional midwives) can be trained for the price of training one nurse or doctor. Because their training is shorter, they can be paid much lower salaries than professionals, and some work unpaid.
   (b) Many health professionals dislike living and working in rural areas, and refuse to spend any length of time in the countryside.
   (c) People in small communities feel more comfortable with someone from their own area, and prefer taking health problems to them than to a professionally trained health worker who may not speak the same language, or know that part of the country, or the habits and customs of the community.

3   *Selective* programmes tend to be vertically organised, and not integrated with other health services; they focus on one health problem, diverting attention and resources away from other, equally or more important, problems; they are

often based on simplistic assumptions about people's behaviour, and do not take into sufficient account the various socio-economic and cultural factors affecting behaviour; they may not be sustainable over the long run; they focus on outputs (numbers of immunisations undertaken, numbers of oral rehydration packets sold), but often cannot say what the impact of the programme has been on the particular problem.

Comprehensive PHC, on the other hand, is based on a broad philosophy about health and disease, which is difficult to put into operation without clear overall government policy. It demands a redistribution of resources across a number of sectors including the environment, education and employment — not only health. Within the health sector, it means building up health services in general, and not focusing only on one or two diseases, although any comprehensive PHC programme will also have a programme of priorities.

4   Health sector reforms emphasised liberalisation, privatisation and decentralisation (i.e. the reduction of the role of the state in health-service provision and devolution to local agencies). Policies such as 'contracting out' of services to the private sector, and a wider range of financing options (e.g. compulsory health insurance and direct charges to users) were widely introduced. Staff numbers were reduced, but pay and conditions were improved. There was a stronger role for management and planning of services, and greater competition between providers.

One lesson learned from the PHC era was that people were willing to pay for inexpensive medicines, but were deterred from using health clinics because they regularly ran out of drugs and other essential supplies. Health sector reform introduced direct charges which provided a 'revolving' drug fund, ensuring better supplies. Initiatives such as these were administered locally, within the community they served, following on directly from the experience of PHC that services were most effective if they were locally accountable and responsive to local needs.

5   The principal force driving the change was the slow-down in the global economic environment in the 1980s, leading to rising debts and falling incomes, which hit the poorest countries the hardest. When they tried to reschedule their debt repayments, financial institutions such as the World Bank and the International Monetary Fund (IMF) insisted on structural adjustments, which included deep cuts in government spending, including on health. A shift in international funding for health programmes occurred, with WHO and UNICEF taking a reduced share, and the World Bank rapidly becoming the dominant provider from 1987 onwards (see Figure 8.14). The Bank insisted on loans for health projects being tied to health sector reforms.

Chapter 9

1   There is a broad association between national income and health spending, as shown for example in Figure 9.1. However, there are many instances of countries spending more or less than might be predicted on the basis of their national income, as Figure 9.1 makes clear. In addition, the chapter suggested (Figure 9.2) that, as national income increases, countries tend to devote a higher *proportion* of it to health care.

2   The UK is unusually reliant on general taxation to fund health care, which contributed 74 per cent of the total expenditure in 1999 (see Table 9.3); only Canada comes close to this level. Other EU countries raise less than 10 per cent of their health expenditure from government sources, and are primarily social insurance-based schemes. In the UK, social insurance (a proportion of the National Insurance contribution is earmarked for the NHS) forms a relatively small part of health-care funding. The USA is more divided between social insurance and private-for-profit insurance, which plays a very small part in the funding of UK health services. The contribution from out-of-pocket expenses is similar at 10–12 per cent in the UK, France and Germany, which is about 5 per cent less than in North America. However, from the mid-1970s onwards, the broad trends in Britain show a gradual increase in private spending on health (either through private health insurance or services bought directly), as the policy emphasis shifted towards the private sector and direct charges, which now provide the source of over a quarter of health-service funding.

3   Researchers have suggested the existence of a phenomenon known as supplier-induced demand: doctors can in effect decide how much of their own services to 'demand'. If financial incentives exist to increase the amount of care provided, as where fee-for-service payment operates, the phenomenon may be reinforced. Thus attempts to overcome a 'shortage' of doctors by increasing their numbers could result in even more demand being generated for their services, and the 'shortage' continuing.

4   It is broadly true that pharmaceutical companies concentrate on areas where a market exists. Unfortunately many of the commonest diseases, especially infectious and parasitic diseases, are found in developing countries, where markets are small because incomes are low. This leads to a lower research priority in pharmaceuticals to treat these conditions, which in turn reduces the likelihood that appropriate drugs will be developed for particular health problems in such countries. The most compelling example of available but unaffordable treatments relates to the new generation of drugs to treat HIV and AIDS, which have increased life expectancy for infected people in the USA and Western Europe, where less than 10 per cent of cases are found. Until 2001, the pricing of these drugs put them beyond the reach of people in Asia and Africa where annual death rates are numbered in millions; then the pharmaceutical companies conceded to international pressure and allowed South Africa to import cheaper generic versions of these drugs.

Acknowledgements

Grateful acknowledgement is made to the following sources for permission to reproduce material in this book:

Figures

Figure 1.1 Käthe Kollwitz Museum, Berlin; *Figures 1.2, 8.2, 8.7, 8.15* Giacomo Pirozzi/ Panos Pictures; *Figures 1.3a, 1.3b, 1.3d, 1.3e* Dr A. Batty Shaw; *Figure 1.3c* Norfolk Museums Service, Norwich Castle Museum; *Figures 1.3f, 7.3a, 7.3b, 7.17a, 7.17b, 7.21, 7.23* Mike Levers/Open University; *Figure 1.3g* Photo: Standley, P. J. (1989) *Norwich: A Second Portrait in Old Picture Postcards*, S. B. Publications, Market Drayton, Shropshire; *Figure 1.4 'Aus dem Kommissionsbericht der Übersichtigen'* drawing by Ernst Barlach, 1907 © Ernst und Hans Barlach GbR, Lizenzverwaltung, Ratzeburg; *Figure 1.5* Jeremy Hartley/Panos Pictures; *Figure 1.6* Lithograph by A. F. Tait *c*. 1850 Science and Society Picture Library; *Figure 2.1* Bibliothèque Nationale, Paris; *Figures 2.2, 3.3b, 4.17* Mary Evans Picture Library; *Figure 2.3 De Luizenjacht*, by Gerard ter Borch (1617–1681) © Royal Cabinet of Paintings, Mauritshuis, The Hague; *Figures 2.4, 2.9, 2.11* Reproduced from Medicine and the Artist (*Ars Medica*) by permission of the Philadelphia Museum of Art; *Figures 2.5, 2.10, 3.5, 3.9, 3.10, 4.10* Wellcome Library, London; *Figure 2.6* From Robert Fludd 'Medicina Catholica', Frankfurt 1631; *Figure 2.7* From Johannes Wechtlin, Bloodletting points on the human body, 1540, *The Art Archive*; *Figure 2.8a Dorfbaderstube*, by Adriaen Brouwer © Alte Pinakothek, Munich, photo: Artothek; *Figure 2.8b Chirugijn Jacob Fransz Hercules met zijn familie*, by Egbert van Heemskerck, 1669 © Amsterdam's Historisch Museum; *Figures 2.12, 3.4, 4.18, 6.12, 6.16* Hulton Getty Picture Collection; *Figure 2.13* Peabody Museum, Harvard University; *Figure 2.14a, 2.14b* The Bridgeman Art Library; *Figure 2.15* British Museum; *Figure 3.1* The Potteries Museum and Art Gallery, Stoke-on-Trent; *Figures 3.2a, 3.2b* Mitchell, B. R. and Deane, P. (1971) *Abstract of British Historical Statistics*, data, on death rates England and Wales 1838–1883, Cambridge University Press (as used in graphs appearing in: Dupree, M. W.: Family Structure in the Staffordshire Potteries, 1840–1880, Oxford University Press); *Figure 3.3a Punch*, 25 September 1852; *Figure 3.6a The Londoners*, The Pilot Press; *Figure 3.6b* University College London; *Figure 3.7* A. F. H. Fabre, *Némésis médicale illustrée*, revised edition, Paris, 1840; *Figure 3.8* Reproduced from a series by Daumier, *Tout ce qu'on voudra*, Paris, 1847; *Figure 3.12* Archives and Local Studies Unit, Manchester Central Library; *Figure 3.13* North West Metropolitan Regional Hospital Board Report, 1948–1968; *Figure 3.15* British Library, London; *Figure 3.16 Punch*, July 1898; *Figures 4.3 and 4.5* Royal Pharmaceutical Society of Great Britain; *Figure 4.4* Royal Holloway and Bedford New College, University of London; *Figure 4.6* Courtesy of the family of Thomas Leonard Harrison; *Figure 4.7* Gwynedd Archives Service; *Figure 4.9 Illustrated London News; Figure 4.11 Punch*, 4 August 1855; *Figure 4.13 Supplement to the Nursing Record*, 20 December 1888; *Figure 4.14* lithograph by J. A. Bonwell, from Graves, C. (1947) *The Story of St. Thomas's 1106–1947*, Faber and Faber Ltd; *Figure 4.15* Imperial War Museum, London; *Figures 4.16, 5.7a, 5.7b, 5.14, 5.15* London Metropolitan Archives; *Figure 4.19 Punch*, 4 August 1895; *Figure 4.21* Courtesy of London School of Hygiene and Tropical Medicine; *Figure 4.22* Church Missionary Society; *Figure 4.23* Bodleian Library, Oxford; *Figure 5.1* © The Estate of Abram Games, by kind permission; *Figure 5.2* G. A. Paddon/The Pilot Press; *Figure 5.3* Prochaska, F. K. (1992) *Philanthropy and the Hospitals of London, The King's Fund, 1897–1990*, Clarendon Press, Oxford; *Figure 5.4* Topham Picturepoint; *Figures 5.5, 5.6, 6.3, 6.4, 6.5, 6.6, 6.8* Crown copyright material reproduced under Class Licence Number C01W000065 with the permission of the Controller of HMSO and the Queen's Printer for Scotland; *Figure 5.8* Royal College of Midwives; *Figure 5.9* The Boots Company, plc, Nottingham; *Figure 5.10* Loudon, I. (1991) 'On maternal and infant mortality, 1900–1960', *Social History of Medicine*, 4(1), © Society for Social History of Medicine, Oxford University Press; *Figure 5.11* Allan, J. (1992) *Berthold Lubetkin: Architecture and the Tradition of Progress*, RIBA, London, by kind permission of John Allan; *Figure 5.12* M'Gonigle, G. and Kirby, J. (1936) *Poverty and Public Health*, Victor Gollancz;

Figure 5.16 Dorien Leigh/The Pilot Press; *Figure 5.17* Ross, J. S. (1952) *The National Health Service in Great Britain*, Oxford University Press; *Figure 5.18* Graves, C. (1947) *The Story of St. Thomas's 1106–1947*, Faber and Faber Ltd; *Figures 5.19 and 5.22* Sorsby, A. (1944) *Medicine and Mankind*, Watts and Co; *Figure 5.20* Balfour, A. and Scott, H. H. (1924) *Health Problems of the Empire*, Collins; *Figure 5.21* Courtesy of the Rockefeller Archive Center; *Figure 6.1* Reprinted by permission of Transaction Publishers, from *The Development of the Welfare States in Europe*, by Peter Flora and Arnold Heidenheimer. Copyright © 1981 by Transaction Publishers; *Figure 6.2* Photo by Mr and Mrs Holliman, from Graves, C. (1947) *The Story of St Thomas's 1106–1947*, Faber and Faber Ltd; *Figure 6.7a* Erich Auerbach/Hulton Getty Picture Library; *Figure 6.7b* Peter Townsend, from Townsend, P. (1962) *The Last Refuge*, Routledge and Kegan Paul; *Figure 6.9* Royal London Hospital Archives; *Figure 6.10* Jean Mohr; *Figure 6.11* Paul Schatzberger; *Figure 6.13* Brook Advisory Centre; *Figure 6.14* Science and Society Picture Library; *Figure 6.15a* WHO/photo by P. N. Sharma; *Figure 6.15b* WHO/photo by Erich Schwab; *Figure 6.17* Diesfeld, H. J. and Hecklau, H. K. (1978) *Kenya: A Geomedical Monograph*, Springer-Verlag; *Figure 7.1* Robert Moore; *Figure 7.2* Geoff Tompkinson/Science Photo Library; *Figure 7.5* Custom Medical Stock Photo/Science Photo Library; *Figure 7.6* Ed Young/Science Photo Library; *Figure 7.7* London Aerial Photo Library; *Figure 7.10* Roger Hutchings/Network; *Figure 7.12* Barry Lewis/Network; *Figure 7.13* Judy Harrison/Format Photographers; *Figure 7.14* Courtesy of Milton Keynes ADHD Support Group, photo Andy Noble; *Figure 7.15* John Birdsall Photography; *Figures 7.16, 7.19, 7.20b* Tony Woodcock; *Figure 7.18* John Paul Agency, Inverness; *Figure 7.20a* John Callan/Shout; *Figure 7.22a* Health Promotion England; *Figure 7.22b* The British Heart Foundation; *Figure 7.24* Courtesy of Professor John R. Ashton, NHS Executive North West; *Figure 7.25* Reuters/Popperfoto; *Figures 8.1, 8.5* Julio Etchart; *Figures 8.3, 8.9, 9.11* WHO/HPR/TDR/photo by A. Crump; *Figure 8.4* WHO/TDR/photo by O. Martel; *Figure 8.6* Sheldur Netocny/Panos Pictures; *Figure 8.8* WHO/TDR/photo by M. D. Gupte; *Figure 8.10 (left)* Manjit Kaur; *Figure 8.10 (right)* courtesy of ECHO International Health Services, Ltd; *Figure 8.11* Sean Sprague/Panos Pictures; *Figure 8.12* WHO/UNICEF: UCI Reports, cited in UNICEF, 1990, *The State of the World's Children*, Oxford University Press; *Figure 8.13* Philip Wolmuth/Panos Pictures; *Figure 8.14* Buse, K. (1994) 'Spotlight on international organizations: The World Bank' *Health Policy and Planning*, **9**(1), pp. 95–99, Oxford University Press; *Figure 8.16* Philip Ojisua/AFP; *Figure 8.17* John Maier/Still Pictures; *Figure 9.9* Michel Bergsma; *Figure 9.10* Joan Russell/Guzelian; *Figure 9.12* Obed Zilwa/Associated Press.

Tables

Tables 3.1 and 3.2 Flinn, M. W. (ed.) (1965) *Report on the Sanitary Condition of the Labouring Population of Great Britain 1842*, by Edwin Chadwick, Edinburgh University Press; *Table 4.3* Scull, A. (1993) *The Most Solitary of Afflictions: Madness and Society in Britain 1700–1900*, Yale University Press; *Table 5.1* Reprinted by permission of the publishers from *The English Health Service: Its Origins, Structure, and Achievements*, by Harry Eckstein, p. 75, Cambridge, Mass., Harvard University Press, Copyright © 1958 by the President and Fellows of Harvard College, renewed 1986 by Harry Horace Eckstein; *Table 7.1 Compendium of Health Statistics*, Office of Health Economics; *Table 7.3* Fisher, P. and Ward, A. (1994) 'Medicine in Europe: Complementary medicine in Europe', *British Medical Journal*, **309**, No 6947, 9 July 1994; *Table 9.1* Emmerson, C., Frayne, C. and Goodman, A. (2000) *Pressures in UK Health Care: Challenges for the NHS*, Institute for Fiscal Studies.

Text

Box 8.5 Cassels, A. (1995) 'Health sector reform: Key issues in less developed countries' *Journal of International Development*, Special Issue **7**(3).

Cover

Index

Entries and page numbers in orange type refer to key words which are printed in **bold** in the text. Indexed information on pages indicated by *italics* is carried mainly or wholly in a figure or a table.

A

Abel-Smith, B., 121

abortion, in Soviet Union, 137

Abortion Act (1967), 191

Abortion Law Reform Association, 191

Abrams, P., 181

absolutist states, 88, 89

acclimatisation (to tropical conditions), 93–4

Acheson Report (1988), 241

Acheson Report (1998), 244, 249

Acheson, Sir Donald, 241, 244

Ackerknecht, Erwin A., 89

Acquired Immune Deficiency Syndrome *see* AIDS

Action on Smoking and Health (ASH), 191, 242

activity rates, 305

acupuncture, 228, *229*, 230

acute hospital sector, 173–4, 201, 334
    see also secondary health care

administrative and clerical hospital staff, 205

advertising, 102, *103*, 277–8

Africa
    armed conflicts, 281
    effect of direct health charges, 314–15
    'great campaigns', 161–2
    imperial expansion in, 125–30
    indigenous health-care workers, 162
    inequalities in, 255
    malnutrition in, 163
    slave trade, 55–6
    'white man's grave', 57

agency relationship (doctor/patient), 317

agriculture
    effects of improvements, 65
    and environmental health, 41

ague *see* malaria

AIDS (Acquired Immune Deficiency Syndrome), 221, 226, 247, 255, 285–6, 287, 315, 324
    caring networks, 226

air pollution, 22, *24*, *25*, *63*, 189–90, 256

alcohol, 105, 243

Alcoholics Anonymous (AA), 227

Alma Ata Declaration *see* Declaration of Alma Ata

almshouses, 18

alternative medicine, 228
    see also CAM (complementary/alternative medicine)

American Development Bank, 283

Amman, Joost, drawing, *39*

amputation, *48*

ante-natal clinics, 137

antibiotics, 192–3
    resistance, 203, 247

apothecaries, *48*, 53, 54, 69, 76, 78
    see Worshipful Society of Apothecaries; Licence of the Society of Apothecaries

Apothecaries' Society, 78

'applied physiology', 150

apprentices, 76

approved societies, 123, 140

area health authorities, 177

Ariès, Philippe, 37

Armstrong, D., 186, 187

Arnold, David, 92

Arusha Declaration, 258

ASH (Action on Smoking and Health), 191, 242

Ashton, John, 246

aspirations to health, 148

asthma, expenditure on research, 323

asylums, 80, *84*, 86–7, 119–20, 220
    admission of elderly to, 106
    management, 104

pre-industrial, 18–19, *20–1*

Athlone Committee, 158

Austoker, J., 203

Austria, health services, 137

Auto-Icons, *73*

auxiliary health workers, 260

ayurvedic medicine, 57, 160

AZT, 226

Aztecs, *55*, *57*

B

Baby Friendly Hospital Initiative, 278

bacteriology, 100, 111–12, 127

Balfour, A., *160*

Balint, Michael, 186

Bamako Initiative, 284

Banerji, Debabar, 257

Bangladesh
    baby-food advertising, 277
    family planning, 262
    oral rehydration programme, 277–8

Bannington, B. G., *111*

barber-surgeons, 46–8, 53, 76

Barber-Surgeons' Company of London, 54

barbers, 46

barefoot doctors, 259–60, 267

Barlach, Ernst, cartoon, *22*

basic health services, 257–61

basic needs targets, 262

bathing, 40

Bayly, C. A., *89*

Bazalgette, Joseph, *107*

'bed blocking', 224

beds, in NHS hospitals, 207–8, 211
    in residential care, 221–2

Beecham, Thomas, 102

Belgian Congo
    appeal for medical missionaries, *130*
    sleeping sickness campaigns, 161, 162

Belize, breast-feeding campaign, 277

Bender, E., 227

Benin, inequalities in, 255

Bentham, Jeremy, 72, *73*

Benthamites, 72–5, 92

beri-beri, *164*

Berlin, health services, 137

Bethel Hospital, Norwich, *21*

Bethnal Green, life expectancy and social class, *66*

Bevan, Aneurin, 142, 170, 171, 187

Beveridge Report, 142

Beveridge, William, 168, 170

Bhore Commission, 194

bilharzia (schistosomiasis), 192, 260

Bill and Melinda Gates Foundation, 291–2

Bills of Mortality, 35

Birmingham, hospitals, 81

birth control/family planning, 105, 148, 190, 262–3, 273

birth rates, 105, 148

Bismarck, Otto von, 122

Black Report, 244, 339

Black, Sir Douglas, 244

Blair, Tony, 311

blood-letting, 46, *47*

Bloom, Gerald, 260n., 283–4

BMA *see* British Medical Association

BMJ see British Medical Journal

Boards of Guardians, 72

Boer War, army recruits, 100

Bombay
    medical services, 90, 91
    mortality among troops, 91

bonesetters, 48

Bonwell, J. A., lithograph, *114*

Booker, B., 273

Boot, Jesse, 102

Boots the Chemist, 147

Borch, Gerard ter, painting, *37*

Bosanquet, N., *156*, 234

Botswana, life expectancy, 285

bovine spongiform encephalopathy (BSE), 203, 247, 248

Bowlby, John, 190

Boyd Orr, Sir John, 151–2

'brain drain', 195

Brazil
    health clinic, *271*
    infant feeding, 278
    urban slums, 289
    water supplies and sanitation, *256*

breast-feeding, 274, 275, 277–8

Briggs Report, 237

British Army
    death rates, 57, 91
    health of recruits, 100
    Indian medical services for, 90–1

British Diabetic Association, 227

British Heart Foundation, 191

British Medical Association (BMA), 79, 123, 141, 155, 214
    and complementary medicine, 230

British Medical Journal (*BMJ*), 79–80, 233

Brockington, C. F., 109

Brookes, Barbara, 190

BSE *see* bovine spongiform encephalopathy

Buchan, William, 68–9

Bunker, J., 307

bureaucracy, 26
    bureaucratisation, 233, 330
    medical, 26, 27

Burgess, M., 278

Buse, K., *282*

Bush, George W., 291

C

Caesarean section, 182, 305

Calcutta
    hospital, 90
    medical services, 91

Caldwell, J. C., *261*

Calman–Hine review of cancer services, 202–3, 219

CAM (complementary/alternative medicine), 226–30, 330

Cameroon
    literacy class, *14*
    segregated housing, 129

Canada, Lalonde Report, 242

cancellation of operations, 207–8

Cancer Act (1939), 150

cancer services, 202–3

capitation fees, 123, 143

Carers' (Recognition and Services) Act (1995), 226

Caring about Carers strategy, 226

Carracci, Annibale, cartoon, *50*

Cartwright, A., 183, 186

cash limits, 208–9

Cassels, A., *283*

cataracts, 129

Cave Committee, 138

censuses, 36, 77

Chadwick, Edwin, 72, 73, 75, 86, 106
    on deaths of paupers, *74*
    on life expectancies, *66*
    and role of MOH, 109
    and sewerage, 108

charges for health services *see* direct health charges

Charity Organisation Society, 106

Charles, HRH, Prince of Wales, 230

Chest and Heart Association, 191

CHI *see* Commission for Health Improvement

child mortality
    in developing countries, 255
    see also infant mortality

childbirth, *39*, 149, 181–2, 184

children
    care of, 37, 145–6
    health care for, in colonial countries, 162–3
    see also paediatric intensive care; School Medical Service

Children's Minimum Council, 153

China
    access to pharmaceuticals, 322–3
    health services, 259–60, 283–4
    infant feeding, 278

chiropody, 155

chlorodyne, *103*

cholecystectomy, 305

cholera, 65, 68, 75, 90, 135

Chowdhury, M., 277

Christianity, influence on health care and welfare, 329–30

chronic hospital sector, 176, 179, 220

chronic sickness, 102

CHWs *see* community health workers

'Cinderella services', 176, 333

Cipolla, C. M., 43, 45

classical tradition, 13, 329

Clean Air Act (1956), 189–90

cleanliness, 39–43

clinical audit, 210, 218, 232, 233

clinical directorates, 231

clinical governance, 233, 235

clinical trials, 226, 229

Clowes, William, 49–50

coffee, 43

Colatrella, B. D., 288

collectivisation, 26

colonialism, 25, 54, 89–94

commercialisation, 32, 102

Commission for Health Improvement (CHI), 218

communicable diseases, 247
    see also infectious diseases

communities
    care within, 38
    contributions to health-care costs, 36, 50–4

community care, 178, 179–81, 215, 220–8

community health workers (CHWs), 268–71, 284

community medicine, 174, 188, 189

community physicians, 240

companies, 42, 53

competitive tendering, 210–11, 216

complementary medicine, 228
    see also CAM (complementary/ alternative medicine)

comprehensive primary health care, 274

Comte, Auguste, 98

consensus management, 208, 210, 236

constipation, 147

consultants, 231–2
    see also hospital clinicians; specialist medical practitioners

Consumers Association, 191

'continued fever', 71–2

contraceptive pill, 190

convergence in health care, 16–17, 335

Cook, Albert, *129*

Cook Islands, nurse training programmes, 162

Cooper, Bransby, *79*

Corfield, P. J., 71, *82–3*

Cornia, G. A., 315

corporate towns, 33
    hospitals, 81

cost recovery programmes, 314–15

Costa Rica
    health expenditure, 299–300
    health services, 260

cottage hospitals, 18, 157

Creutzfeldt–Jakob disease (vCJD), 203, 248, 287

Crimean War, *114*

Crosby, Alfred, 54

cryptococcal meningitis, 286

Cuba, health services, 260

Cullen, L., 224–5

Currie, Edwina, 243

D

Dagenham, housing estate, *153*

Dakar, segregated housing, 128

Dare, Rev. Joseph, 110

Darwinism, 98

Daumier, Honoré, *76*

Davies, Celia, 237

Dawson Report, 137, 335

Dawson, Sir Bertrand, 165

day surgery, 157

DDT, 193, 194

de Morgan, S. E., 64

death certification, 108

death insurance, 146

decentralisation, 284

Declaration of Alma Ata, 234, 265–6

deforestation, 289

demand-led services, 208–9

Denoon, D., 25

dentists
    charges, 209, 248, 311
    private practice, 204
    state registration, 154

Department of Health and Social Security, 177

developing countries
    access to pharmaceuticals, 286–8, 322–4
    emigration of health workers, 195, 240, 258, 319–21, 337
    evolution of health policy, 257–66
    expansion of 'scientific' medicine in, 192–5
    health expenditure, *297*, 298, 302, 306
        distribution, 303
        sources, 314–15
    health service access, 298
    hospitals, 334
    imports, 338
    mission hospitals/dispensaries, 129–30, 314, 315
    pace of modernisation in, 62
    poverty in, *23*
    primary health care in, 16, 254, 259–61, 264–73
    variation in health profiles, 255–6

Diagnosis Related Groups, 318

diarrhoea, 277

Diesfeld, H. J., 195

Digby, A., 116, *156*

Dingwall, Robert, 184

direct health charges, 171, 283, 284, 311–12, 314–15
    see also prescription charges

dispensaries, 18, 84–5
    African, 129
    French and German, 122–3
    Indian, 91, 92, 163

district general hospitals, 18, *173*, 200, *201*, 211, 334

district nurses, 113, 222, 235, 236

District Visiting Societies, 113

Djukanovic, V., 264

doctors *see* consultants; general practitioners; hospital clinicians; junior doctors; medical practitioners

Doll, Sir Richard, 242

domestic and ancillary hospital staff, 205, *206*

domiciliary services, 179, 181, 222

Donaldson, L. J., 233

Doyal, L., 101

Draper, P., 245

druggists, 69–70

drugs, 257
 against HIV/AIDS, 226, 286, 324
 against other infections, 287, 323–4
 from New World, 34, 57–8
 'magic bullets', 112, 192–3
 provided by Squire, 68
 sale by GPs, 117
 sale by health centres, 284
 see also pharmaceutical industry

Dufferin Fund, 163

Dunn, C. L., *142*

Dunn, S., 332

Dunnell, K., 183

E

E. coli, 203, 247, 248

East India Company (EIC), 89–92, 93–4

Eckstein, H., *139*

economic liberalism, 67

Economy Act (1926), 138

education, 14, 100
 female, 14, 261
 nurses, 236–7
 see also medical education

elderly people, 104, 106, 209, 307, 308
 assistance under NHS, 171
 care within extended family, 145, 224–5
 community care, 178–9, 221, *222*
 isolation, 224
 in mental hospitals, 176
 mortality in World War I, 124
 in pre-industrial England, 33, 36
 in residential care, 179–81, *221*, 309

elephantiasis, 324

Elias, Norbert, 40, 48

elite/elitism, 26, 70

Elliott-Bins, Christopher, 226–7

Elphinstone, Lord, 92

Emergency Medical Service, 141, *142*

enclosure of common land, effects, 65

Engels, Friedrich, 24, 66, 339

'English sweat', 34

Enlightenment, 68, 72

enrolled nurses, 158

environmental factors, 15, 41–3, 99, 112, 150, 289–91
 see also cleanliness; pollution

environmental health officers, 189, 240

epidemics, 34, 40–1, 73–4, 135
 see also AIDS

epidemiological exchange, 54, 56–8

Epidemiological Society of London, 108

equality, 23

equity, 23, 266

ethical concerns, 330

eugenics, 98, 148

evidence-based medicine, 17, 218, 233

evolution by natural selection, 98

expert reference groups, 218

extended families, 33

Exxon, 291

eye tests *see under* opticians

Eyler, J. M., 98

F

families, 33, 38, 104, 145, 182

Family Doctor's Charter, 187

Family Health Services, 209

family planning, 262
 see also birth control/family planning

Family Planning Association, 148, 190, *191*

family practitioners, 213
 exclusion from cash-limits system, 208–9

Farr, James, 42, 43

Farr, William, 98, *99*, 106, 108

fee-for-service payments, 317, 318

feldschers, 260

female education, 14, 261

fertility rates, 98, 99

fever, 71–2

fever hospitals, 72, 80

'fever nests', 65, 75, 93

financing of health care, 23, 121–3, 135–6, 138, 139, 140, 332
 in developed countries, 308–13
 in developing countries, 314–15
 from taxation, 23, 204, 309, 332
 in India, 159
 pre-industrial, 50–1
 public and private, 309–13
 in USA, 310, 318
 World Bank policy, 282
 see also health expenditure; Private Finance Initiative

Finkel, D., 286n.

Finsbury Health Centre, *134*, 150, *151*

fistulae, 48

Flexner, Abraham, 117

Flinn, M. W., *66*, *74*

Flora, P., *169*, 199

fluconazole, 286

Fludd, Dr Robert, *45*

fluoridation, 248–9, 330

Flynn, R., 215

folk medicine, 226
 see also indigenous medical systems

food, adulteration, 108, *109*

food poisoning, 203, 243, 247, 248

Food Standards Agency, 248

foot-and-mouth disease, 203,

Fores, S. W., cartoon, *77*

formal health-care system, 14, 26, 38–9, 154–8
 definitions of health care, 304

former socialist economies of Europe (FSEs), 296

Forsyth, G., 174–5

Foundation for Integrated Medicine, 230

France, health expenditure distribution, 303

Frank, Johann Peter, 88

Friendly Societies, 70, 102, *103*, 140

Fulham and Hammersmith workhouse, *67*

funding of health care *see* financing of health care

G

Garrett, Thomas, 286n.

Gates, Bill and Melinda, 291

GDP *see* Gross Domestic Product

General Board of Health, 75

General Household Survey (1995), 225

general management, 210, 231

General Medical Council, 116, 162, 233

general practitioners, 49, 75–6, 76–80, 121, 233–5, 316
    fundholders *see* GP-fundholders
    group practices, 188, 234, 235
    independent contractors, 143, 185
    midwifery practised by, 117
    NHI panel practices, 123, 137, 155–6
    in NHS, 174, 185–7
    Primary Care Groups, 217, 246
    remuneration, 156–7, 317

generic drugs, 324

genetically modified crops, 290

germ theory of disease, 100

Germany
    health services, 137
    hospital funding, 318
    impact of World War I, 124
    medical education in, 117
    poverty in, 12
    preventive medicine, 148
    sickness insurance in, 122–3
    social welfare schemes, 136

Gilbert, Bentley, 123

Gillam, S., 239

GlaxoSmithKlein, 322

Global Climate Coalition, 290

Global Initiative on AIDS, 285

global warming, 290–1, 339

globalisation, 17, 337

Gluckman Commission, 194

GNP *see* Gross National Product

Goa, indigenous medical systems, 58

GOBI interventions, 274–80

Godber, Sir George, 137, 172–3

GP-fundholders, 214, 215, 217, 231–2
    management costs, 216

Graham, Hilary, 224

Grant, C. J., lithograph, *70*

Granville, J. M., 104, 120

Graves, C., *170*

Gray, N., 144

Great Hospital, Norwich, *20*

'greenhouse gases', 290

Greek medical tradition, 13, 329

Griffiths Report (1983), 210, 231, 236

Griffiths Report (1988), 215, 221

Griffiths, Sir Roy, 210, 221

Gross Domestic Product (GDP), 297–9

Gross National Product (GNP), 297–8

growth monitoring, 274, 275, 276

Guatemala, rural health services, 260

guilds, 42n., 53, 70, 78

Guillebaud Report, 172

H

Haines, A., 289

Hanwell Asylum, 120

Hardoy, J., 290

Hartlepool Engine Works, 110

Haynes, B., 110

HCHS *see* Hospital and Community Health Services

HDA *see* Health Development Agency

Health Action Zones, 219, 248

'Health for All by the Year 2000' programme, 246, 264–5, 267, 339

Health Authorities, 214, 217, 218

health care, 12
    definitions, 304
    see also inequalities in health care

health-care systems, 329
    convergence, 16–17, 335
    diversity, 17–18, 333, 335, 337
    historical background, 12, 13, 16–19, 328–30
    levels of organisation, 16
    pluralism, 330
    see also formal health-care system; informal health-care system; National Health Service

health care assistants, 236

health centres, *134*, *137*, 143, 150, 175, 187, 188, 335

Health Development Agency (HDA), 244–5

health education, 242–4, 246

health expenditure, 199, 200, 296–304, 300–1
    distribution, 303–4
    through NHS, 170, 171–2, 174, 205, 300, 301–2
    variations between countries, 304–7
    variations over time, 308
    see also financing of health care

Health Improvement Programmes/Plans (HImPs), *217*, 218, 246

health insurance, 17, 100, 123, *309*
    in Germany, 122–3
    private, 204, 310
    see also National Health Insurance; 'provident' dispensaries

Health Maintenance Organisations (HMOs), 316

health management, 118, 183
    see also National Health Service management reforms

Health of the Nation initiative, 215, 247–8

health promotion, 174, 245, 246

health sector reforms, 280, 282–4, 291–2, 335

health service access, 298

Health of Towns Association, 75

health visitors, 106, 146, 188

health workers
    migration, 195, 240, 258, 319–21, 335, 337
    see also headings such as medical practitioners; nurses; village health workers; volunteer health workers; etc

Healthy Cities campaign, 246

healthy eating campaigns, 242, 243

Healthy Living Centres, 219, 239

Heath, Edward, 203, 213

Hecklau, H. K., 195

Heclo, Hugh, 199

Heggenhougen, K., 259, 270

Heidenheimer, A. J., 169, 199

Hellesdon Mental Hospital, Norwich, 21

Helman, C., 226

herbalism, 69
    anti-depressant remedy, 229

Hercules, Jakob Fransz, 47

hierarchy of resort, 26–7

Hill, A. Bradford, 242

HImPs see Health Improvement Programmes

Hindu medicine see ayurvedic medicine

Hippocrates, 19

HIV (Human Immunodeficiency Virus), 285–6, 287

HMOs see Health Maintenance Organisations

Holland, H., 163

Holloway, Thomas, 102

home-help service, 179

homelessness, 22, 221, 247

homoeopathy, 69, 117, 228, 229

Horder, John, 187, 235

Horn, Joshua, 259

hospice care, 230, 308–9

Hospital and Community Health Services (HCHS)
    cash limits on, 208, 209
    PCTs responsible for, 218

hospital doctors, 27, 231–3
    clinicians, 231–2
    junior, 232, 239

hospital matrons, 183, 236

Hospital Plan, 172, 174, 200

Hospital Sunday/Saturday Funds, 122, 139

hospitals, 118, 120–1, 333–4
    acute sector, 173–4, 201, 334
    chronic sector, 176, 179
    contributory schemes, 139, 157
    cottage, 18, 157
    district general, 18, 173, 200, 201, 211, 334
    fever, 72, 80
    funding of, 205, 318
    hierarchical structures in, 183–4
    historical background, 18–19, 20–1
    Indian, 90, 91, 92
    inter-war period, 138–9
    long-stay, 220
    mission, 129–30, 314, 315
    modernisation, 200
    municipal, 139
    in NHS, 175
        see also nationalisation of hospitals
    numbers of beds, 206–8
    out-patient departments, 121
    pre-industrial, 51–2, 77
    resource management, 209–10
    scandals, 203, 220, 240
    specialist, 85
    staff, 205–6
    teaching, 177, 334
    see also voluntary hospitals

houses of correction, 52

housing, 22, 63, 108, 153, 192, 289

Howard, John, 71

Huddersfield, 64

Human Immunodeficiency Virus (HIV), 285–6, 287

humanism, 32, 35

hunger marchers, 153

hydropathy, 69

I

IMF see International Monetary Fund

immunisation, 275, 278–80, 336, 338

imperialism, 125–30

Inchcape Commission, 160

income redistribution, 262

independent contractors, GPs as, 143, 185

India
    Bhore Commission, 194
    Central Research Institute, 128
    health care for women, 163
    Indian Mutiny, 94
    indigenous medical systems, 57, 58, 160–1, 316
    infant feeding, 278
    in inter-war years, 159–6
    malaria eradication, 193
    malnutrition in, 163, 164
    medical education, 162
    traditional midwife training, 272–3
    under East India Company, 89–94

indigenous medical systems, 57–8, 91, 160–1, 193, 256, 257, 316

Indonesia, forest fires, 289

Industrial Revolution, 24–5

industrialisation, 24–5, 42, 62–4, 67, 256

inequalities in health care, 22–4, 64–7, 151–2, 244–5, 248–9, 256, 298, 302, 303, 321, 322–4, 332–3, 338
    see also postcode lottery

infant formulas (breast-milk substitutes), 277–8
    see also breast-feeding

infant mortality, 63, 64, 99, 105, 124, 306
    in colonial countries, 162
    in developing countries, 255, 261

infectious diseases, 34, 110, 247, 287–9, 336
    effects of public-health measures, 125
    epidemics, 34, 40–1, 73–4, 135
    excluded from voluntary hospitals, 84
    hospitals for, 120
    multifactorial approach, 112
    notification, 108
    spread through slave trade, 56
    see also immunisation

influenza pandemic, 135

informal health-care system, 14, 26, 51, 101, 224–8
    see also lay care

inoculation (smallpox), 41, 56

institutionalisation, 104, 106

insurance *see* death insurance; health insurance; social insurance

integrated care, 216–19, 241

intensive care services, 207
    paediatric, 219, 237

Intermediate Care service, 224

internal market in health care, 210, 213, 214–6, 231, 241

International AIDS Vaccine Initiative, 287

International Conference on Population and Development, 263

International Conference on Primary Health Care (Alma Ata), 264–6

International Health Commission, *161*

International Labor Organization (ILO), 262, 266

International Monetary Fund (IMF), 199, 281, 337

International Panel on Climate Change, 290

international standard-setting, 135

Internet, 17, *227*, 228, 319

Invalid Care Allowance, 225–6

Ireland
    emigration from, 65
    fevers, 72

Islamic medicine, 57, 329

Italy
    public health, 43
    social welfare schemes, 136
    surgeon-physicians, 45

itinerant medical practitioners, 48, 77

ivermectin MSD (Mectizan), 288

J

Jeffery, P., 272–3

Jefferys, Margot, 186, 187

Jejeebhai, Sir Jamsetji, 92

Jenner, E., 64n.

Jenner, M., 40, 42, 43

Jewell, T., 241

Jiminez, E., *303*

Johns Hopkins School of Medicine, 117

Johnson, James, 94

Johnson, Samuel, 71

Jones, William, 91

Jordan, B., 273

journals *see* medical journals

Julian Hospital, Norwich, *21*

junior doctors, 232, 239

K

Kaleeba, N., 286

Katz, A., 227

Kelleher, D., 227

Kendal, life expectancy and social class, *66*

Kenya
    effect of direct health charges, 314
    hospitals, *195*
    primary health care, *259*

Keynes, John Maynard, 168

King, Maurice, 258

Kirby, J., *152*

Kirkwood, Tom, 328, 336

'kitchen-physic', 38

Kitching, G., 280

Kollwitz, Käthe, lithograph, *10, 12–13*

Kruif, Paul de, 328

Kyd, J. G., *82–3*

Kyoto Protocol on International Climate Change, 291

L

lady visitors, 81, 106

Lalonde Report, 242

Lambert, S. M., 162

Lambeth Conference, 190

Lancet, The, 79, 120, 278

Larkin, Gerald, 154, 185

Lawrence, C. J., 69

lay care, 37, 38–9, 51, 68–70, 101–6, 144–5, 178–83, 224–8
    see also headings such as community health workers; village health workers; *etc.*

lay control, 104, 118, 331

Laybourne, K., *153*

Lazar House, Norwich, *20*

League of Nations, 135, 163

Leech, John, cartoon, *65*

Leeds
    life expectancy and social class, *66*
    Quarry Hill Flats, 153

leprosy, 129

'less eligibility' (principle of), *67*, 332

Lewis, J., *116*, 150, 151, 187–8

Liberia, AIDS campaign, 285

lice, *37, 145*

Licence of the Society of Apothecaries (LSA), 78

licences to practise (pre-industrial), 53, 76, 78

life expectancy
    Elizabethan, 33
    and social class, 66–7
    see also longevity

lithotomy, 48

Liverpool, 65
    life expectancy and social class, *66*

Liverpool School of Tropical Medicine, 127, 128

living standards, 22, 62, 84, 106, 338

Llewellyn Davies, M., *105*

local authority services, 100, 104, 213, *214*, 240, 331
    health promotion, 246
    inter-war years, 136, 137, 139, 146, 150
    pre-industrial, 71
    residential homes, *221*
    within NHS, 143, 187–8, 189
    in World War I, 124

Local Government Act (1929), 139, 150

locality commissioning of health services, **215, 217**

London, 33, 44
   'great smog', 189
   hospitals, 52, 80, 81, 113, *138*, *170*
   housing, 153
   sewer system, *107*, 110
   workhouse, *119*

London Fever Hospital, 80

London School of Tropical Medicine, 127

longevity, 328

low-cost interventions, 274–5

Lubetkin, Berthold, *151*

lunatic asylums *see* asylums

lung cancer, 191, 242

Lyons, M., 162

M

MacCarrison, Robert, 163

MacFarlane, A., *149*, *182*

Mach, E. P., 264

McKeown, Thomas, 125, 242

Maclean Committee, 138

Macleod, Iain, 190

McMichael, A., 289

McNamara, Robert, 262

McPake, B., 284

McVie, Gordon, 202, 203

Madras
   medical services, 91
      in inter-war years, 159
   Royal Naval Hospital, 90

Maggs, C. J., *114*

'magic bullets', 192

magnetic resonance imaging (MRI), *202*

Mahler, Halfdan, 246, 264

malaria, 192, 287, 288
   in African populations, 129
   eradication programmes, 193–4, 263, 287–8
   expenditure on research, 323
   in India, *159*
   oil company's donation for treatment, 291
   in pre-industrial England, 41
   in primary health-care programmes, 274

Malaysia, traditional midwives in, 271–2

malnutrition, 151–2
   in colonial countries, 163

Malthus, Thomas; Malthusianism, 62, 62n., 98

man-midwives, 77

management reforms *see under* National Health Service

Manchester, hospitals, 81, *84*

Manchester and Salford Sanitary Association, 106

Manchester Statistical Society, 108

Manchester Unity Friendly Society, *103*

manipulative therapies, 229

markets, 42

Marks, S., 194

Marland, Hilary, 64, 68, 69, 84, 85, 101

marsh fever *see* malaria

Marylebone Workhouse, *119*

maternal mortality, 149
   in colonial countries, 162
   in low-income countries, 273

maternity benefits, 122, 123

Maternity and Child Welfare Act (1918), 124, 146

maternity and child welfare clinics, 146, 150

Mbugua, J. K., 315

'meals on wheels', 179

means-tested payments, 223–4

Mectizan (ivermectin MSD), 288

Medical Act (1858), 79, 116, 117

medical assistants, 258

medical audit *see* clinical audit

medical auxiliaries, 258

medical botany, 69

medical directories, 78–9

medical education, 117, 174
   in developing world, 194

medical journals, 79–80, 127

medical manuals, 68–9, 91

medical missions, 129–30

Medical Officers of Health (MOHs), 75, 88, **109**–10, 188, 240

medical police, 87–**88**

medical poor relief, **51**, 68, 85–6

medical practitioners, **43**–4
   control of services by, 104, 118
   emigration from developing countries, 195, 258, 319–21
   erosion of power, 183, 335
   and introduction of NHS, 142
   pre-industrial, 38–9, 43–50
   private practitioners, 316
   public trust and confidence, 19, 22
   qualifications, 117
   regular and irregular, 76–7
   regulation, 53–4, 77–8, 116–17
   remuneration, 118, 156–7, 306, 317–18
   training *see* medical education
   see also community physicians; general practitioners; hospital doctors; medical education

Medical Reform movement, 79

medical research, 117, 127, 128, 139

Medical Research Committee, 123

Medical Research Council, 123

medical societies, 53–4

medical topography, 94

medicalisation, **15**

Medicare, 318

'medicine men', 57, *58*

MENCAP, 191

'mental handicap', 176n.

mentally ill/mentally handicapped people, 179, 223
   residential facilities, *221*

Merck & Co, 288

mesmerism, 69

Metropolitan Asylums Board, 120

metropolitan hospitals, 88

Metropolitan Poor Act (1867), 120

Mexico
   malaria eradication, *193*
   midwife training, 273

Mexico City, air pollution, 256

M'Gonigle, George, 152

midwives, 39, 116, 146, 184, 236
    male GPs as, 117
    man-, 77
    training of traditional, 271–3
    working in NHS hospitals,
    205–6
Midwives Act (1902), 116, 146
migration of health workers, 195,
240, 258, 319–21, 335, 337
Milburn, Alan, 203
Mills, A., 282
MIND, 191, (subsequently, Mind),
332
Ministry of Health, 134, 144, 158
    envisaged by Simon, 108
Ministry of Labour, 179
mission hospitals/dispensaries,
129–30, 314, 315
Mitchell, B. R., *82–3*
modernisation, 25–6, 62, 330
Modernisation Agency, 219
MOHs *see* Medical Officers of Health
Monsanto, 290
Montagu, Lady Mary Wortley, 41
moral economy, 67
morbidity, 101
    difficult to measure, 67
    early twentieth-century, 125
More, Sir Thomas, 43
Morison, James, *70*
Morley, David, 195, 258
Morrell, D., 329
mortality, 33, 34, 99, 101, 307
    early twentieth-century, 124–5
    in European colonies, 57
    and poverty, 152
    and social class, 66–7
    see also infant mortality;
    maternal mortality
Moryson, Fynes, 45
Mozambique, structural
adjustments, 281
Mugford, M., *149, 182*
municipal hospitals, 139
Muraleedharan, V. R., 159
mutualism, 103
myalgic encephalomyelitis, 229

N

Nairobi, Kenyatta National Hospital,
195
National Ankylosing Spondylitis
Society, 227
National Association for the
Prevention of Tuberculosis, 191
National Audit Office, 208
National Beds Inquiry, 208
National Birth Control Council, 148
National Birthday Trust Fund, 148
National Health Insurance scheme,
101, 117, 122, 123, 135–6, 137,
138, 140, 310
    compared with NHS, 171
    GP panel practice, 123, 137,
    155–6
    tuberculosis treatment
    included, 124
National Health Service, 18, 134,
136–7, 142–4, 169–77, 300, 311,
331–3
    beds, 207–8, 211
    direct health charges, 171,
    283, 284, 311–12, 314–15
    hierarchies of health workers,
    231–40
    inertia in, 201–4
    integrated care, 216–19, 241
    internal market, 210, 213–16,
    231, 241
    management reforms, 208–19,
    231, 236, 241
    privatisation of services, 206,
    210–11
    public health responsibility, 241
    reorganisation (1974), 176–7,
    213
    staff numbers, shortages,
    205–7, 232, 237–8
    tripartite system, 143, 176
National Institute for Clinical
Excellence (NICE), 218
National Service Frameworks
(NSFs), 217, 218–19
    for mental health, 223
National Society for Smoke
Abatement, 189
nationalisation of hospitals, 142,
143, 144, 176, 187
Native Americans, medicine men,
57, *58*

neo-Malthusianism, 98
Neumann, Salomon, 88
New Deal, 136
New NHS (White Paper), 216, 218
New Poor Law, *67–8*, 72, 73, 86–7,
104
new public health, 245–6
new public management, 212,
217, 218, 231
Newell, K., 260, 263, 264, 274
Newsholme, Sir Arthur, 146
NHS and Community Care Act
(1990), 221
NHS Direct, 219, 239
NHS Plan, 216, 218, 219, 223–4,
232, 233, 236, 238
NHS Trusts, 214, 215, *217*
NICE (National Institute for Clinical
Excellence), 218
Nightingale, Florence, 106, 113, *114*
Norwich
    census (1570), 36
    hospitals, *20–1, 201*, 211, 329
'nuisance', 42–3, 108
Nurse Consultants, 238, 239
nurse practitioners, 238
nurses, 304
    education, 236–7
    emigration from developing
    countries, 195, 240, 320–1
    enrolled, 158
    hospital matrons, 183, 236
    lay, 37
    in management, 236
    managerial structure for, 184
    professionalisation, 112–15
    recruitment crisis, 239–40
    registration, 115, 154, 157
    specialist, 27, 237–8
    unregistered, 236
    visiting, 106
    working in hospitals, 205–6
    see also district nurses;
    Nurse Consultants; nurse
    practitioners; practice nurses;
    Project 2000; VAD
nursing assistants, 205, 236
nursing auxiliaries, 184, 205, 236
nursing homes, *221*

Nursing and Midwifery Council, 237

nutrition, 125, 135, 163, *164*
    diet of mothers, 148–9

nutritional standards, 135

O

obstetric intervention, trends, 182
    see also Caesarean section

occupational diseases, 25

occupational health, 108

odours, 40

OECD *see* Organisation for Economic Cooperation and Development

oil companies, 290–1

oil price crisis of 1973, 198–9, 336–7

old-age pensions, 104

Old Poor Law, 36, 85–6

onchocerchiasis (river blindness), 288

OPEC *see* Organisation of Petroleum Exporting Countries

opticians
    charges for services, 209, 311–12
    state registration, 154–5, 184

oral rehydration, 274, 275, 276–7

Organisation for Economic Cooperation and Development (OECD), 198, 296, *300*, 301, 312

Organisation of Petroleum Exporting Countries (OPEC), 198

Our Healthier Nation programme, 248–9

out-door relief, 52, 86

out-of-pocket expenses, health care funding from, *309*, 311, 314

out-patient care, 121

over-the-counter drugs, 257, 311

Oxford Institute of Social Medicine, 153

P

paediatric intensive care, 219, 237

panaceas, 48

Papua New Guinea, industrialisation, 25

parasitology, 127

parishes, poor relief, 36, 51, 52, 331

part-time nurses, 158

part-time practitioners, 38, 49, 50

Pasteur, Louis, 111

patent remedies, 70, 102

Patient's Charter, The, 212

pauperism, 68, *74*, 86, 120

pay beds, 122, 139, 157

payments
    to doctors, 317–8
    for hospitals, 318

PCGs *see* Primary Care Groups

PCTs *see* Primary Care Trusts

penicillin, 192

Pennell, I., 101

People's League of Health, 149

PEP *see* Political and Economic Planning

per diem payments, 318

Percival, Thomas, 72

Performance Assessment Framework (PAF), 219

performance reviews/indicators, 210, 219
    see also Commission for Health Improvement

personal responsibility for health, 100–1, 112, 151, 164, 224, 242

Peru
    child nutrition, *276*
    'Children's workshop', *263*

PFI (Private Finance Initiative), 18, 208, 211

pharmaceutical industry, 70, 102, 257, 286, 321–4
    anti-HIV drugs, 226, 286, 324
    private spending on drugs, 204, 257

pharmacists, 147–8

PHC *see* primary health care

philanthropy, 80–7

Philippines, emigration of health workers, 195, *320*

physical fitness, 148

physicians, 44–5

physiotherapy, 155

Picken, R. M. F., 150–1

Pickstone, J. V., 146, 147–8

Pierce, G. L., 156–7

Pilgrim, A., 203

plague, 34, *35*, 41, 43, 128

'polyclinics', 122–3, 260

poliomyelitis, 279

Political and Economic Planning (PEP), 141, 146

pollution, 22, 25, 42–3, *63*, 75, 189–90, 256

poor law *see* New Poor Law; Old Poor Law

Poor Law nurses, 115

Poor Law Unions, 67, 72, 86

poor rate, 36, 57

poor relief, 85–6, 331
    see also medical poor relief

population
    age-structure of Elizabethan, 33
    density, 99
    growth, 262

Porter, Roy, 19

postcode lottery, 201, 203, 216, 332

potatoes, 58

Potter, A. R., 255

poverty, *10*, 12–13, 33, 35–6, 65–7, 105, 106, 152, 291–2, 337–9

PPP *see* purchasing power parity

practice nurses, *234*, 235, 236, 238

practitioners of physic, 44

prescription charges, 209, 311
    see also direct health charges

pressure groups, 75, 79, 189–91, 227–8

preventable diseases, 75, 195

preventive medicine, 148, 150–1, 174, 242–4, 258

priest-physicians, 88

Primary Care Groups (PCGs), 217, 246

Primary Care Trusts (PCTs), *217*, 218

primary health care, 16, 121, 174, 195, 234–5, 263–6, 283, 284, 291–2, 334–5
    decline in developing countries in 1990s, 280–1
    in developing countries, 267–73
        comprehensive *v.* selective, 274–80, 289
    WHO definition, 256–6
primary health-care approach (PHC), 234–5, 264–6
Pringle, M., 235
Private Finance Initiative (PFI), 18, 208, 211, 334
private funding for health care, 309, 310–12, 313
private health insurance, 204, 310
private spending on health, 310–11
Prochaska, F. K., 81, *138*
profession, 15
professionalisation in health-care services, 15, 27, 38
    health visiting, 106
    medical practitioners, 116–18
    midwifery, 149
    nursing, 112–16
professions supplementary to medicine, 154–5, 184–5
Project 2000, 237
proprietary remedies, 70
Protestantism, 52n.
'provident' dispensaries, 84–5
Provincial Medical Directory, 78
Provincial Medical and Surgical Association, 79
provision of health care, 308–9, 316–17
    pre-industrial, 50–1
public funding for health care, 309–10, 312–13, 314
    in developing countries, 314
public health, 15, 71–5, 125, 135, 189–92, 240–9, 331, 336, 338
    alarms in recent years, 203
    and communicable diseases, 247
    fragmentation of responsibility, 240–1
    and health inequalities, 244–5
    Health of the Nation initiative, 215, 247–8

    and health promotion, 245–7
    in India, 92, 93–4
    Our Healthier Nation programme, 248–9
    and preventive medicine, 242–4
    sanitarian movement, 75, 99, 106–12
    see also new public health
Public Health Act (1848), 75
public-health inspectors, 188, 189
public-health profession, 150–3, 187–8
public–private partnership, 288, 289
purchaser–provider split, 214, 215–16
purchasing power parity (PPP), 297, 306
putrefaction, 41

Q

'quacks', 50
quality of life, 307

R

racial segregation, 128–9
radiography, 155
randomised controlled trials (RCTs), 229
Rather, L. J., 338
Rees, D. C., *127*
Reformation, 52n., 329
regionalisation of health services, 144, 177
registered nurses, 157
registration (births, marriages, deaths), 35
Reidy, A., 280
relapsing fever, 71
religious belief, 68, 76
religious institutions, 88, 113, 330, 331
    see also medical missions
Renaissance, 19, 32, 329
reproductive health, 263

research
    medical, 117, 127, 128, 139
    pharmaceutical, 321
residential care, 179–81, *221*, 222–3, 309
Resource Management Initiative, 210, 231
Rhodes, Cecil, *125*
river blindness (onchocerchiasis), 288
Roberts, Elizabeth, 144–5, 146, 147–8
Roberts, Ffrangcon, 170, 171
Roberts, Robert, 147
Robinson, J., 236
Rockefeller Foundation, 135, 161–2, 163, 192
Rogers, A., 203
Roosevelt, F. D., 136
Ross, J. S., *158*
Ross, Ronald, 127–8
Rowntree, Seebohm, 178
Royal College of General Practitioners, 187
Royal College of Nursing, 115, 158
Royal College of Physicians, 77–8, 228, 242
Royal College of Physicians of London, 54
Royal College of Surgeons, 77–8
Royal Commission on Long Term Care, 223–4
Royal Commission on Mental Illness, 179
Royal Commission on National Health Insurance, 138
Royal Holloway College, *102*
Royal Society of Medicine, 186
rural societies, 65, 255, 256, 259–60
    environmental health, 41
    health expenditure distribution in, 303
    health services in, 258–9
    physicians in, 44
    primary health care in, 234
Ryle, John, 153

S

Sachs, Hessie, 186, 187

St Andrew's Mental Hospital, Norwich, *21*

St Thomas's Hospital, 113, *170*
Nightingale Training School, *158*

Salisbury, C., 234

Salmon Report, 184

Salmonella, 203, 240, 243, 247

salvarsan, 112

Salvation Army, 331

sanatoria, 122

sanitarianism, 75, 99, 106–12

sanitary inspectors, 108, 188, 189

sanitary movement, 68, 72–5
in India, 92

sanitation, *256*

Scally, G., 233

Scharlieb, Mary, 105

schistosomiasis (bilharzia), 192, 260

School Medical Service, 118, 145

scientific and technical hospital staff, 205, *206*

Scotland
health system, 134
hospitals, *82–3*
medical organisation, 46
National Health Service, *143*

Scott, H. H., *160*

Scull, A., 104, *119*, 120

secondary health care, 16

secularisation, 25, 330, 331

Seebohm Committee, 188, 240

selective primary health care, 274, 276–8

self-governing NHS Trusts, 214, 215, *217*

self-help groups, 227–8

self-help systems, 69–70, 102

self-medication, 147–8, 182–3, 226–7

Seveso accident, 290

sewers, *107*, 108, 110

sexually transmitted diseases, 34, 48, 101, 124, 193

Seymour, Howard, 246

Shaw, M., 249

Shellard, P., 110

Sheridan, R. B., 56, *57*

sickness insurance *see* health insurance

Sigerist, Henry, 338, 339

sight tests, 311

Simon, Sir John, 73, 79, 88, 100, 106, *107*, 108–9, 110–11, 117

single-issue campaigns, 189–91, 242–4

slave trade, 55–6

sleeping sickness, 128, 161, 162

slum clearance, 153

smallpox, 34, 41, 54, *55*, 92–3, 336
see also vaccination

'smog', 189

smoke pollution *see* air pollution

smoking, 242–3, 248, 249

Snell, K. D. M., 65

Snow, John, 75n.

social class, 64–7, 151–2
medical practitioners, 117
nurses, 113, 115

social Darwinism, 98

social insurance, 168, 169, *309*, 310

social medicine, 88, 137, 153, 338

social science, 98, 108

social welfare systems, 136–7, 304

social workers, 188, 189

Socialist Medical Association, 141

socio-economic environment, 245–6

Sorsby, A., *159*, *164*

South Africa
costs of anti-AIDS drugs, 324
Gluckman Commission, 194
'good health train', 281n.
health expenditure, 299–300

Southwood Smith, Thomas, *73*

Soviet Union, health services, 136, 137, 260

spa towns, 40, *69*

specialist hospitals, 85, 334

specialist medical practitioners, 48, 117, 157, 172–3, 183, 334

specific remedies, 48

Spens Committee, 156

Sri Lanka, health services, 260

Stacey, M., 183

Starr, Paul, 100

statistical methods, 108

Stevens, Rosemary, 121, 157, 185, 300

Stewart, F., 315

Stockport, 24–5

Stoke-upon-Trent, death rates, 62–4

Stone, Lawrence, 37

Stopes, Marie, 148

Strong, P. M., 236

structural adjustment policies, 281

Summers, Anne, 113

superior health achievers, 260n.

supplier-induced demand, 317–18

surgeon-apothecaries, 44, 48

surgeons, 45–6, 48

surgical interventions, 305, 318

'survival of the fittest', 98

Swaan, A. de, 25, 26, 168

Swaziland, effect of direct health charges, 315

Sweden, social welfare schemes, 136, 169

syphilis, 34, 41, 56–7, 112

Szreter, Simon, 125

T

Tait, A. F., lithograph, 24

Tanzania
Arusha Declaration, 258
health service reforms, 258–9, 270
structural adjustments, 281

targets, for health improvement, 247–8, 249

Task Force for Child Survival, 278

taxation
concessions for health insurance, 310–11
health care funding from, 23, 204, 309, 337

Taylor, D., 269

Taylor, P., 243

Teaching Hospitals, 177, 211, 334

tertiary health care, 16

Thackrah, C. T., 66, 67

thalidomide, 191, 257

Thatcher, Margaret, 199, 210, 211, 244

Third World *see* developing countries

Thomas, K., 229

Thompson, E. P., 62, 66

'three-quarters rule', 194, 258, 303

tobacco, 58
    advertising, 248, 249
    and lung cancer, 190
    see also smoking

tobacco industry, 242–3

Todd Report, 188

Torbay Hospital, *173*

Townsend, Peter, 179, *180*, 181, 244

**traditional midwives, training,
271–3**

Trapham, Thomas, 56–7

**tripartite division of medicine,
44–8**

**tripartite system of health care,
143, *176***

triumphalist fallacy, 19, 22, 328

tropical hygiene, 92–4

**tropical medicine, 56–7, 126–30,
161, 192**

TSO (The Ugandan AIDS Support
Organisation), 286

tuberculosis (TB), 123, 124, *159*,
247, 287, 336
    sanatoria, 122

Tudor Hart, Julian, 186

typhoid, 71

typhus, 34, 71, 135

U

Uganda, AIDS in, 285, 286

UKCC (United Kingdom Central
Council for Nursing, Midwifery and
Health Visiting), 236, 237

unani medicine, 57, 160

unemployment, 135, 151, 152

UNICEF (United Nations Children's
Fund), 193, 263, 264–5, 266, *272*,
276, 278, 284

United Kingdom Central Council for
Nursing, Midwifery and Health
Visiting (UKCC), 236, 237

United Nations Population Fund,
266

urban areas
    effect of sanitarian movement,
    106–11
    health expenditure in, 303
    housing conditions, 289–90
    pollution control, 42–3

**urbanisation, 25, 33, 64, 65, 256,
289–90**

USA
    elimination of general practice,
    121, 185
    health funding in, 310
    Health Maintenance
    Organisations, 316
    hospital funding, 318
    hospital management, 118
    medical education in, 117
    New Deal, 136
    social insurance, 168
    specialisation by medical
    practitioners, 157

utopias, 43

V

vaccination, 64, 88, 92, 274, 275,
336
    see also immunisation

vaccines, 193, 247, 275, 287

vagrant poor, 35

vCJD *see* Creutzfeldt–Jakob disease

Vaughan, J. P., 277

Vaughan, Megan, 161

vehicle exhaust emissions, 191

venereal diseases (VD) *see* sexually
transmitted diseases

Venezuela, rural health services, 260

Verkade, Olivia, 286

vertical programmes of health-care
interventions, **263**

Vickers, A., 229, 230

Vienna
    General Hospital, 88
    health services, 137

Viet Nam, travelling doctors, *265*

**village health workers, 258, *259*,
267**
    see also community health
    workers

Vincent, D., 178

Vincent-Priya, J., 271–2

Virchow, Rudolph, 88–9, 338

Vogel, R., 315

Voluntary Aid Detachments (VADs),
115

**voluntary hospitals, 18, *21*, 72,
80–3, *84*, 121–2, 137, 138–9**

volunteer health workers, 269, 312

W

Wakefield, 64, 65, 69

Wakley, Thomas, 79–80

Walk-in Centres, 219, 239

Wallace, Alfred Russel, 98

Wallington, Nehemiah, 'A judgement
of God', 40

Walsh, J., 274

Walt, G., 270

Wandsworth School Treatment
Centre, *145*

Warren, K., 274

water supplies, 108, 110, *256*
    fluoridation, 248, 249

Waterton, Charles, 68

wealth redistribution, 262

Webster, Charles, 140, 171

Wechtlin, Hans, illustrations, *46*, *48*

**welfare state, 16, 101, 168, 192,
198–200, 300**

Wellcome Trust, 323

Werner, David, 268

Wesley, John, 68

West Norwich Hospital, *20*, 201

Western health-care systems, 17

Western society, 13
    expansion, 16–17, 24, 54–8, 89–94, 125–30, 338

Westminster Infirmary, 80

Whitehead, Margaret, 244

WHO *see* World Health Organisation

Williams, G., 215

Willmott, P., 183

Wiltshire, life expectancy and social class, *66*

Winslow, Charles, 329

Winter, Jay, 124

Woelk, H., 229

Wohl, A. S., *107*

women
    carers, 13, 14, 37, 51, 101, 105, 178, 179, 224, 225–6
    diet of mothers, 148–9
    education, 14, 261
    and health care for families, 100
    health care for, in colonial countries, 162–3
    Indian, 92
    medical practitioners, 49, 118, 233, 235
    in nursing, 112–15
    sickness among childbearing, 151
    see also childbirth; maternal mortality; maternity benefits; maternity and child welfare clinics

Women's Co-operative Guild, 106, 148

Women's Institutes, 148

Woodward, J., *82–3*

Woolworths, 147

Worboys, Michael, 128, 163

Workhouse Infirmary, Norwich, *20*

workhouse test, 67

workhouses, 18–19, 52, *53*, 67, 85–6, *87*, 104, 119, 220
    infirmaries, *20*, 120, 137, 139

working class, 64

Working for Patients (White Paper), 214

World Bank, 266, 281

World Development Report, 261

world health-care system, 296, 325

World Health Organisation (WHO), 193, 245, 246, 263–5, 266, 272, 278, *279*, 280, 338, 339

World War I
    army recruits, *100*
    impact on health/health services, 101, 124, 134, 159
    Voluntary Aid Detachments, 115

World War II, 134, 193
    impact on health services, 141–2

Worshipful Society of Apothecaries of London, 54

X

Xingyuan, Gu, 260n., 283–4

Y

yaws, 192

Yemen, midwife training, *272*

Yoder, R. A., 315

Young, M., 183, 224–5

Young, Sir George, 242–3

Yudkin, John, 243

Z

Zambia
    health sector reforms, 283
    immunisation campaign, *279*

Zimbabwe
    HIV-positive women in, 285
    midwife training, 273

Zollman, C., 229, 230

Zwi, A., 281, 282